The Shift

The Dramatic Movement Toward Health Centered Dentistry

DeWitt C. Wilkerson, DMD
With E. Shanley Lestini, DDS

Foreword by Peter Dawson, DDS & Brad Bale, MD

Widiom Publishing llc.
ISBN-10: 0-9985336-2-9
ISBN-13: 978-0-9985336-2-9

The Shift
The Dramatic Movement Toward Health Centered Dentistry
First edition
Copyright © 2019 by Widiom Publishing llc

ALL RIGHTS RESERVED. No part of this publication may be reproduced, distributed, or transmitted in any form or by any means, including photocopying, recording, or other electronic or mechanical methods, without the prior written permission of the publisher, except in the case of brief quotations embodied in critical reviews and certain other noncommercial uses permitted by copyright law. For permission requests, write to the publisher, addressed "Attention: Permissions Coordinator," at the address below.

Widiom Publishing, LLC.
1 Beach Drive SE, #1106
St.Petersburg, FL 33701
www.WidiomPublishing.com

ISBN-10: 0-9985336-2-9
ISBN-13: 978-0-9985336-2-9

Dedication

To all you *shifters,* who will experience the health benefits that come from an anti-inflammatory lifestyle, better breathing, and better oral health.

To our Great Creator, who designed us to experience both better health and daily joy.

∗ ∗ ∗

"For you created my inmost being;
you knit me together in my mother's womb.
I praise you because I am fearfully [reverently]
and wonderfully made;
your works are wonderful,
I know that full well.
My frame was not hidden from you
when I was made in the secret place,
when I was woven together in the depths of the earth.
Your eyes saw my unformed body;
all the days ordained for me were written in your book
before one of them came to be.
How precious to me are your thoughts, God!
How vast is the sum of them!"

Psalm 139
King David of Israel

TABLE OF CONTENTS

Acknowledgements..iii
How to use this book...vii
Foreword by Peter Dawson, DDS...ix
Foreword by Brad Bale, MD..xv

Part 1 – The Shift and Integrative Dental Medicine
1. Why *The Shift*?...3
2. A New Model...9
3. An Introduction to Integrative Dental Medicine............................15

Part 2 – The Great Fire: Inflammation and Infection
4. Inflammation as a Central Theme in Integrative Dental Medicine..27
5. Inflammation & Infection – History: Signs and Symptoms..........33
6. Inflammation & Infection – Evaluation/Screening & Testing.....67
7. Inflammation & Infection – Treatment...73
8. Frequently Asked Questions about Inflammation and IDM...93
9. A Conversation with Steven Masley, MD.....................................105

Part 3 – The Great Awakening: Airway, Breathing, & Sleep
10. "Dentistry's Great Awakening" 117
11. Airway, Breathing, & Sleep – History: Signs and Symptoms.......129
12. Airway, Breathing, & Sleep – Evaluation/Screening & Testing...149
13. Airway, Breathing, & Sleep – Treatment......................................161
14. Treatment of Airway and Breathing Disorders: A Key Focus of Integrative Dental Medicine for Patients of All Ages...............177
15. *The Shift:* A Pediatric Perspective, by Kevin Boyd, DDS, MS...185

Part 4 – The Great Imposer: T.M.D. & Occlusion Disorders
16. T.M.D. & Occlusion Disorders and Integrative Dental Medicine..195
17. T.M.D. & Occlusion Disorders – History: Signs and Symptoms..199
18. T.M.D. & Occlusion Disorders – Evaluation/Screening & Testing..215
19. T.M.D. & Occlusion Disorders – Treatment................................233

Part 5: Integrative Dental Medicine's 7 Key Questions
20. Integrative Dental Medicine's 7 Key Questions.......................255

Part 6: In Closing
21. A Look Back, A Look Ahead, by Gary Kadi...........................267
22. Personal Reflections, by Witt Wilkerson, DMD......................271
23. Personal Reflections, by Shanley Lestini, DDS......................275

Part 7: Appendix
24. The Disease of Caries – Intervention and Disease Treatment, by Kim Kutsch, DDS..281
25. A Medical Model for Diagnosing and Treating Periodontal and Peri-implant Disease, by Thomas Nabors, DDS, FACD............299
26. ADA Policy Statement: The Role of Dentistry in the Treatment of Sleep-Related Breathing Disorders..331
27. Ozone Therapy, by Rachaele Carver Morin, DMD.................335
28. Books Referenced in Inserts.......................................341
29. Endnotes..345

ACKNOWLEDGMENTS

This project is the result of many years of sitting at the feet of great teachers, mentors, and coaches. Many are my dearest lifelong friends.

In the beginning…there was Mom! My mother, Dorothy Collins Wilkerson Templet, is an inspiration to all who know her. She has always exemplified a life committed to total health. My earliest memories include her daily routines of juicing carrots and celery, hands full of vitamins, weighing on the bathroom scales, jogging, biking, golf, Bible reading, and much prayer for her kids. This goes back to the 1960s! Thank you, Mom, for being such a great role model and cheerleader. I'm your biggest fan and love you so much.

Then there was Pat! My wife is such a special person – super talented, beautiful inside and out, eternally optimistic, and fully committed to every relationship in her life. She has taught me about all aspects of balance and love that have shaped our family and my career. Patty, you are my hero, role model, best friend and the love of my life. Thank you for believing in this project because you believe that everyone deserves to experience a life filled with health and joy. Our children – Todd, an Integrative Health coach; Whitney, an educator; and Ryan, a medical technologist – have each provided great feedback and support and have made me a very blessed and proud father.

Dr. Pete Dawson mentored me even before I entered dental school. We first met as family friends. When he learned I had been accepted into dental school, he immediately gave me a copy of his textbook and invited me to attend his three advanced dental seminars, as his guest. This was just the beginning of the many years of incredible influence Pete has had in my life. Thousands of dentists around the world join me in thanking Pete for leading a revolution from "usual and customary" to being the very best we can be, both professionally and personally. Upon graduation from the University of Florida College of Dentistry, I was invited to join Pete in his private practice, along with Dr. Pete Roach and Dr. Glenn DuPont. I'm grateful for the many years we've worked together.

Dr. David Hildebrand taught me so many lessons about life, inspirational leadership, and seeing the very best in other people – David, you will always be the best!

This book is divided into three major areas of focus: (1) Inflammation/Infection, (2) Airway/Breathing/Sleep Disorders, and (3) TMD/Dental Occlusion Disorders. I would like to thank the following individuals, who have been instrumental in influencing my learning in each area:

- Inflammation & Infection:
    - Steven Masley, MD, Brad Bale, MD, Amy Doneen, DNP, ARNP, Michael Roizen, MD, Caldwell Esselstyn, MD, Tom Nabors, DDS, David Seaman, DC, MS, Covert Bailey, MS, Jeff Novick, MS, Isabelle Simon, MA, Colin Campbell, PhD, Mark Hyman, MD, Joel Fuhrman, MD, Mehmet Oz, MD, Robert Lustig, MD, Doug Thompson, DDS, Mark Cannon, DDS, Susan Maples, DDS, Michael Schuster, DDS, Jamie Koufman, MD, FACS, Charles Whitney, MD, Elizabeth Board, MD, Gary Kadi, and Ron Kobernick, DDS, MScD
- Airway/Breathing/Sleep Disorders:
    - John Tucker, DDS, Richard Bonato, PhD, Rose Nierman, RDH, Barry Glassman, DDS, Tom Colquitt, DDS, Ben Miraglia, DDS, Kevin Boyd, DDS, Barry Raphael, DDS, Marianna Evans, DDS, MS, Steven Park, MD, Christian Guilleminault, MD, John Remmers, MD, Jeff Rouse, DDS, Scotty Bolding, DDS, MS, Lance Manning, MD, Gy Yatros, DMD, Jim Metz, DDS, Patrick McKeown, Roger Price, BSc, Pharm, William Hang, DDS, MSD, and David Gozal, MD, and Keith Thornton, DDS
- TMD & Dental Occlusion Disorders:
    - Peter Dawson, DDS, Mark Piper, DMD, MD, Parker Mahan, DDS, Terry Tanaka, DDS, Henry Gremillion, DDS, Bill Arnett, DDS, Ormand Ware DDS, Robert Corruccini, PhD, Jerome Rose, PhD, Weston Price, DDS, and Richard Roblee, DDS, MS

A very special thanks, with much gratitude, to each one of you!

I would also be remiss if I did not thank Aramelys Canales (DMD, Cuba), my clinical assistant for 23 years. Your competency, attention to detail, and spirit is invaluable. I would also like to thank Greg Sitek, whose technical expertise has helped us complete this manuscript. Amy Trumbull Harmon, my super talented niece and graphic artist, designed the cover – thank you, Amy!

Finally, from the bottom of my heart, let me thank Shanley Lestini, my co-author. You are one very special person. Your commitment to excellence, in all areas of your life, is an inspiration to all who know you. I'm so proud of your incredible contribution to this project. You have worked tirelessly and joyfully every step of the way. I could not have done it without you, nor would I have wanted to. The Wilkersons consider you part of our family and love you very much. Now rest!

– Witt Wilkerson

* * *

I am grateful for the opportunity to echo my thanks to the professionals and friends Dr. Wilkerson has already named. It has been a privilege to learn from your teaching, advice, and examples. I know that patients around the world are receiving more excellent care because of your tireless efforts and the excellent work to which you are each committed. You will never know how much your training has impacted me, and I am excited to continue learning from all of you!

Specifically, Dr. Dawson, I will never forget the conversation we had during lunch at one of your seminars shortly after I finished dental school, when we talked about my hopes and goals. Your time, advice, and encouragement meant so much to me. Also, your readiness to share about the difference your personal relationship with Jesus has made in your life greatly encourages me. I am very grateful for the privilege of learning so much from you and the other incredible faculty at the Dawson Academy! The training and encouragement I have received at the Dawson Academy have enabled me to better serve my patients in countless ways, and I look forward to continue benefiting from your exceptional teaching and commitment to excellence.

In addition, I would like to thank Drs. Richard and Amy Hunt. Working with you and our wonderful team is such a blessing! You are both such incredible dentists and teachers, and I thank the Lord for the gift of having you both as amazing mentors and as dear friends. Thank you also for introducing me to the Pankey "family"! I so appreciate the training and friendships I have found at the Institute. It is inspiring to witness the leadership and spirit of service in the men and women of the Pankey Institute!

I would also like to thank my parents, Bill and Stephanie, for their love, encouragement, and support. Thank you for pointing me to the Lord, the Great Physician, and for instilling in me a love for His Word. You were the first to share with me about a relationship with Jesus, and it is because of my relationship with Him that I have true joy and purpose. In addition, Dad, your example as a physician, who always served his patients with excellence and compassion, inspires me every day! Mama, thank you for the time and energy you have poured into our family and for your tireless support and encouragement. I would also like to thank my sister, Lysandra, for her support throughout this project. Lysandra, I am so proud of you for pursuing your passion for painting portraits, but I am also glad that we share a passion for dentistry!

Finally, I am grateful to the Wilkersons for their years of friendship and encouragement. All of you mean so much to me! Dr. Wilkerson, thank you for the incredible privilege of getting to be a part of this project. The principles of *The Shift* have changed the trajectory of my life and the lives of countless other dentists and patients. I will never forget the conversation we had on the ServingHIM mission trip in Romania when you shared with me about all the ways the profession of dentistry can bring about restoration and healing in people's lives. That conversation launched my personal and professional life on this amazing path, and I can't wait to witness the transformation of more and more lives through this message. Thank you for being an incredible mentor and an example of someone who serves the Lord and other people wholeheartedly. I could not be more grateful that you have given me the opportunity to be a part of spreading the message of *The Shift*!

– Shanley Lestini

How to use this book:

<u>If you are a dentist</u>…it is our hope that this book will inspire and assist you in implementing health-centered dentistry and the message of *The Shift*. Your desire to provide your patients with the best care possible motivates and encourages us as we continue on this journey.

<u>If you are a physician</u>…your collaboration is key to the success of the mission of *The Shift*. The tireless efforts of the experts in your fields give us hope that our patients truly can live lives of genuine health and not just settle for the absence of disease. We welcome your input in these efforts and thank you for your assistance in providing patients with optimal care.

<u>If you are a member of a dental or medical team</u>…we are grateful for your invaluable contributions toward empowering patients to adopt the strategies they need to maintain health for a lifetime. *The Shift* would not be possible without you.

<u>If you are a patient</u> desiring to improve your health or the health of those you love…we applaud you for your efforts to seek out true health for a lifetime. We invite you to use this book in whatever ways are most helpful. We have sought to communicate the research and recommendations of *The Shift* in a way that is approachable, and we have also included inserts of several quotations from a variety of professionals whom we respect. Your personal successes and goals give us hope that we are indeed entering a new era of health care. It is because of you that we are committed to continuing on this exciting journey.

FOREWORD, by Peter E. Dawson, DDS

The shift from "tooth dentist" mentality has evolved to recognition that acceptable care of dental patients requires more than just repair of teeth.

The masticatory system is one of the most complex systems in the body, and dentists are the only health professionals who are trained (or should be) in the many aspects of health that are directly or indirectly affected by disharmony or disease within the masticatory system.

Dentists must be physicians of the total masticatory system. But that does not downplay the importance of teeth. Teeth are composed primarily of neurogenic origin. They act as exquisite sensors to the neuromuscular system that controls the function and comfort of the muscles of the jaw. They have a major influence on the musculature of the face and cranium.

Teeth are almost always a factor that must be considered in patients with orofacial pain, including tension headaches and TMJ disorders. Symptoms caused by disharmony between the dental occlusion and the temporomandibular joints (*occluso-muscle pain*) is the most prevalent cause of facial pain as well as damage and pain to the teeth and the TMJs. But sadly, it is also the most missed diagnosis.

Misalignment of teeth can affect the airway. The effects of a crowded dentition or arch deformity can be diagnosed and corrected at an early age to avoid later serious problems of obstructive airways that lead to major health issues.

As a rule, dentists see their patients on a regular schedule and typically spend more time per office visit than physicians do. Thus they are in an ideal situation to partner with physicians as gatekeepers for observing early signs or symptoms of disease or behavioral issues affecting maintenance of general health.

There is a growing trend for dentist/physician collaboration that requires expertise and reliability on the dentists' part. A major responsibility is to be accurate in determining if a masticatory system disorder contributes in any way to a patient's disease or discomfort. In the complex analysis of orofacial pain, as an example, physicians must be able to rely on the dentist to correctly diagnose if a masticatory system disorder is responsible for all of the pain, some of the pain, or none of the pain.

Dentists must accept that responsibility and avail themselves of advanced training if their diagnostic skills fall short of this new norm. Physicians must recognize the importance of collaboration with dental expertise when it is appropriate.

Dentistry has gone through a number of shifts starting with a major shift in the 1960s in which the importance of occlusion opened new frontiers in diagnosis and treatment. In the 1970s advancements in periodontics and restorative dentistry got major attention. This was followed by new knowledge about implantology that made it a practical alternative to full dentures or partials. In the 1990s, new restorative materials plus adhesive dentistry changed the way dentistry was practiced. Then in the 2000s computer-guided technologies opened new doors to diagnosis through advanced imaging capabilities as well as actual treatment options.

As advancements at all levels of practice became the norm, none of them negated the importance of the basic principles of stable occlusion or the recognition of the goal of TMJ health and stability in harmony with the occlusion. Occlusal disease remains a focus of every dental practice. The shift to Integrative Dental Medicine does not in any way diminish the principles of sound practice that have evolved through the years. It is additive to those advancements. Concerns about the general health of every patient must become an integrative inclusion into the concept of complete dentistry.

So what is the next frontier shift in dental medicine?

I believe it is the utilization of our well-established oral health model as a foundation to look more closely at the whole person with emphasis on complete health. That requires development of an expanded Integrative Dental Medicine model of care. Complete dentists must routinely address critically important issues that are often ignored in our busy healthcare system.

Let's look at some examples of what complete dentists should be observing:
- Dentists are in a unique position to observe systemic inflammation that may be reflected in periodontal inflammation, elevated blood sugar levels, pre-diabetes or even full-blown diabetes that exacerbates periodontal disease but is often ignored by patients.
- Gastric reflux that visibly destroys tooth enamel but is also associated with a high risk for esophageal cancer, the fastest-growing cancer in the Western world.
- Nasal allergies and upper airway restrictions that promote mouth breathing and improper tongue positioning. This leads to altered neutral zones that affect arch contours that, in turn, crowd the tongue into airway obstruction. Any alteration of the neutral zone can also affect craniofacial growth and development, altered dental occlusions, neuromuscular imbalance and potential TMD signs and symptoms.
- Observable signs of airway obstruction can lead to disordered breathing that can affect sympathetic dysregulation with increased chronic stress hormone production such as cortisol. The effects of this harmful body-wide stress during waking hours or during sleep should be noticeable enough during a complete dental examination to alert the dentist to seek answers that may require collaboration with medical specialists. The solution may require a dental solution such as changes in arch form to allow proper positioning of the tongue.
- Upper Airway Resistance Syndrome (UARS) and Obstructive Sleep Apnea (OSA) are major health risks experienced by millions of people of all ages. Visible signs may include dental occlusal wear, crowded dental arches, soft tissue obstruction in the throat and scalloping of the tongue. These disorders are commonly associated with gastric reflux. Other frequently occurring signs may include fatigue, poor sleep quality, snoring, attention deficit, morning headaches and sore muscles.

The opportunity for dental professionals to contribute to primary care assessment and intervention is extensive. This will require a shift for both dentists and physicians to appreciate the vital role of dentists, dental hygienists and team members to save not only smiles but to potentially save lives.

This new focus of care is defined by understanding both the nature and scope of oral-systemic connections and how best to treat these newly appreciated relationships between infection, inflammation, breathing, airway, TMD and dental occlusion. This requires an in-depth search of the scientific literature and extensive clinical experience.

I know of no one better equipped to undertake the challenge that lies ahead than Dr. Witt Wilkerson, my practice partner since 1982. Witt brings to the table the needed broad perspective required to resolve the challenging interplay of restorative, occlusal, and TMD problems with the complex relationships to general health issues. Through his association with the Dawson Academy for Advanced Dental Study as a senior faculty member, he has taught thousands of dentists the fundamentals of dental occlusion and diagnosis and treatment of TMJ disorders. With this background, he can bring to the profession a logical insight into integrating these concepts with a new and better correlation with the general health of dental patients.

Dr. Witt Wilkerson is an outstanding professional innovator and leader. He has served as the president of the American Equilibration Society (AES), the largest Academy dedicated to TMJ disorders and occlusion. He is also currently serving as president of the American Academy for Oral and Systemic Health (AAOSH).

In this well-researched and very readable text, Witt has beautifully illuminated dentistry's next frontier. Every dentist who is dedicated to optimum patient care must make a serious effort to seek the necessary education to incorporate these concepts into every-day practice.

Peter E. Dawson, DDS

* * *

Pete Dawson is considered by many to be the most influential clinician and teacher in dentistry in the United States – and the world. He is known globally for his contributions to the fields of occlusion and restorative dentistry and for his concepts on the diagnosis and treatment of temporomandibular disorders. Dr. Dawson authored the #1 best-selling dental text, <u>Evaluation, Diagnosis and Treatment of Occlusal Problems</u>, which is published in 13 languages. He has also authored <u>Functional Occlusion: From TMJ to Smile Design</u>, <u>The Complete Dentist Manual</u>, and <u>A Better Way</u>.

He is the Past-President of the American Equilibration Society, the American Academy of Restorative Dentistry and the American Academy of Esthetic Dentistry. In 2016, Dr. Dawson was awarded the American Dental Association Distinguished Service Award.

Dr. Dawson and Dr. Wilkerson have been partners in private practice, in St. Petersburg, Florida, since 1982.

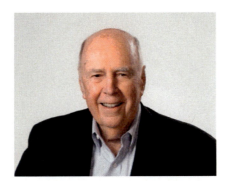

FOREWORD, by Brad Bale, MD

Whether you are reading this book from the perspective of a medical or dental professional or simply as a recipient of our overloaded health care system, it is clear that we as a society currently face critical issues of health and disease. As one of the developers (with Amy Doneen, DNP, ARNP) of the Bale/Doneen Method® for the prevention of heart attacks and strokes, I feel that this book represents a critical bridge between past practices and the future of health and wellness in medicine and dentistry. As a medical professional, I emphatically believe that a strong partnership with our dental colleagues is of the utmost importance for our patients' well-being. To help convey this truth, it is necessary to fully understand the reality of the medical crisis in which we find ourselves.

Heart attacks remain the number one killer in this country, and strokes are the number one cause of disability. Cardiovascular disease (CVD) ranks number one for healthcare expenditures and may single-handedly destroy the solvency of America's healthcare system. In light of this, CVD is the most costly healthcare issue from a humanitarian and fiscal standpoint. Every thirty-four seconds, someone has a heart attack, and every minute someone dies from one. Sudden Cardiac Death (SCD) is responsible for more years of productive life lost (YPLL) than any single cancer. It is currently estimated that every year SCD will claim 2 million YPLL from men and 1.3 million YPLL from women. Strokes occur every forty seconds, and someone dies from a stroke every four minutes. The current annual combined direct and indirect cost of CVD is $315 billion and is projected to reach $1.2 trillion by 2030. Whether you are a patient or a practitioner, these numbers are incredibly alarming.

We can no longer tolerate this degree of human suffering and monetary expenditure. We need to migrate to a platform of preventing arterial disease or, at a minimum, treating it before it leads to a heart attack or stroke. The wonderful news is that we now possess the technology and knowledge to do exactly that. We now have painless, inexpensive tests which can identify patients who have silent but potentially deadly arterial disease lurking in their arteries. Furthermore, it is now known that inflammation initiates the formation of such disease and then drives the progression of it. Arterial disease fueled with enough inflammation *will* culminate in a heart attack or stroke. Extinguishing this arterial 'fire' will halt this disease, allowing it to stabilize prior to causing devastating damage to the heart or brain. To eradicate the inflammation, a holistic approach is needed and, within this approach, a critical factor is maintaining a healthy mouth. Oral health will play a critical role in removing cardiovascular disease from "Number One" on the billboard of death and disability. Therefore, whether you are a patient seeking to maintain your oral health or a dental/medical professional aiming to provide the best care possible, it is imperative to internalize this truth and the message of *The Shift*.

To further understand the reasons behind this, a deeper look at how oral health can optimize cardiovascular health is helpful. To begin with, examining the role of periodontal disease (PD) is critical, as PD is a big dog in the cardiovascular arena of healthcare. The most revered organization in the CVD arena, the American Heart Association (AHA), has concluded that PD is extremely important. In healthcare, there are two things that must be achieved in order to have no doubt that an issue is important, and each one is difficult to establish. Firstly, "level A" evidence needs to be obtained. This type of evidence provides the highest degree of scientific confidence. It must be produced from multiple populations and include conclusions derived from numerous randomized clinical trials or meta-analyses. Secondly, "independent association status" bolsters assurance; however, it is extremely difficult to obtain. It refers to the process by which the investigators make adjustments for numerous other factors known to be associated with the outcome in question in order to see if the issue being studied remains significantly predictive of the outcome. The AHA did indeed conclude that there is level A evidence that periodontal disease is independently associated with arteriosclerotic vascular disease (ASVD). The independent association status was achieved after they adjusted for the following: age; ethnicity; sex; socioeconomic status (income and/or education); smoking habits; diabetes (presence or duration/hemoglobin A1c); hyperlipidemia (or low-density lipoprotein cholesterol and/or high-density lipoprotein cholesterol and/or triglycerides); hypertension (or systolic and/or diastolic blood pressure); body mass index or waist/hip ratio or obesity; alcohol consumption; physical activity; marital status; microalbuminuria; C-reactive protein; fibrinogen; diet; vitamin E intake; statin intake; history of ASVD; family history of ASVD; current access to dentist; renal disease; papillary bleeding score; dependent living; hypertension medication; frequency of dental visits; oral hygiene; missing teeth; DMFT index (decayed, missing, filled teeth); family history of diabetes; and family history of hypertension. This 2012 publication by the AHA rendered a verdict that is exceptionally powerful, acknowledging that periodontal disease is very important in cardiovascular disease. Therefore, we can be confident that oral health plays a vital role in the maintenance of healthy arteries and in the stability of diseased arteries. As such, it is important that both patients and practitioners make decisions with this in mind.

Inflammation plays a key role in the intersection between oral and systemic health. Over 150 years ago, Dr. Rudolf Virchow proposed that inflammation was the cause of arterial disease. Large, genetically-based studies confirmed this theory in 2012. The potential sources of arterial inflammation are numerous. They include the following: poor diet, lack of exercise, lack of sleep, anxiety, nicotine, cholesterol, auto-immune diseases like rheumatoid arthritis, low vitamin D, pre-diabetes, hypertension, genetic predispositions, infectious diseases and oral disease (both periodontal and endodontic disease). If such oral disease persists, the resulting inflammation will contribute to the progression of arterial disease. In 2013, Dr. T. Pessi published an excellent study indicating a significant number of heart attacks may be triggered by oral infection, including endodontic infection (Pessi, 2013). We know inflammation initiates and propagates ASVD. It also appears to trigger CV events. With the understanding that oral disease can create arterial inflammation, it is mandatory that periodontal and endodontic disease be effectively managed to reduce CVD risk. With this in mind, efforts to substantially reduce the current burden of CVD must include the world of dentistry. The abilities of the entire professional oral health team and the engagement and participation of the patient are critical to effectively assess and manage periodontal and endodontic disease in order to avoid arterial inflammation.

The Bale/Doneen Method® was developed for the prevention of heart attacks and strokes. The method advanced to the degree that we began 'guaranteeing' our work several years ago. That guarantee is grounded in being able to extinguish arterial inflammation. We have had (and will continue to have) many cases that required eradication of periodontal and endodontic disease in order to quell inflammation. Some cases have been emergent, which necessitated the awareness of both the patient and his/her dental practice's front office staff to understand the significance of the oral-systemic connection to appreciate the urgency. To the dental team members reading this book, we applaud you for your interest in this subject and your commitment to offer the best treatment possible to those within your care. We appreciate and rely on a close collaboration with our dental colleagues for our success with patients. To the patients reading this book at the recommendations of their dental care providers, we want to encourage you: the fact that you are reading *The Shift* indicates that you are currently in a dental practice that understands the significance of sustaining excellent oral health in order to minimize cardiovascular risk. Please follow all of their advice. If you have periodontal disease, it can be successfully treated and maintenance therapy can keep it at bay. This will reduce your chance of having a heart attack or stroke. If you have infected teeth, the infection can be eradicated. This will also reduce your cardiovascular risk. You are fortunate to be with this dental team. Thank you for reading this material and for joining us in the effort to reduce the number of heart attacks and strokes. Together, as patients and providers alike, we can anticipate the healthier future that *The Shift* can provide.

Works Cited

1. Stone NJ, Robinson J, Lichtenstein AH, Merz CNB, Blum CB, Eckel RH, et al. 2013 ACC/AHA Guideline on the Treatment of Blood Cholesterol to Reduce Atherosclerotic Cardiovascular Risk in Adults: A Report of the American College of Cardiology/American Heart Association Task Force on Practice Guidelines. Circulation. 2013.
2. Lockhart PB, Bolger AF, Papapanou PN, Osinbowale O, Trevisan M, Levison ME, et al. Periodontal disease and atherosclerotic vascular disease: does the evidence support an independent association?: a scientific statement from the American Heart Association. Circulation. 2012;125(20):2520-44.
3. Pessi T, Karhunen V, Karjalainen PP, Ylitalo A, Airaksinen JK, Niemi M, et al. Bacterial Signatures in Thrombus Aspirates of Patients With Myocardial Infarction. Circulation. 2013;127(11):1219-28.
4. Wang J, Liu H, Sun J, Xue H, Xie L, Yu S, et al. Varying Correlation Between 18F-Fluorodeoxyglucose Positron Emission Tomography and Dynamic Contrast-Enhanced MRI in Carotid Atherosclerosis: Implications for Plaque Inflammation. Stroke. 2014.
5. Stecker EC, Reinier K, Marijon E, Narayanan K, Teodorescu C, Uy-Evanado A, et al. Public Health Burden of Sudden Cardiac Death in the United States. Circulation: Arrhythmia and Electrophysiology. 2014;7(2):212-7.
6. Go AS, Mozaffarian D, Roger VL, Benjamin EJ, Berry JD, Blaha MJ, et al. Heart disease and stroke statistics--2014 Update: A Report from the American Heart Association. Circulation. 2014;129(3):e28-e292.

DeWitt C. Wilkerson, DMD

* * *

Brad co-founded the Bale/Doneen Method® and the Heart Attack & Stroke Prevention Center. He is a principal instructor in the Bale/Doneen Method®, training other medical providers across the country.

He has a private clinical practice in Nashville, Tennessee. He also serves as the medical director of the Heart Health Program for Grace Clinic in Lubbock, Texas, Adjunct Professor for Texas Tech Health Sciences, School of Nursing, Clinical Associate Professor for Washington State University College of Medicine, and Assistant Professor at the University of Kentucky, College of Dentistry. Dr. Bale serves on the Board of Directors of the American Academy for Oral Systemic Health (AAOSH).

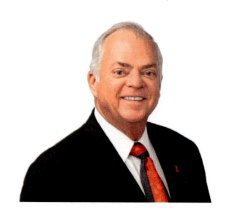

Part I:
The Shift and
Integrative Dental Medicine

**As you change the way you look at the world,
the world you look at changes.**

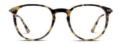

1. WHY "*THE SHIFT*"?

The Shift began in my family as early as the 1940s. My dear mom, Dottie, was raised in rural North Carolina. She observed obesity and poor health throughout her family and community. Relatives all around her were experiencing severe health problems at relatively young ages. Diabetes, strokes, heart attacks, cancer, and early deaths were all too common.

She made a decision at a young age to stay fit and healthy, if at all possible. She began researching and seeking answers. She followed the advice of others, such as the nationally-known nutritionist Adelle Davis who taught, *"We are indeed much more than what we eat, but what we eat can nevertheless help us to be much more than what we are. As I see it, every day you do one of two things: build health or produce disease in yourself."* That made sense to my mom.

She made the *shift*. She chose a very disciplined daily lifestyle of whole foods, juicing, Vitamin C and supplements, limited sugars and white bread, daily exercise, controlled weight, and "walking by faith", believing that God loved her and had a wonderfully positive plan for her life.

As a child, I remember watching her juice carrots in the kitchen, drinking so much carrot juice that her feet and hands would turn orange! When my sisters, DeAnne and Kitty, or I caught a sniffle, my mother would fill a syringe with B12 that she kept in the bathroom medicine cabinet and give us shots in the bottom! It was both an entertaining and traumatic childhood, but that was our mom... and it worked!

Fast forward 70 plus years, and despite many apparent genetic predispositions and disadvantages, my mother has not suffered from osteoporosis, or diabetes, or cancer, or heart attack, or stroke, or Alzheimer's or any other chronic illness. In fact, she recently told me that prior to a recent broken bone, the last time she was hospitalized was the day I was born, over 60 years ago!

She remains vibrant, independent, and mentally strong – working out two times a week with a personal trainer, walking on a treadmill 30 minutes each day, driving her car, traveling, and wearing high heels well into her mid-90's! She looks like she's in her mid-70's. She thinks and acts like she's in her mid-60's! She is a super-hero to all who watch her in stunned amazement, admire her, and want her secret! Her secret is the message of *The Shift*!

Personally, I've been interested in nutrition for years, but not sure which "diet" was best. Many years ago, I was diagnosed with high total cholesterol, hovering ominously around 300. I was prescribed by a cardiologist not one but two statin prescriptions daily for several years, making my muscles feel weak. I've had four surgeries on my right knee over the past few years, which was a great excuse not to exercise. My sweet wife, Pat, threatened not to take me back if I had a fatal heart attack due to lack of exercise! Furthermore, my father died from leukemia, at the young age of 63. Did I inherit a cancer gene? Do I have cardiovascular disease? All this left me worried and with no real, solid answers. It was like a black cloud hovering ominously over my head as I approached 60.

In June 2012, I was invited to attend the meeting of the newly formed American Academy for Oral Systemic Health (AAOSH), held that year at the Cleveland Clinic. The theme, heralded by the physicians leading the world-renowned Cleveland Clinic Wellness Institute, is the same theme that describes *The Shift*: you can take control of your own health, through your lifestyle choices.

The following are some of the messages they shared:
- Michael Roizen, MD, Chief Medical Officer, Cleveland Clinic Wellness Institute, stated, *"Aging is a process that you can control. Research has demonstrated that lifestyle choices and behavior have a far greater impact on longevity and health than heredity."* He pointed out that though our genetic makeup is significant, DNA research is showing that nearly 80% of our genes act like "switches" that turn on or off the other 20% of expressive genes that can

cause disease. He explained that these switches are largely controlled by diet, physical activity, stress, and smoking (toxins). Therefore, our health is not all inherited. That's great news, and it's a great explanation of the focus of *The Shift*.

• Caldwell Esselstyn, MD, former Chief of Surgery at the Cleveland Clinic, reviewed the epidemiological research for coronary artery disease that established it as primarily a diet-controlled illness. He examined the method and result of nutritional changes that may halt and reverse coronary artery disease. He spoke of one patient who had undergone 20 arterial stent procedures, quadruple bypass surgery, and was experiencing angina so severely he couldn't walk to the kitchen without being exhausted. He was not a candidate for further surgery because his vascular system was literally collapsed. He was a dead man walking. He enrolled in a pilot program at the Cleveland Clinic run by Dr. Esselstyn, described in his book, <u>Prevent and Reverse Heart Disease</u>. This program was based on evidence which showed that a diet rich in plants, which produce nitric oxide when digested, dilate the arterial system and shrink plaque. 20 years later, the patient was still alive and thriving. That's *The Shift* in action!

• Brad Bale, MD, co-author of <u>Beat the Heart Attack Gene</u>, explained the connection between vascular health and inflammation. Heart attacks and ischemic strokes are triggered by an inflammatory process that can be initiated and exacerbated by periodontal (gum) disease, as well as poor diet, physical inactivity and stress – another key point of *The Shift*.

• Anthony Iacopino, DMD, PhD, Dean of the University of Manitoba, College of Dentistry, reviewed recent evidence that supports systemic inflammation as the most reliable link between periodontitis and various systemic diseases/conditions, such as diabetes and cardiovascular disease. Diabetes and periodontal disease have similar effects on systemic inflammation. Inflammation is a key theme in *The Shift*, as is the role that oral bacterial pathogens entering the bloodstream can play.

• Mladen Golubic, MD, PhD, prominent researcher at the Cleveland Clinic, explained that the root causes for the development and progression of type 2 diabetes in most people are lifestyle factors, including poor diet, lack of physical activity and unmanaged stress. Lifestyle interventions for this reversible disease positively impact the health of all tissues, including those in the oral cavity. Therefore *The Shift* includes potentially life-changing information for diabetics, including their dental health!

The two days I spent at the AAOSH meeting in 2012 forever changed my understanding of true health and solidified my commitment to learn all I could about *The Shift*, both for my own health as well as for the dental patients that I serve every day.

Following the AAOSH meeting, I sought out Steven Masley, MD, former Medical Director of the famed Pritikin Longevity Center in Miami, Florida and author of <u>Ten Years Younger</u>, <u>The 30-Day Heart Tune-Up</u>, <u>Smart Fat</u>, and <u>The Better Brain Solution</u>, plus numerous scientific articles and PBS Specials on television. Dr. Masley is one of the pioneering Integrative/Functional Medicine Physicians in the world, and he has become my primary coach. I underwent a full-day comprehensive evaluation in his clinic. Strictly following his prescription of an anti-inflammatory diet, supplements, exercise and stress reduction dramatically improved my total wellness. Within a few months, my total cholesterol had dropped below 200, my knee pain had improved significantly, my energy level was much higher, my memory had improved noticeably, my testosterone levels had risen 40%, and my blood counts had normalized. Most significantly, based on carotid intima-media thickness testing (CIMT), which is used to diagnose the extent of carotid atherosclerotic vascular disease, my carotid artery showed an increase of 13% lumen diameter after one year. My arterial disease was reversing! I'd become a *Shifter*! At that time and since, my former concerns about heart attacks, strokes, and cancer have turned into excitement about health and wellness, which I share with anyone even remotely interested in their own health – and who isn't?

Now you understand why *The Shift* is such an important project, as we all work together to turn around the health crisis that is affecting all of our lives. This is the foundation upon which we will build the Integrative Dental Medicine model.

"As a functional medicine physician, I would strive to enhance your cardiovascular system through a broad and holistic range of options, which must involve the weblike interactions among your diet, activity level, weight, environmental toxins, hormones, stress, and biochemical factors such as blood sugar control and inflammation levels. My aim, and that of functional medicine, is to lower your blood pressure from elevated, to normal, to optimal with a lifestyle plan that matches your unique needs. Instead of a diagnosis of hypertension, I would likely call this something like: 'not enough exercise, not enough fruits and vegetables in the diet, high emotional stress, and excessive body fat.' The plan wouldn't be to treat the blood pressure problem with a drug, but rather to view the whole matrix of health issues, optimize a new lifestyle plan with customized tools designed for your success, and correct the underlying cause of the high blood pressure once and for all. The result would be a personalized plan that achieves normal blood pressure without medication."

Steven Masley, MD
The 30-Day Heart Tune-Up

2. A NEW MODEL

American physicist and philosopher Thomas Kuhn is credited with introducing the term "paradigm shift" in his 1962 book, The Structure of Scientific Revolutions. A "paradigm", in science or medicine, represents a widely accepted view of how things are and how things happen. For example, in Western medicine, it has been a widely accepted paradigm that our health is primarily determined by our inherited genetic makeup. Therefore, if a person develops Type 2 diabetes and his or her parent was also a Type 2 diabetic, that appears to sufficiently explain the cause and effect relationship at play. Within that paradigm, the course of treatment may be prescription medications to try to limit the damaging effects of the inherited disease. The dose may necessarily increase over time, if the disease progresses.

However, it is possible that something very radical might then occur. *A paradigm shift* could create a fundamental change in the basic concepts and experimental practices of the scientific discipline.

Continuing with our example, a large study could be conducted with a group of Type 2 diabetics. They could be enrolled in a program focused on a prescribed "anti-inflammatory" regimen. Processed and fried foods, refined sugars, and refined carbohydrates would be removed from their diet. Daily supplements of vitamins and minerals could be added, along with daily physical activity, stress management, sleep hygiene, and smoking cessation.

However, as you might have guessed, this example is not hypothetical. Such a study has been done. The results were that within weeks, nearly 90% of the study subjects' blood sugar levels were reduced to within the normal range, even without medications. These findings create *a scientific crisis* of thought that leads to the following questions:
- If repeated, can we validate the findings of the study? In this case, yes.
- Does this invalidate the genetic inheritance paradigm? No, not necessarily.
- Does this add the factors of *lifestyle* and *inflammation* to the paradigm? Yes.
- Does this represent a potential *paradigm shift* or *scientific revolution* of thought and treatment strategy for Type 2 Diabetes? Yes, absolutely.

Michael Roizen, MD, is an Internist, former Chief of Anesthesiology at the world-renowned Cleveland Clinic, and Past-President of the American Society of Anesthesiologists. He currently serves as the Chief Medical Officer for the Cleveland Clinic Wellness Institute. In his keynote address to the American Academy for Oral Systemic Health (AAOSH) in 2012, Dr. Roizen brilliantly explained that America is in the midst of a pandemic health care crisis. The United States ranks #16 in health among the top 16 developed nations in the world. Every year there is a rise in the incidence of childhood obesity and diabetes. Every year there is a rise in the incidence of adult heart attacks, strokes, and dementia. This is the first generation in which the life expectancy of children will be less than that of their parents.

Additionally, the health crisis is rapidly bankrupting the United States economy. Due to crippling health care costs, Dr. Roizen described two options going forward:
- *Ration health care.*

  One way of rationing health care is to limit the allowable expenditures per patient. I was recently on a flight from New York City to Tampa. Seated next to me was a practicing neurologist from New Jersey who worked for a large insurance-based hospital corporation in New York City. He expressed great frustration because of the limitations set for the number of tests he could run each month for his patients. Exceeding the approved number of ordered MRIs, for example, would result in a reduction in his personal salary. What would Hippocrates think of this philosophy of health care? Rising insurance deductibles, exclusions due to age limits for coverage and pre-existing conditions, and paying out of pocket for certain prescriptions are a few of the many ways of rationing health care.

- *Rational self-care.*

    Alternatively, each of us can chose to take personal responsibility for our own good health. Here we see *The Shift* at work: **we are not victims of our bad genes, but rather victors of our proactive choices**. It's no longer good enough to be diagnosed with Type 2 diabetes and simply accept that diagnosis as our fate, taking a prescription medication as our only option. The science and support are available to rationally and proactively take control of our own health. We will at various times need support from physicians, dentists, dental hygienists, health coaches, personal trainers, nutritionists, therapists, clergy, and accountability partners. But in general, **if we are going to be healthy and free of chronic disease, it's primarily up to our own healthy choices, not our health care professionals.** Just like my mother, Dottie, we will need to take proactive responsibility for our mind, body and spirit.

Dr. Roizen concluded his poignant address by pointing out that the average physician is often only able to spend a few minutes every year with his or her patients, due to time constraints related to low insurance reimbursement and high patient volume. Meanwhile, dental visits typically involve an hour or more of chair time, at least two times per year. He also pointed out that dentists and dental hygienists may spend more time with their patients than any other health care providers. He ended his address by figuratively throwing down a gauntlet, openly challenging dental professionals to see the urgent need in front of all of us and to accept the responsibility of becoming leaders in complete health.

I will never forget Dr. Roizen's admonition: *"I believe that dentists* (dental teams) *should be on the front lines, fighting the health care crisis that is destroying our nation."*

I personally knew, at that moment, that the challenge was very personal, and I would spend the remainder of my professional career as a committed champion for complete health through dentistry and oral medicine.

For me, *The Shift* was a professional awakening, and there was no going back!

> "A true health program should have as its thesis the anticipation and prevention of disease rather than mere identification and treatment. At the present time no such formal program exists anywhere in the world...Predictive medicine may be defined as the clinical discipline designed to anticipate disease in man, to foretell illness before it erupts in its classical form. In addition, predictive medicine is concerned with primary prevention of disease — prevention of occurrence...Predictive medicine stresses that environmental influences play a more significant role in the genesis of disease than heretofore held. Thus, far more can be done to prevent disease than most people realize."
>
> E. Cheraskin, MD, DMD, and W. M. Ringsdorf, Jr., DMD, MS
> <u>Predictive Medicine: A Study in Strategy (1973)</u>

The World Health Organization (WHO) defines health as "a state of complete physical, mental and social well-being and not merely the absence of disease or infirmity[1]." **Integrative Medicine** is the discipline of health professionals focused on complete health.

Duke University Health Center, Division of Integrative Medicine, describes the mission of Integrative Medicine as follows: "Integrative Medicine seeks to restore and maintain health and wellness across a person's lifespan by understanding the patient's unique set of circumstances and addressing the full range of physical, emotional, mental, social, spiritual and environmental influences that affect health. Through personalizing care, integrative medicine goes beyond the treatment of symptoms to address all the causes of an illness. In doing so, the patient's immediate health needs, as well as the effects of the long-term and complex interplay between biological, behavioral, psychosocial and environmental influences, are taken into account."[2]

How do we apply the Integrative Medicine model to dentistry? Borrowing from their inspiring mission, we view the mission statement of **Integrative <u>Dental</u> Medicine** to be the following:

> Integrative Dental Medicine "seeks to restore and maintain health and wellness across a person's lifespan by addressing the full range" of influences that affect oral and systemic health. This "goes beyond the treatment" of oral "symptoms to address all the causes" of illness and disease. In doing so, the patient's immediate health needs as well as the effects of the long-term and complex interplay" between oral and systemic influences "are taken into account."[3]

What is *the Shift*?

***The Shift* is a project**, designed to guide the clinical implementation of Integrative Dental Medicine.

***The Shift* is an effect**, for those who receive the benefits of an Integrative Dental Medicine philosophy of care.

***The Shift* is a scientific revolution**, intentionally saving teeth, intentionally saving smiles, and intentionally saving lives, through Integrative Dental Medicine.

Let's intentionally make *The Shift* – and get this revolution started!

"The ultimate goal of any dental treatment should be to provide optimum oral health. The most meticulously executed dental treatment is incomplete if it is not part of a total treatment plan that results in healthy *maintainability* of the teeth and their supporting structures in harmony with the muscles, bones, joints, and ligaments of the mouth and jaws.

There really is no way to isolate the gnathostomatic system and ignore the other components of the system. Whatever affects one part also affects the other parts. Our objective of optimum oral health cannot be achieved unless all the functional components are in harmony with each other. We must achieve a harmonious interrelationship of all the parts, without excessive stress, since stress accelerates the deterioration of the weaker parts of the system.

We cannot stop the oral structures from aging, but normal aging should not concern us. The teeth, their supporting structures, and the bones, joint, and muscles that make them function are made to last a lifetime. It is only when abnormal factors of deterioration are present that accelerated aging takes place. The dentist who is striving for optimum oral health is constantly searching out and correcting *any* factor that speeds up deterioration and prevents maintainability of all the tissues making up the system…"

Peter E. Dawson, DDS
Evaluation, Diagnosis and Treatment of Occlusal Problems
"Chapter 1: The Concept of Complete Dentistry"

3. AN INTRODUCTION TO INTEGRATIVE DENTAL MEDICINE

> Remembering our Mission Statement:
>
> *Integrative Dental Medicine "seeks to restore and maintain health and wellness across a person's lifespan by addressing the full range" of influences that affect oral and systemic health. This "goes beyond the treatment" of oral "symptoms to address all the causes" of illness and disease. In doing so, the patient's immediate health needs as well as the effects of the long-term and complex interplay" between oral and systemic influences "are taken into account."*[4]

"Traditional" Western Medicine

The Western model of medicine has traditionally focused on the role of genetic predisposition in the expression of chronic diseases. For example, a patient develops type 2 diabetes, with a family history of type 2 diabetes. The traditional Western medical perspective typically considers this to be an irreversible, inherited condition, much like eye color. The underlying framework here would follow the following hypothetical responses: *"Your mother and grandmother had diabetes, so now you've got it. The treatment will consist of prescribed diabetes medications and monitoring of blood sugar levels. The dosage will increase if the blood sugar levels continue to rise over the years. In some cases of extreme weight gain, bariatric surgery (to restrict stomach capacity) may be considered."* While physicians are required to maintain continuing medical education credits to stay abreast of medical innovation, the pace of such new information can be overwhelming. Therefore, a not-insignificant percentage of Western non-specialist physicians have a limited knowledge of diabetes and new research findings. They may be unaware of new studies, based on solid research, showing that a specific low-calorie diet causes remission in 90% of trial patients who lose 33 pounds or more, even those who had been diabetic for six years.[5]

The medical model in the U.S.A is also highly influenced by corporate hospital and insurance restrictions. Physicians now receive lower personal reimbursement for their time and expertise. This forces them to see more patients. Currently, the average visit with a primary care physician is less than 15 minutes per patient. The physician's focus is to quickly identify and address the patient's one chief complaint. In this system, there is virtually no time available for general health screening, testing, or secondary patient questions or concerns. In this setting of quick turnover and daily crunch time, it's challenging for primary care physicians to keep up with new studies based on solid research; as such, any significant preventative measures and present health concerns may often go unaddressed.

We also live in an age of tremendous specialization in Western medicine. Doctors spend four years in university, four years in medical school, and often several other years in specialization training before opening their medical practices. Cardiovascular surgeons are super-specialists in open heart surgery. The patients they treat typically have coronary arteries that are severely occluded from years of accumulating arterial plaque and atherosclerosis. They save lives every day and are tremendous servants to society. We are right to treat them with the utmost respect and to applaud them with gratitude. Yet, very important questions remain unanswered. Why is the plaque there in the first place? Is it really all hereditary, like a black cloud hovering over a family? Who is studying the other possible etiologic factors of vascular disease? Is there a way to prevent and even reverse heart disease in a significant percentage of the population? These are critically important questions for Western health care providers.

> "Think back to your own last visit to the doctor's office. Why did you go? What did he do? What was the result? Were you advised as to what you could do to achieve optimal health and how to maintain it? Or did he patch you up with a prescription and perhaps recommend surgery? The chances are that he performed some repair work, or checked you over, found nothing clinically wrong and told you that you were 'all right.' Yet you still felt bad. Your doctor was not to blame. He was doing what he was trained to do — what you expected him to do — and he probably did it well. But it wasn't health care. True health care aims at prevention of future diseases, not their treatment after they've finally developed. A patient who goes to the doctor when he feels good could learn how to keep feeling good for the rest of his life..."
>
> John McCamy, MD, and James Presley
> Human Life Styling (1975)

Three Eras of Medicine

It is helpful to consider these questions within the context of the different historic and future models of medicine. Our medical health care model has evolved through 3 distinct eras[6]:

1. The first era represents the **Infectious Disease Medical Model.** This was an historic time of research breakthroughs, leading to an understanding of bacterial and viral infections. Two examples of these discoveries were Alexander Fleming's antibiotic, penicillin, in 1928, and Jonas Salk's polio vaccine, in 1957. How grateful we are for these brilliant researchers and the many life-saving drugs and vaccines that are available.
2. The second era represents the **Reactive Medical Model.** During this time, technological advancements in medicine led to amazing life-saving procedures for potentially fatal conditions. In 1954, the first successful organ transplant was performed in Boston, when a young boy donated a kidney to his identical twin brother. Liver, heart and pancreas transplants were successfully performed by the late 1960s, while lung and intestinal organ transplant procedures were begun in the 1980s. Millions of lives have

been saved from imminent death due to these mind-boggling procedures and the brilliant surgeons who perform them.
3. The third era represents the **Root Cause Medical Model.** The main principle of this model is, *"Ask WHY until you can't ask WHY anymore"*. In recent years, a number of medical research institutions in the U.S.A. have implemented this model. This philosophy has led to the growing emphasis on taking an integrative approach to each patient's complete health. It is in this context that we can discuss **Integrative Medicine.** Also known as **Functional Medicine,** it is a growing discipline whereby the objective is to understand cause and effect relationships of health and disease. Patients are counseled on how to prevent accelerated aging and chronic degenerative conditions, such as metabolic syndrome, type 2 diabetes and atherosclerosis. At the same time, patients are coached on how they can engage in a lifestyle that can turn back the clock, increase energy, sharpen their minds, make them trimmer, fitter and help them live with more vibrancy and joy.

Charles "Chip" Whitney, MD, a leading Integrative Physician, stated the following in a personal communication; *"3rd Era Medicine is about empowering another person to create personal health. Health is not just the absence of disease. It is a state of vitality where we have the energy, motivation, excitement, and hope of youth!"*

"Your life style is you. You are what you eat, drink, breathe, think and do. Therefore, what you become tomorrow depends upon what you do today. You are the only person in the world who can do what is necessary to make you healthy and happy."

John McCamy, MD, and James Presley
<u>Human Life Styling (1975)</u>

These very same principles can be applied through **Integrative Dental Medicine (IDM)**, by addressing the **4 B's**:
- **B**ite: TMJ, Masticatory Muscles, Dental Malocclusion, Occlusal Orthotics, Headaches
- **B**acteria: Oral Pathogens, Salivary Testing, Probiotics, Periodontal Therapy
- **B**reathing: Sleep Apnea, Disordered Breathing, Nasal vs. Mouth Breathing, Sleep Studies
- **B**ody: Systemic Inflammation, Nutrition, Physical Inactivity, Toxins, Stress, Gastric Reflux

The primary purpose of *The Shift* is to explore how dentistry, as a true medical sub-specialty, can lead in the cause of both oral and complete health.

My mentor and dental practice partner, Peter Dawson, DDS, founder of the Dawson Academy for Advanced Dental Study, has taught the concepts of complete dentistry to thousands of dentists around the world. In his teaching, the main paradigm is that "dentists are the physicians of the masticatory system". Dentists are the primary health providers responsible for managing the health of the teeth, periodontal bone and soft tissues, temporomandibular joints (TMJs or, as I like to call them, "TMJoints"), muscles of mastication, dental occlusion (bite), neuromuscular harmony, and the balance of forces throughout the dynamic system. The Integrative Dental Medicine (IDM) model builds on this solid foundation by exploring the relationship between the masticatory system and the rest of the body. After all, we've all known since childhood that "the head bone's connected to the neck bone!" Dentists are the physicians of the masticatory system – and much more. By shifting the paradigm of dentistry, we can expect to achieve greater predictability in preventing and resolving dental problems as well as associated systemic health concerns.

In developing an Integrative Dental Medicine/Root Cause Model, three areas of major focus were identified:

1. **Inflammation/Infection**
2. **Airway/Breathing/Sleep Disorders**
3. **TMD/Dental Occlusion**

Due to the integrative/interlinked nature of the human body systems, it is very important to note the following regarding our focus of study:

Systemic Inflammation/Infection, Airway/Breathing/Sleep Disorders and TMD/Dental Occlusion are LINKED.

Because of the interconnected nature of these issues, it is important to assess these three concerns side-by-side while developing a diagnosis and treatment plan. Therefore, *The Shift* of focus toward Integrative Dental Medicine requires careful attention to several key factors of oral and systemic health. To simplify an evaluation, it is helpful to concentrate on specific signs and symptoms. To that end, the following **7 Key Questions** should be considered for every patient:

- Does the **DENTAL OCCLUSION** appear unstable?
- Does the patient **BRUX**?
- Does the patient have **SORE MUSCLES**?
- Are there signs of **TMJOINT CHANGES**?
- Could there be an **AIRWAY PROBLEM**?
- Are there signs of local or systemic **INFLAMMATION**?
- Is there an **UNESTHETIC SMILE** concern?

Addressing all of the factors involved in this wide range of topics might seem like a daunting task, especially for a busy practitioner. How are these goals to be achieved within the rhythm of a dental practice?

For the answer, we turn to insight already utilized within the medical field. In his bestselling book, The Checklist Manifesto, Atul Gawande, MD, a surgeon, describes a basic problem in critical situations, such as handling hospital infections or flying commercial airplanes (or integrating dentistry and complete health). The basic problem is human failure. Gawande exposes two primary shortcomings:
- Ignorance: Where you don't know what you don't know (and therefore need more information or education).
- Ineptitude: Where knowledge is applied inconsistently or incorrectly (such as skipping steps in analyzing or solving a problem).

Historically, the solution to these has been, "experience and training". In medicine, extreme complexity has been addressed through super specialization. But as statistics reveal, with many complications (both avoidable and unavoidable) from surgery each year, minimizing any possible complications would be in the best interest of all involved. Even under the best of circumstances and with ideal care being provided, complications can arise. In the cases where surgical complications could have been avoided, it is even more necessary to look beyond relying solely on traditional training and experience.

In a complex environment, common diagnostic and performance failures can be the result of:

1. Fallibility of human memory and attention – especially tasks which are considered mundane and routine.
2. Skipping steps because they don't always matter...until they do.

Question: What's the solution to avoid these important human lapses, systems' shortcomings, and performance failures?
Answer: Checklists.

Checklists can help with memory recall and clearly set out minimum steps necessary in a process. Good checklists are simple, clear and explicit. They offer verification and also produce discipline of higher performance. Implementing checklists can also be a positive vehicle for behavior change that produces much needed predictability.

Gawande discussed a study using a basic checklist to help prevent central line hospital infections. Using the checklist, he established a higher standard of baseline performance. The incidence of infections decreased quickly and dramatically as all hospital personnel followed the exact checklist protocols.

Therefore, because of the significant benefit of a systematic approach, I have developed the **Integrative Dental Medicine (IDM) Checklist** to guide the clinical implementation process, step-by-step. For each of the three areas of focus (**Inflammation/Infection**, **Airway/Breathing/Sleep Disorders**, and **TMD/Dental Occlusion Disorders**), the IDM Checklist will systematically address the following:

1. **History: Signs & Symptoms**
2. **Evaluation: Clinical Signs**
3. **Screening & Testing**
4. **Treatment**

Reviewing the IDM Checklist will complete your introduction to the Integrative Dental Medicine model. The following chapters will then address the IDM Checklist in detail. We have also included a summary chapter (Chapter 20) before the Appendix reviewing the 7 Key Questions; this summary chapter is intended to serve as a guide for dentists seeking to implement the IDM model.

The Shift

	Infection/Inflammation			Airway/Breathing Disorders			TMD/Occlusion Disorders		
History **Signs & Symptoms**	Caries/Toothaches	−	+	Mouth Breather	−	+	Joint Discomfort	−	+
	Bleeding Gums	−	+	Snoring	−	+	Popping/Clicking	−	+
	Oral Sores	−	+	Sleep Apnea	−	+	Limited Opening	−	+
	Tobacco/Toxins	−	+	Daytime Sleepiness	−	+	Sore Muscles	−	+
	High Blood Pressure	−	+	Poor Sleep Quality	−	+	Nerve Pain	−	+
	Pro-inflammatory Diet	−	+	Nasal Congestion	−	+	Bruxism (Grind or Clench)	−	+
	Chronic Pain/Stress	−	+	Forward Head Posture	−	+	Poor Bite	−	+
	Diabetes	−	+	Tongue Tie	−	+	Worn Teeth	−	+
	Gastric Reflux	−	+	Chronic Cough	−	+	Tongue Thrust	−	+
	Physical Inactivity	−	+	Deviated Septum	−	+	Crooked Teeth	−	+
Evaluation **Clinical signs**	Visual Inspection	−	+	Neck Circumference >16"	−	+	ROM Atypical	−	+
	Periodontal Probing	−	+	Mallampati Score >2	−	+	Muscle Palpation	−	+
	Oral Lesions	−	+	Scalloped Tongue	−	+	Joint Palpation	−	+
	Lymph Nodes	−	+	40% Tongue Restriction	−	+	TMJ Load Testing	−	+
	Swollen Tonsils	−	+	Nasal Stenosis	−	+	CR to MIP Slide	−	+
				Skeletal Profile		+			
Screening & Testing	Radiographic Imaging	−	+	Overnight Pulse Oximetry	−	+	Doppler Auscultation	−	+
	Hb A1c Testing	−	+	Home Sleep Test	−	+	Imaging (CBCT/MRI)	−	+
	Salivary Testing	−	+	Heart Rate Variability(HRV)	−	+	Dawson Photo Series		
	Oral Cancer Screening	−	+	Polysomnogram(PSG)	−	+	Diagnostic Study Models		
	Reflux Symptoms Index (RSI)						Dawson Wizard Analysis		
Differential Conclusion	− Negative		+ Positive	− Negative		+ Positive	− Negative		+ Positive

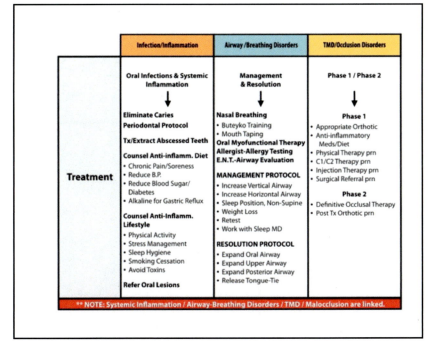

	Infection/Inflammation	Airway/Breathing Disorders	TMD/Occlusion Disorders
Treatment	**Oral Infections & Systemic Inflammation** ↓ **Eliminate Caries** **Periodontal Protocol** **Tx/Extract Abscessed Teeth** **Counsel Anti-inflamm. Diet** • Chronic Pain/Soreness • Reduce B.P. • Reduce Blood Sugar/ Diabetes • Alkaline for Gastric Reflux **Counsel Anti-Inflamm. Lifestyle** • Physical Activity • Stress Management • Sleep Hygiene • Smoking Cessation • Avoid Toxins **Refer Oral Lesions**	**Management & Resolution** ↓ **Nasal Breathing** • Buteyko Training • Mouth Taping **Oral Myofunctional Therapy** **Allergist-Allergy Testing** **E.N.T.-Airway Evaluation** **MANAGEMENT PROTOCOL** • Increase Vertical Airway • Increase Horizontal Airway • Sleep Position, Non-Supine • Weight Loss • Retest • Work with Sleep MD **RESOLUTION PROTOCOL** • Expand Oral Airway • Expand Upper Airway • Expand Posterior Airway • Release Tongue-Tie	**Phase 1 / Phase 2** ↓ **Phase 1** • Appropriate Orthotic • Anti-inflammatory Meds/Diet • Physical Therapy prn • C1/C2 Therapy prn • Injection Therapy prn • Surgical Referral prn **Phase 2** • Definitive Occlusal Therapy • Post Tx Orthotic prn

** NOTE: Systemic Inflammation / Airway-Breathing Disorders / TMD / Malocclusion are linked.

> "There is a vacuum in health care now. Only a few, perhaps a few hundred, are actively teaching true health care in this country. We need to start redistributing medical training funds, in order to provide more true health training. We need fewer persons trained in disease treatment and more in preventative medicine, until there is at least a fifty-fifty balance.
>
> It is also hoped that each of our large clinics in this country will add a preventative medicine section. This would enable each patient to have not only an excellent disease work-up but also competent dietary, exercise and stress evaluations. These could be explained to the patient, with his risk factors spelled out clearly – compared to the normal, not the average. Total-health centers are needed, so that people can go and learn total-health living and doctors can be trained there to teach it…
>
> As a profession, dentists are far ahead of physicians in preventative techniques…"
>
> John McCamy, MD, and James Presley
> Human Life Styling (1975)

Part II:
The Great Fire
Inflammation and Infection

4. INFLAMMATION AS A CENTRAL THEME IN INTEGRATIVE DENTAL MEDICINE

Dr. Bale's *Foreword* clearly describes the primary role of systemic inflammation in cardiovascular disease. The current research in all fields of medicine are reporting the same findings. The Mayo Clinic Health letter states, "Inflammation is the new medical buzzword. It seems as though everyone is talking about it, especially the fact that inflammation appears to play a role in many chronic diseases."[7]

Dental professionals are very familiar with the most common chronic inflammatory disease in the human body: periodontal disease. Inflamed periodontal tissues appear red, swollen and bleed easily. There are multiple reasons for this appearance, including bacterial acidic biofilms, decreased salivary flow, reactions to medications, smoking, a compromised immune system, hormonal changes, elevated blood sugar levels, poor nutrition, vitamin and nutritional deficiencies, chronic mouth breathing and gastric reflux. As we can see, periodontal inflammation is a multi-factorial, oral-systemic disorder. It appears as a localized concern but actually concerns the whole body. The astute dentist, as a physician of the masticatory system who addresses periodontal disease, must take an integrative medicine approach to treatment decisions.

Whether one is considering periodontal tissues, blood pressure, cholesterol levels, arterial plaque, blood sugar levels, heart health, brain health, gut health, weight control, sleep hygiene or aging, inflammation is a major concern.

> ### "What is the effect of diabetes on oral health and glycemic control?
> Diabetes, especially if poorly controlled, affects oral health by increasing the risk for periodontal disease and tooth loss....On the other hand, periodontitis can adversely affect glycemic control and increase the risk for complications such as cardiovascular disease and end-stage renal disease in patients with type 2 diabetes.
>
> ### What is the biologic plausibility of the association between oral health and diabetes?
> The bidirectional relationship between diabetes and periodontal diseases is most likely related to the increased level of systemic inflammation each disease causes. This heightened systemic inflammation results in insulin resistance, poor glycemic control, and aggravated destruction of periodontal tissues.
>
> ### What is the appropriate message to give to the public about the association between oral health and diabetes?
> The message for the public is that diabetes, especially if poorly controlled, is an important risk factor for periodontal disease. Tooth loss is also increased twofold in patients with diabetes, and this loss often leads to poor nutrition, which can make dietary control of diabetes more difficult. People with diabetes can also suffer from xerostomia [dry mouth] or burning mouth syndrome and are more susceptible to fungal infections.
>
> ### What is the biologic plausibility of the association between oral health and cardiovascular disease?
> Oral microbes colonize atherosclerotic plaque via bacteremia, and they may contribute to the eventual destabilization of the plaque. They may also lead to myocardial infarction or ischemic stroke. Also, oral microbes contribute to the cumulative burden of systemic inflammatory responses that may lead to atherosclerosis."
>
> <u>The Oral-Systemic Health Connection</u>
> Edited by Michael Glick, DMD

What are some of the common factors of local and systemic inflammation that can be identified through a thorough health history, clinical evaluation, screening, and testing in a general dental or medical setting? The following areas deserve our focus in this discussion:
- **Oral Pathogens**
- **Tobacco & Toxin Exposure**
- **Pro-inflammatory Diet**
- **Blood Sugar Dysregulation & Insulin Resistance**
- **Gastric Reflux**
- **Stress**
- **Physical Inactivity**
- **Biochemical Imbalance**
- **Disordered Breathing & Disrupted Sleep**

To examine these, let's direct our attention to the Integrative Dental Medicine (IDM) Checklist in order to organize our discussion of **Inflammation** and **Infection**.

We will follow the IDM Checklist sequentially as follows:
1. **History:** Signs & Symptoms
2. **Evaluation:** Clinical Signs
3. **Screening & Testing**
4. **Treatment**

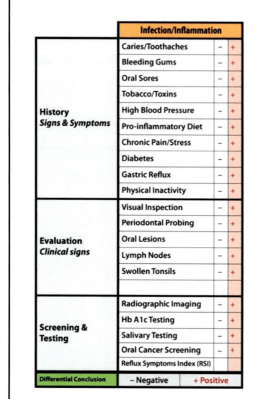

"Doctors cannot give you health. Doctors can only remove symptoms or causes of symptoms; they cannot make you healthy. Becoming healthy is the job of the individual. We all have to be our own personal healthcare practitioners. We are the only ones who can do it. We do this with proper nutrition, exercise, getting adequate sleep, and by managing the stressors in our lives. If we fail ourselves in these endeavors, then we become sick or unwell. If we do not reverse this process by correcting our behaviors, we eventually become diseased. All chronic diseases are diseases of chronic inflammation, which is why [we are] focused on reducing inflammation, or 'DeFlaming.'

With the above in mind, having health insurance will not make you healthy. And from a terminology perspective, 'health insurance' is another inaccurate term. In truth, there is no such thing as health insurance. It is really a type of financial insurance or protection for when we become sick, diseased, or injured. My suggestion is to become 'DeFlamed' and healthy so you can avoid the need to use insurance and hopefully pass through life in a disease-free fashion without becoming a burden on family or society.

[Our focus is] how to pursue a healthy 'DeFlamed' state with nutrition. The opposite is what most people do — they pursue chronic inflammation, sickness and disease with an inflammatory diet and then somehow expect medications and surgery to make them healthy. This is a physiological impossibility. Only we can make ourselves healthy. We are our only true 'healthcare' practitioners, and we practice healthcare by DeFlaming our bodies."

David R. Seaman, DC, MS
<u>The DeFlame Diet: DeFlame Your Diet, Body, and Mind</u>

5. INFLAMMATION & INFECTION – HISTORY: SIGNS AND SYMPTOMS

**Inflammation/Infection:
History:** *Signs & Symptoms*
1. Caries and Toothaches

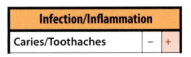

"Caries" is Latin for "rottenness", a disease of teeth that is most common in the developed world, due to an increased consumption of refined sugars. Early childhood caries (ECC) represents a major health concern. Approximately 56% of U.S. children, aged 6-8, have dental caries, making it one the most common infection conditions in children.[8]

Risk factors for childhood caries include early exposure to cariogenic bacteria such as the mutans streptococci (MS) group. These bacteria adhere to enamel and metabolize fermentable carbohydrates; this process produces acids which lower the enamel pH, promote demineralization, and result in carious decay. MS in infants is commonly acquired from the caregiver (most often the mother) through infected saliva.[9]

Poor feeding habits, such as the consumption of fermentable carbohydrates and snacks, will lower the pH in the presence of MS and increase the risk for caries. Interestingly, the prevalence of caries in dogs is low, having been documented at 5% in a study of 435 dogs.[10] Caries in cats is almost nonexistent. These pets typically have high salivary pH, diets low in refined carbohydrates, a low MS incidence, and shallow pit and fissure grooves in their molars.

The immediate effects of ECC are pain and infection. These can affect the child's ability to eat, with findings showing that children with ECC are at risk of weighing less than 80% of their ideal weight, representing a true "failure to thrive". Nutritional deficiencies in a growing child may have lifelong, systemic health implications on both growth and cognitive development. Normal growth and development may be delayed due to pain and sleep disturbances.[11]

Dental caries represents the earliest of localized infections that can have systemic affects. But there's more. The NIH reports that 92% of adults between the ages of 20 and 64 have caries in their permanent teeth.[12]

In all ages of life, dental caries is associated with both local and systemic infection and inflammation when the pulpal tissues (nerves and blood vessels) within the tooth abscess. Drainage out of the tooth causes a breakdown of bone with the formation of a pus-filled infection site and access to the bloodstream. We will discuss the systemic implications of this in the next section.

Inflammation/Infection:
History: *Signs & Symptoms*
2. Bleeding Gums (Periodontal Disease)

Infection/Inflammation		
Caries/Toothaches	−	+
Bleeding Gums	−	+

A localized inflammation or infection can be characterized as reddened, swollen, hot, and often painful tissue, resulting from an immune reaction to an injury or infection. Periodontal disease (a.k.a. gum disease) is a set of inflammatory conditions affecting the tissues surrounding the teeth. In the early "gingivitis" stage, the gums become swollen and red, and may bleed easily. In the more serious "periodontitis" stage, the gums can separate from the teeth, bone can be lost around the teeth, and the teeth may loosen and eventually fall out. Periodontal disease is generally due to the presence and effects of acid-producing bacteria in the mouth, which significantly lowers the oral pH; this also results in an imbalance of the oral bacteria, which negatively affects the body's immune system response and leads to infection and inflammation of both hard and soft tissues around the teeth.[13]

Sig Socransky, DDS (1934-2011), a revered oral microbiologist, and his research team at Harvard University and the

Forsythe Institute in Boston, revolutionized our understanding of oral microbiology with a focus on the etiology and treatment of periodontal infections. In his words,

> Studies in experimental animals have added considerable support to the hypothesis of the significant role of microorganisms in the etiology of periodontal disease. Germ-free animals are essentially free of periodontal destruction...with minimal observable inflammation or pocket formation. The use of antibiotics or antiseptics in a variety of animal model systems controls the soft tissue pathology and most of the hard tissue destruction in these animals. Periodontal disease can be transmitted from an animal harboring the disease to one initially free of it by caging diseased and disease-free animals together or by the implantation of plaque or specific microorganisms derived from the plaque of diseased animals.[14]

In addition to the role of microorganisms in periodontal disease, risk factors can include smoking, diabetes, HIV/AIDS, family history of periodontal disease, and certain medications.[15]

According to a recent National Institutes of Health (NIH) Human Microbiome Project estimate, 90% of cells in and on the human body are bacterial, fungal, or otherwise non-human. Incredibly, "the microbes that live inside and on us (the microbiota) outnumber our somatic and germ cells by an estimated 10-fold."[16]

More than 700 different bacterial species have been identified in the human oral cavity, with the majority of them being associated with dental plaque. Extensive animal and clinical research indicates that the oral microbial flora is responsible for two important human diseases: dental caries (tooth decay) and periodontitis (gum disease). According to UCLA researcher Xuesong He, PhD, and cohort, "...more recent studies have shown that, instead of a single pathogen, periodontitis may be a poly-microbial infectious disease caused by potentially pathogenic microbial communities, in which microorganisms interact in a synergistic or cooperative manner, leading to pathogenesis."[17]

Meanwhile, hundreds of different types of "good" bacteria play a very important role in our health by processing fiber and producing certain vitamins (such as B vitamins, vitamin K, and other nutritive substances); playing essential roles in digestion; and in bolstering the immune system. These health-promoting bacteria are called **probiotics** and are normal inhabitants of the human gastrointestinal tract. Bacterial **probiotics** may be thought of as the right bacteria, in the right place, at the right time. Bacterial

pathogens on the other hand may be thought of as the wrong bacteria, in the wrong place, at the wrong time.

There are two ways bacteria can harm the human body:
- **Toxicity** – the bacteria produce toxins which damage specific tissues in the body.
- **Invasiveness** – the bacteria multiply rapidly at the site of infection and overwhelm the body's defense mechanisms. The bacteria may then spread to other parts of the body.

This raises an important question in the study of Integrative Dental Medicine: *are the oral bacteria that influence periodontal and periapical tooth disease only <u>localized</u> sources of infection and inflammation?*

There is an increasing body of evidence that the pathogenic bacteria which cause periodontal disease and dental caries can have serious, detrimental influences beyond the mouth. Let's review several examples from the research literature.

***Fusobacterium nucleatum* (Fn)** is a gram negative oral bacteria that is abundantly present in periodontal plaque and which is implicated in periodontal and periapical disease.[18] Yiping Han, PhD, has focused her research efforts at Case Western Reserve and Columbia University largely on the role of Fn, regarding both its role as a periodontal pathogen and its implications within several significant systemic issues. Dr. Han's studies associate this oral bacteria with adverse pregnancy outcomes (such as chorioamnionitis, preterm birth, stillbirth, neonatal sepsis, preeclampsia), GI disorders (such as colorectal cancer, inflammatory bowel disease, appendicitis), cardiovascular disease, rheumatoid arthritis, respiratory tract infections, Lemierre's syndrome and Alzheimer's disease. [19]

Another study which Dr. Han co-authored revealed that when Fn moves from the gum tissues into the bloodstream, it can increase permeability of the arterial endothelium (inner lining), allowing other bacteria originating in the mouth to penetrate from the bloodstream through the arterial wall.[20] Arteries have an endothelial lining that is one cell layer thick, similar to chimney stacks lined by bricks that are one layer thick. The bricks are held together by "grout", just as the endothelial cells are held together by biologic "grout". Fn essentially weakens the endothelial grout, making it more permeable for circulating bacteria in the bloodstream to seep out through the arterial wall. This leads to another important possible association found in other studies –

periodontal pathogens (gum disease bacteria) found in arterial plaque.

"Atheroma" is the medical term for the "plaque" buildup in the lining of arteries, which consists of deposits of fat, cholesterol, calcium, connective tissue, and inflammatory cells. An "endarterectomy" is a surgical procedure to remove an atheroma. Endarterectomies are commonly performed to "clean out" blocked carotid arteries in the neck as a preventative measure against strokes.

A 2009 endarterectomy study of 44 subjects at the University of Sao Paulo, Brazil, produced the following significant report:

> *Oral pathogens, including periodontopathic bacteria, are thought to be aetiological factors in the development of cardiovascular disease. In this study, the presence of* **Aggregatibacter actinomycetemcomitans *(Aa)*, Fusobacterium nucleatum–periodonticum–simiae group *(Fn)*, Porphyromonas gingivalis *(Pg)*, Prevotella intermedia *(Pi)*, Prevotella nigrescensv *(Pn) and* Tannerella forsythia *(Tf)*** *in atheromatous plaques from coronary arteries was determined by real-time PCR. Forty-four patients displaying cardiovascular disease were submitted to periodontal examination and endarterectomy of coronary arteries...Total bacterial and periodontopathic bacterial DNA were found in 94.9 and 92.3%, respectively, of the atheromatous plaques from periodontitis patients, and in 80.0 and 20.0%, respectively, of atherosclerotic tissues from periodontally healthy subjects. All periodontal bacteria except for the F. nucleatum–periodonticum–simiae group were detected, and their DNA represented 47.3% of the total bacterial DNA obtained from periodontitis patients. Porphyromonas gingivalis, A. actinomycetemcomitans and Prevotella intermedia were detected most often. The presence of two or more periodontal species could be observed in 64.1% of the samples...**The significant number of periodontopathic bacterial DNA species in atherosclerotic tissue samples from patients with periodontitis suggests that the presence of these microorganisms in coronary lesions is not coincidental and that they may in fact contribute to the development of vascular diseases.***[21]

It is important to note that six different bacteria from the mouth associated with periodontal disease were found in significant concentrations in carotid artery plaque.

In 2017, Drs. Bale and Doneen published a summary article citing numerous studies, including the one above, with the following conclusions:

> *Periodontal disease (PD) is generated by microorganisms. These microbes can enter the general circulation causing a bacteraemia. The result can be adverse systemic effects, which could promote conditions such as cardiovascular disease. Level A evidence supports that PD is independently associated with arterial disease. PD is a common chronic condition affecting the majority of Americans 30 years of age and older. Atherosclerosis remains the largest cause of death and disability. Studies indicate that the adverse cardiovascular effects from PD are due to a few putative or high-risk bacteria:* **Aggregatibacter actinomycetemcomitans, Porphyromonas gingivalis, Tannerella forsythia, Treponema denticola or Fusobacterium nucleatum**. *There are three accepted essential elements in the pathogenesis of atherosclerosis: lipoprotein serum concentration, endothelial permeability and binding of lipoproteins in the arterial intima. There is scientific evidence that PD caused by the high-risk pathogens can influence the pathogenesis triad in an adverse manner.* **With this appreciation, it is reasonable to state PD, due to high-risk pathogens, is a contributory cause of atherosclerosis. Distinguishing this type of PD as causal provides a significant opportunity to reduce arterial disease.**[22]

From this report we can gather the following significant clinical lessons:

➢ Periodontal disease, due to high-risk pathogens, can adversely influence atherosclerosis and may be considered to be a contributory cause of arterial disease.

➢ The dental community has a significant interventionary role in cardiovascular disease, through effective management of periodontal disease due to high-risk pathogens.

Further research points out that a potentially even-greater cardiovascular risk may come from oral **periapical disease** (abscessed teeth due to dental decay). In 2013, Tanja Pessi, PhD, and research cohort at Tampere University Medical Center, Finland, completed a research project evaluating a common hypothesis: infectious agents, especially bacteria and their components originating from the oral cavity or respiratory tract, can contribute to inflammation in the coronary plaque, leading to rupture and the subsequent development of coronary thrombus (blood clot/heart attack). The study measured bacterial DNA in thrombus aspirates (removed and evaluated the oral bacterial levels in the blood clot) of subjects immediately following acute myocardial infarction (heart attack), assessing a possible association between bacterial findings and oral pathology.[23]:

> *Findings: 101 subjects were evaluated following acute myocardial infarction. The obstructing thrombi and arterial blood in the vessels were analyzed for oral/periodontal pathogenic bacteria. The bacterial load in the thrombi averaged 16 times greater than in the arterial blood. Bacterial DNA typical for endodontic infection (mainly oral viridans streptococci) was measured in 78.2% of thrombus aspirates, and periodontal pathogens were measured in 34.7%.*
>
> *Conclusions: The study confirms earlier studies and suggests that dental infections are implicated in the inflammation and rupture of vulnerable plaques. Repeated transient bacteremia after dental procedures or other bacterial infections (such as periodontal disease, periapical disease and "leaky gut") during the lifetime may cause entrapment of pathogens in vulnerable atherosclerotic plaques.*[24]

They concluded that "dental infection and oral bacteria are associated with the development of acute coronary thrombosis (heart attack). Dental health and dental care should be one major element in efforts to prevent heart attacks."[25]

"What's the link between periodontal disease and CVD [cardiovascular disease]? Very sophisticated studies have demonstrated a strong similarity between the amount of inflammation in our gums and the amount of inflammation in the major arteries of the neck and the heart's largest artery, the aorta. That's dangerous because inflammation is the key player in destabilizing plaque in the artery walls, explaining why some people with relatively little build up experience plaque rupture and subsequent strokes or heart attacks, while others with substantial deposits never suffer these events. Studies are now revealing that most plaques in the carotid artery actually contain many of the germs known to cause periodontal disease (PD)."

Bradley Bale, MD, and Amy Doneen, DNP, ARNP
<u>Beat the Heart Attack Gene</u>

As we systematically continue through the IDM Checklist, we will discuss clinical evaluation and treatment considerations for periodontal and periapical disease. For now, keep the words of Dr. Brad Bale's *Foreword* in the forefront of your mind: ***"All cardiovascular prevention programs must include an oral-systemic component. Dentistry is a big dog in the cardiovascular wellness arena!"***

The important role oral pathogens can play extends to all parts of the body. "Gum disease" has been identified as the body's most abundant source of chronic low-grade inflammation and has been described as "a smoldering fire in your body where the alarm bell is not answered." **The American Academy of Periodontology, American College of Obstetricians and Gynecologists and other reputable sources** list the following research findings connecting periodontitis to systemic inflammation and various systemic diseases:

SYSTEMIC INFLAMMATION:
"Research has shown that periodontal disease is associated with several other diseases. For a long time it was thought that bacteria was the factor that linked periodontal disease to other disease in the body; however, more recent research demonstrates that inflammation may be responsible for the association. Therefore, treating inflammation may not only help manage periodontal diseases but may also help with the management of other chronic inflammatory conditions."[26]

STROKE:
"Studies have pointed to a relationship between periodontal disease and stroke. In one study that looked at the causal relationship of oral infection as a risk factor for stroke, people diagnosed with acute cerebrovascular ischemia were found more likely to have an oral infection when compared to those in the control group."[27]

DIABETES:
"Diabetic patients are more likely to develop periodontal disease, which in turn can increase blood sugar and diabetic complications. Severe periodontal disease can increase blood sugar, contributing to increased periods of time when the body functions with a high blood sugar. This puts people with diabetes at increased risk for diabetic complications."[28]

PREGNANCY COMPLICATIONS:
"*Oral inflammatory burden and preterm birth*: [In a study of] 328 Finnish women with singleton births, 77 had preterm births and 251 had full-term births. Gingival bleeding on probing, probing depth, and the presence of dental calculus and mouth ulcers were recorded; the oral inflammatory burden index (OIBI) was constructed based on these clinical findings. Conclusion: The combined effects of multiple oral infections were significantly associated with preterm birth."[29]

STILLBIRTH
In 2010, the Journal of the American College of Obstetricians and Gynecologists reported a "case of stillbirth caused by Fusobacterium nucleatum, which originated in the mother's mouth." She had gum disease, developed an upper–respiratory infection, and experienced a stillbirth a few days later. "F. nucleatum was isolated from the placenta, baby, and subgingival plaque... Conclusion: F. nucleatum may have moved from the mother's mouth to the uterus when her immune system was weakened by the respiratory infection."[30]

PANCREATIC CANCER
"A new study has found significant associations between antibodies for multiple oral bacteria and the risk of pancreatic cancer, adding support for the emerging idea that these seemingly unrelated medical conditions are linked. The study of blood samples from more than 800 European adults, published in the journal *Gut*, found that high antibody levels for one of the more infectious periodontal bacterium strains of Porphyromonas gingivalis were associated with a two-fold risk for pancreatic cancer. Meanwhile, study subjects with high levels of antibodies for some kinds of harmless 'commensal' oral bacteria were associated with a 45-percent lower risk of pancreatic cancer. In response to these results, Brown University epidemiologist Dominique Michaud, the paper's corresponding author, had this to say: 'The relative increase in risk from smoking is not much bigger than two. If this is a real effect size of two, then potential impact of this finding is really significant.' Pancreatic cancer, which is difficult to detect and kills most patients within six months of diagnosis, is responsible for 40,000 deaths a year in the United States. These findings are therefore very important; additionally, several researchers, including Michaud, have found previous links between periodontal disease and pancreatic cancer."[31]

With all of this in mind, it is clear that oral pathogens, whether from periodontal or periapical disease, appear to be much more significant prognosticators of multiple health complications than ever imagined. Dental teams are the medical specialists equipped to evaluate, diagnose and treat the etiologic bacteria, in order to both prevent and reverse disease.

Inflammation/Infection:
History: *Signs & Symptoms*
3. Oral Sores

Infection/Inflammation		
Caries/Toothaches	-	+
Bleeding Gums	-	+
Oral Sores	-	+

Oral sores can have multiple sources related to both local and systemic causes. **Canker sores (apthous ulcers)** are commonly seen in the dental office due to tooth and denture irritations and hard foods. Evidence suggests that canker sores often result from an altered local immune response associated with stress, trauma, or irritation. Acidic foods such as tomatoes, citrus fruits, and some nuts are known to cause irritation in some people. They appear quickly and typically heal within 7-14 days.

Fever blisters (cold sores) are also common and result from a dormant herpes simplex virus that becomes active. The virus is often activated by conditions such as stress, fever, temperature change, trauma, hormonal changes, and exposure to sunlight. They begin with a sensation of heat, swelling and then blistering, often in the same location, with intermittent frequency for years. They typically heal within 14 days.

Oral cancer typically appears more gradually, producing a firmer mass, often discolored, with a raised border and a depressed center. **Kaposi's Sarcoma lesions** appear as purplish intraoral masses associated with HIV infections.

Additionally, sore throats, hoarseness, and chronic cough can be present with the sexually-transmitted **Human Papilloma Virus (HPV),** the new leading cause of throat cancer.

Mouth swelling, sore throats, coughing, hoarseness, post nasal drip, heartburn, tongue soreness and worn teeth can result from **Gastro-Esophageal Reflux Disease (GERD).** GERD plays a significant role in Barrett's Esophagus (chronic inflammation of the esophagus) and esophageal cancer, which is reportedly the fastest growing cancer in the modern Western world.[32]

Oral outbreaks can reflect other systemic conditions such as **viral** infections. **Fungal or yeast infections** (candidiasis) are often associated with antibiotic usage (which decreases normal bacteria in the mouth), a compromised immune system, and dry mouth (which is a common side effect of many medications).

Inflammation/Infection:
History: *Signs & Symptoms*
4. Tobacco/Toxins

Infection/Inflammation		
Caries/Toothaches	−	+
Bleeding Gums	−	+
Oral Sores	−	+
Tobacco/Toxins	−	+

Tobacco use is a risk factor for many diseases, especially those affecting the heart, liver, and lungs, as well as many cancers, including oral cancer. In 2008, the World Health Organization named tobacco as **the world's single greatest preventable cause of death**. In the 20th century, the tobacco epidemic killed 100 million people worldwide. During the 21st century, it could kill one billion.

The nicotine in any tobacco product is quickly absorbed into the blood when a person uses it. In the bloodstream, nicotine immediately stimulates the adrenal glands to release the hormone epinephrine (adrenaline). **Epinephrine stimulates the central nervous system** and **increases blood pressure**, **breathing**, and **heart rate**. This is a stressor to the autonomic (involuntary) nervous system. As with drugs such as cocaine and heroin, nicotine activates the brain's reward circuits and also increases levels of the chemical messenger dopamine, which reinforces rewarding behaviors. Tobacco smoking can lead to **lung cancer**, **chronic bronchitis**, and **emphysema**. It increases the risk of **vascular disease**, which can lead to **stroke** or **heart attack**. Smoking has also been linked to other cancers, including **leukemia; cataracts**; and **pneumonia**. It **impedes healing** and **reduces blood** flow, which is a fact well-known by dentists, who observe a high rate of failure of osseointegration of dental implants placed in patients who use tobacco. It is safe to assume that it is virtually impossible for a tobacco abuser to live a life free of chronic, systemic inflammation.

Exposure to toxins is very pervasive for those living in highly-congested city environments, especially given the many modern conveniences in such places. In an urban setting, there is a tremendous usage of fossil fuels such as gasoline, oil, and natural gas. Their effects are increasingly significant to the quality of the air we breathe, and therefore to our health. The United States holds less than 5% of the world's population but uses more than 25% of the world's supply of fossil fuels (due to large houses, private cars, etc.).[33]

Combustion of fossil fuels also produces air pollutants, such as nitrogen oxides, sulfur dioxide, volatile organic compounds and heavy metals. Additionally, polluted air contains other pollutants such as concrete dust from building construction, pesticides from lawn maintenance, pollen, microbes, allergens, dust, pet dander, and human germs. All of these can be possible sources of allergies that produce respiratory health concerns.

The food we eat can also be a source of toxicity. North Carolina State University's Department of Applied Ecology released the following statement in 2018:

> Mercury is the most common pollutant in North Carolina's freshwater fish. Mercury is released when coal is burned to produce electricity, and mercury eventually makes its way into lakes and rivers, where it builds up in fish. The entire state of North Carolina has a fish consumption advisory for mercury, meaning that in every waterbody in the state, at least some of the fish have been polluted with mercury. Avoiding eating larger, predatory fish can reduce the amount of mercury you might be exposed to when eating fish from North Carolina waterbodies…Our bodies remove mercury very slowly and do not show symptoms of mercury exposure right away. Mercury affects our nervous systems and various other parts of our bodies, impacting both adults and children. Mercury is most dangerous, even at low levels, for children and infants. Women can pass mercury in their bodies on to unborn children.[34]

This is a serious issue of which many people are unaware and which necessitates an increase in education regarding these risks.

Presently, 45 states in the United States have fish consumption advisories for mercury. According to the 2018 Florida Fish and Wildlife Conservation Commission report,

> Largemouth bass and other long-lived predatory fish have higher concentrations of mercury; however, smaller largemouth bass have less mercury than larger individuals. In marine waters, shorter lived species such as striped mullet, Florida pompano, sheepshead, common dolphin, gray snapper, gulf flounder, and southern flounder generally have much lower concentrations while king mackerel, swordfish, and sharks tend to have the highest concentrations. Ultimately, **mercury concentrations in fishes depend on diet and lifespan: those that consume other fish and live longest have the highest mercury concentrations.**[35]

Another source of food toxicity concerns the way the natural presentation of fruits, vegetables and proteins are modified by farmers, ranchers, and the food industry. Hormones, antibiotics, pesticides, preservatives, chemical additives, and genetic modifications can produce toxic effects in some people.

A subject of tremendous controversy for many years has been the question of the toxicity of silver mercury dental fillings. The position of the American Dental Association is that scientific studies show the health risk is minimal. Other researchers strongly disagree and believe that harmful mercury vapors are continuously released from silver fillings, producing systemic injury, and the fillings should be removed. At the present time, the controversy continues, with no governmental restrictions in existence for the placement of silver mercury fillings.

"Action Steps: Step 1 – Take Care of Your Teeth"

"A habit that takes five minutes a day can add years to your life and also reduces risk for heart attacks, strokes, diabetes, colds, flu, and even arthritis. A 2012 study found that one of the simplest — and cheapest — ways to a long life is brushing and flossing your teeth daily. Conversely, neglecting your chompers can actually be fatal, the researchers reported.

Just how much impact does good oral heath have? California researchers tracked 5,611 seniors for 17 years and found that:

*Never brushing at night boosted the risk for death during the study period by 20 to 25%, compared to brushing every night.

*Never flossing hiked mortality risk by 30%, versus daily flossing.

*Not seeing a dentist in the previous 12 months raised the risk of death by up to 50%, compared to getting dental care two or more times a year.

Another startling finding: One major predictor of early death was missing teeth, even after other risk factors were taken into account, the study reported. That's powerful motivation to see your dentist regularly and fight heart disease with a toothbrush and floss…"

Bradley Bale, MD, and Amy Doneen, DNP, ARNP
<u>Beat the Heart Attack Gene</u>

Inflammation/Infection:
History: *Signs & Symptoms*
5. High Blood Pressure

Infection/Inflammation		
Caries/Toothaches	−	+
Bleeding Gums	−	+
Oral Sores	−	+
Tobacco/Toxins	−	+
High Blood Pressure	−	+

High Blood Pressure (Hypertension) can be a cardinal sign of systemic inflammation in the body. The presence of **hypertension** means that the pressure at which your arteries pump blood from your heart to the rest of your organs and throughout your body is excessively elevated. This abnormal vascular pressure is what contributes to dangerous stress and inflammation levels in the vascular system and heart.

It is estimated that **"about 75 million American adults (29%) have high blood pressure – that's 1 in every 3 American adults."**[36] Anyone, including children, can develop high blood pressure. It greatly increases the risk for heart disease and stroke, the first and third leading causes of death in the United States, respectively.

Blood pressure is a baseline measurement that should be recorded during every dental visit. Normal blood pressure is now considered **115 / 75,** for a lifetime. If a patient has an elevated blood pressure, or it is found to be gradually increasing, this should be cause for concern and action.[37]

Blood Pressure Categories

BLOOD PRESSURE CATEGORY	SYSTOLIC mm Hg (upper number)		DIASTOLIC mm Hg (lower number)
NORMAL	LESS THAN 120	and	LESS THAN 80
ELEVATED	120 – 129	and	LESS THAN 80
HIGH BLOOD PRESSURE (HYPERTENSION) STAGE 1	130 – 139	or	80 – 89
HIGH BLOOD PRESSURE (HYPERTENSION) STAGE 2	140 OR HIGHER	or	90 OR HIGHER
HYPERTENSIVE CRISIS (consult your doctor immediately)	HIGHER THAN 180	and/or	HIGHER THAN 120

©American Heart Association

heart.org/bplevels [38]

Blood pressure monitoring is a significant service provided in the Integrative Dental Medicine practice. Let's study the reasons for high blood pressure and the significance of hypertension.

Thirteen commonly-known factors that can elevate blood pressure (including, but not limited to):

1. A Pro-inflammatory Diet

A poor diet stimulates the production of biochemical inflammatory mediators in cells throughout the body, which results in vascular inflammation. Vascular inflammation can, in turn, increase the pressure within the blood vessels, increase levels of unstable plaque and atherosclerosis, increase the constant work load on the heart, and, therefore, increase the risk of cardiovascular events such as heart attacks and strokes.

An example of a pro-inflammatory diet is the daily ingestion of refined sugars, refined grains, refined omega-6 seed oils, and trans fats. These foods can all increase blood pressure; they can also result in elevated levels of LDL cholesterol, increased systemic inflammation, weight gain, a higher diabetes risk, unstable arterial plaque and atherosclerosis.

2. High Salt Diet

According to the American Heart Association, excessive levels of salt (sodium intake of more than 1,500 milligrams per day) can lead to high blood pressure, diabetes, and cardiovascular diseases. Interestingly, some studies have raised questions about the true role of sodium alone as a factor of elevated or reduced blood pressure. It does appear that an increase in calorie-rich refined foods, often heavily salted, do play a significant role in elevating blood pressure, along with increasing weight gain. It appears the prudent action is to reduce the intake of highly-processed, pro-inflammatory foods – and the salt they contain – to reduce blood pressure.[39]

3. Sleep Apnea

Decreased oxygen saturation levels occur when breathing ceases during sleep. This oxygen deprivation stimulates an internal emergency, code blue, "fight or flight" response of "Hey, we're choking to death!" The sympathetic nervous system responds by stimulating the release of adrenal stress hormones (such as cortisol) in order to increase the heart rate and immediately deliver more oxygen throughout the body. If these apneic (ceasing breathing) events are chronic, they can induce chronic high blood pressure and cardiac arrhythmias.

The American College of Cardiology describes Sleep Apnea and High Blood Pressure as "a dangerous pair".

There's a wealth of research suggesting that sleep apnea and high blood pressure are a dangerous pair. Obstructive sleep apnea, which occurs when breathing is briefly and repeatedly interrupted during sleep, has been shown to increase risk for high blood pressure. Research also shows that high blood pressure, often referred to as the 'silent killer,' can cause sleep apnea or worsen breathing in patients already affected by sleep apnea. Sleep apnea and high blood pressure have both been linked to significantly increased risk for serious complications, such as stroke and heart attack. [40]

4. Medications, Drugs & Alcohol

The American Heart Association offers the following advice regarding the consumption of alcohol and its effect on high blood pressure and overall health:

If you drink alcohol, including red wine, do so in moderation. Heavy and regular use of alcohol can increase blood pressure dramatically. It can also cause heart failure, lead to stroke and produce irregular heartbeats. Too much alcohol can contribute to high triglycerides, cancer, obesity, alcoholism, suicide and accidents. If you drink, limit consumption to no more than two drinks per day for men and one drink per day for women. Generally, one drink equals a 12-ounce beer, a four-ounce glass of wine, 1.5 ounces of 80-proof liquor, or one ounce of hard liquor (100 proof).[41]

Additionally, many prescriptions, over the counter medications, and illegal drugs can raise blood pressure. These include:

* Pain medications – including non-steroidal anti-inflammatories (NSAIDs)
* Antidepressants
* Hormonal birth control
* Caffeine
* Cold medicine/decongestants
* Herbal supplements
* Immunosuppressants
* Stimulants – including methylphenidate (Ritalin)
* Illegal drugs – including amphetamines, cocaine, anabolic steroids

"Government studies estimate that nearly 75% of Americans are either overweight or obese. If you aren't overweight, you're in the minority. And obesity-related illness, like heart attacks, strokes, high blood pressure, diabetes, and even certain cancers, has become the number one preventable cause of early death in the United States.

We continue to see the rise and fall of fad diets. No-fat, no-carb, low-carb, Jenny Craig, Nutrisystem, Sugar Busters, Atkins, South Beach...the more we diet, the fatter we get. Studies have shown that about 98% of people who lose weight on a diet will regain the weight or even more within five years.

Why? Hormonal imbalance.

If you want to be part of the 2% of dieters who experience permanent weight loss, your hormones have to be balanced. Through hormonal balance, you will be able to lose weight and keep it off forever.

What is hormonal balance? It depends on whom you ask. A gynecologist will tell you it's about the female hormones – estrogen, progesterone, and prolactin. A urologist will tell you it's all about testosterone. A diabetologist will tell you it's about balancing your insulin, glucagon, and blood sugar. An endocrinologist will tell you that it is having all your hormones balanced. This is because all your hormones affect one another. It's one big circle. When one hormone is out of balance, it has profound effects on all your hormones. They are all connected. Hormonal balance means having the right amount of every hormone. It means having a body that's healthy and resilient."

Scott Isaacs, MD, FACP, FACE
<u>Hormonal Balance: How to Lose Weight by Understanding Your Hormones and Metabolism, 3rd Edition</u>

5. Hormonal Imbalance

MedStar Washington D.C. Hospital, Endocrinology Research Center explains hormonal imbalance related elevated blood pressure as follows: *"Endocrine hypertension is a type of high blood pressure caused by a hormone imbalance. Most often these disorders originate in the pituitary or adrenal gland and can be caused when the glands produce too much or not enough of the hormones they normally secrete."* Additionally they state that *"there are several types of endocrine hypertension, including:*

> *-**Primary hyperaldosteronism:** a hormonal disorder that leads to high blood pressure when the adrenal glands produce too much aldosterone hormone, which raises sodium levels in the blood.*
> *-**Pheochromocytoma**: a rare endocrine tumor originating in the medulla, the inner part of the adrenal gland; causes the release of excessive amounts of hormones that control responses to stress, heart rate and blood pressure.*
> *-**Paraganglioma:** a tumor that originates from the cortex, the outside of the adrenal glands; most often these are located in the head and neck region, heart, bladder, spine, chest, abdomen, or pelvis and produce excessive amounts of the catecholamine hormone, which can lead to high blood pressure. Most often, treatment for endocrine hypertension focuses on the cause of the high blood pressure. Sometimes, additional blood pressure medication may be prescribed."*[42]

6. Kidney Disease

Kidney disease may include the restricted flow of fluids. This backup can elevate blood pressure. Reciprocally, high blood pressure is one of the major causes of kidney failure in the United States, at 28.4%.[43]

7. Diabetes

As of 2018, "about 25% of people with Type 1 diabetes and 80% of people with Type 2 diabetes also have high blood pressure."[44] It is clear that "having diabetes raises your risk of heart disease, stroke, kidney disease and other health problems. Having high blood pressure also raises this risk".[45]

8. Nutrient Deficiency

At least 4 nutrient deficiencies have been identified as being related to high blood pressure, including:
* Potassium
* Magnesium
* Coenzyme Q10
* Omega-3 Fats[46]

> "Despite what you might have heard, diabetes is not a lifelong condition. It does not have to shorten your life span or result in high blood pressure, heart disease, kidney failure, blindness, or other life-threatening ailments. In fact, most diabetics can get off medication and become 100 percent healthy in just a few simple steps."
>
> Joel Fuhrman, MD
> <u>The End of Diabetes: The Eat to Live Plan to Prevent and Reverse Diabetes</u>

9. Thyroid Problems

Thyroid problems can be a possible cause of high blood pressure. For example, hypothyroidism can lead to an increase in blood pressure. One theory for why this might be the case is that low amounts of thyroid hormone can slow the heartbeat, which can affect pumping strength and blood vessel wall flexibility. Both may cause a rise in blood pressure.

10. Stress

Stress can be produced by a pro-inflammatory diet, physical inactivity, smoking, obesity, sleep apnea, drugs & alcohol, hormonal imbalance, kidney disease, diabetes, nutrient deficiency, thyroid problems, medication side effects, and the personal challenges of life.

The interaction between the mind, body, emotions, and personality has a tremendous effect on the health of every cell in our body. "Stress" can save our lives when we face a "flight or fight" situation, and we find an internal super-power for that moment. Adrenaline and cortisol flood our bodies with strength, speed and aggression we didn't know we possessed. However, if we move beyond the emergency and continue replaying the trauma and fear it produced, we can remain in a "fight or flight" state chronically, which can effectively kill us long after the real danger is gone. It appears that humans are the only living beings on the earth that can live in a chronic state of mental and thus physical stress. This is a major factor of chronic systemic inflammation and high blood pressure.

> "Scientists are finding that the same parts of the brain that control the stress response, for example, play an important role in susceptibility and resistance to inflammatory diseases such as arthritis. And since it is these parts of the brain that also play a role in depression, we can begin to understand why it is that many patients with inflammatory diseases may also experience depression at different times in their lives. Thus, the psychosomatic notion that inflammatory and allergic diseases originate in a disordered upbringing and repressed emotions can now be reexamined in more precise physiological terms. Rather than seeing the psyche as the source of such illnesses, we are discovering that while feelings don't directly cause or cure disease, the biological mechanisms underlying them may cause or contribute to disease. Thus, many of the nerve pathways and molecules underlying both psychological responses and inflammatory disease are the same, making predisposition to one set of illnesses likely to go along with predisposition to the other."
>
> Esther M. Sternberg, MD
> <u>The Balance Within: The Science Connecting Health and Emotions</u>

11. Physical Inactivity

Regular physical activity makes your heart stronger. A stronger heart can pump more blood with less effort. If your heart can work less to pump, the force on your arteries decreases, thus lowering your blood pressure.

There is also an important relationship between physical activity and the immune system. Physical inactivity inhibits proper immune function. Quoting Australian Massage Therapist, Lynne Gillogly,

> *Lymph is a colourless fluid which is the waste disposal system of the tissues and the lymph nodes are the battle fields in the body where most infections are fought. It works to maintain healthy immunity, to drain stagnant fluids, regenerate tissues and detoxify the body by filtering out foreign substances and toxins. 'Sluggishness' in the lymphatic pathways can affect your ability to concentrate and make you feel vague and 'foggy headed', disorientated and tired, and experience a feeling of 'un-wellness' without knowing why…Exercise or activity*

(doing things you love while you are in motion) is critical to keeping your lymph system open and flowing. When your muscles are moving this also helps move and pump the lymph within its vessels. Walking, running, swimming, bike riding, yoga etc, stretching and strength training are great ways to keep the lymph flowing.[47]

12. Smoking

The nicotine in cigarette smoke is a big part of the problem with smoking. It raises the blood pressure and heart rate, narrows the arteries and hardens their walls, and makes the blood more likely to clot. It stresses the heart and is a set up for a heart attack or stroke.

13. Obesity/Weight

When there is increased weight, it takes more pressure to move the blood around a body that is most often also suffering from vascular deterioration due to a pro-inflammatory diet, physical inactivity, sleep apnea, hormonal imbalance, kidney disease, diabetes, nutrient deficiency, thyroid problems, medication side effects, and the personal challenges of life. One of the very best strategies for complete, long-term health is to maintain the weight of most people's lean teenage weight, throughout adulthood. When the circumference of the waistline is equal to or less than the circumference of the hips, it is rare to find metabolic syndrome – the precursor to type 2 diabetes.

* * *

High Blood Pressure is a huge red flag of **The Great Fire** of inflammation within. Therefore, any practitioner who would seek to provide care within an Integrative Dental Medicine model must be aware of its causes, its effects, and the interplay between it and both oral and systemic diseases.

> **"Chronic Systemic Inflammation [CSI]:**
> In CSI, the body's immune response doesn't work as it should. Instead of quickly striking and resolving an insult, your immune system continues to release white blood cells and biochemical byproducts that damage your tissues, especially the linings of your blood vessels.
>
> Drs. Bradley Bale and Amy Doneen, authors of <u>Beat the Heart Attack Gene</u>, call this a 'fire' in the blood vessels. This weakness lets traveling oral bacteria from gum disease penetrate the blood vessel wall. There the bacteria can build a nest, reproduce and eventually erupt — triggering a clot that could cause a heart attack or stroke.
>
> The chemical mediators that are part of inflammation may also reach the liver, activating the production of proteins there. That's why one way to measure CSI is with a blood test called HsCRP (High Sensitivity C-Reactive Protein). This test will tell you if you're experiencing inflammation in the body, although it won't tell you where. But given the relationship between inflammation and cardiovascular disease, physicians use the HsCRP test to determine the risk of heart attack and stroke.
>
> In addition to cardiovascular disease, uncontrolled CSI can lead to a litany of ailments from diabetes to pregnancy complications to periodontitis. That's why reducing levels of inflammatory markers may help reduce the risk of systemic diseases."
>
> Susan Smallegan Maples, DDS, MSBA
> and Diana Kightlinger DeCouteau, MA
> <u>Blabbermouth!: 77 Secrets Only Your Mouth Can Tell You to Live a Healthier, Happier, Sexier Life</u>

Inflammation/Infection:
History: *Signs & Symptoms*
6. Pro-Inflammatory Diet

Infection/Inflammation		
Caries/Toothaches	–	+
Bleeding Gums	–	+
Oral Sores	–	+
Tobacco/Toxins	–	+
High Blood Pressure	–	+
Pro-inflammatory Diet	–	+

Caldwell Esselstyn, MD, former Chief of Surgery at the world-renowned Cleveland Clinic, resigned from his prestigious (and most certainly lucrative) position to study nutrition's role in cardiovascular disease. He found that by emphasizing a strict anti-inflammatory diet, he was able to clinically observe reversal of atherosclerosis with angiogram imaging. He subsequently recorded his research findings in his book entitled Prevent and Reverse Heart Disease, a New York Times bestseller. A very powerful documentary film featuring Dr. Esselstyn's work, Forks Over Knives (Monica Beach Media, 2011), is another valuable educational resource. It reveals the severe health crisis that we face, due to our very dangerous Western lifestyles of processed fast-food, which has created a cardiovascular tsunami.

I've been privileged to attend Dr. Esselstyn's *Farms to Forks* weekend retreat, which he teaches with his wife, Ann, his son, Rip, and his daughter, Jane. One of Dr. Esselstyn's famous quotes while speaking is *"Cardiovascular disease is a paper tiger; it's completely controlled by what you eat, and I can prove it!"* He has proven the truth of this statement over and over again, both scientifically and in the lives of hundreds of patients he has personally treated at the Cleveland Clinic Wellness Institute over the past 25+ years.

Let me repeat a wonderful story from Dr. Esselstyn that I shared in the opening chapter, because it is so dramatic and impactful. I want you to always remember it! A patient was brought into the Cleveland Clinic in a wheelchair. He had a history of 20 arterial stents and quadruple bypass surgery, and he still experienced angina so severely that he couldn't walk to his kitchen. His family asked if the doctors at the Cleveland Clinic could save his life. His vascular system was completely shut down. No surgery could correct his problem. No medication could reverse the damage and inflammation. In fact, he was the embodiment of inflammation. He was literally a dead man (not) walking. Dr. Esselstyn enrolled him in his pilot program, focused on a strict plant-based, anti-inflammatory diet. Within months, there was visible arterial improvement. The patient went on to live many more years with a dramatic reversal of symptoms and quality of life.

Could it be that the body's immune system is powerful enough to protect our complete health...if it is free of the insults introduced through a pro-inflammatory lifestyle? There is an increasing body of evidence that points to (1) **the harm** that can be caused by a pro-inflammatory diet filled with empty calories, refined sugars, refined carbohydrates, refined omega-6 seed oils and trans fats (not to mention additives, food coloring, pesticides, hormones and preservatives) *and*, conversely, (2) **the benefits** of instead adopting an anti-inflammatory diet.

This is obviously a critical point of emphasis as we consider an Integrative Dental Medicine model of complete health care. Thank you, Dr. Esselstyn, for your brave contribution and determination to find the truth. You have pioneered the Third Era Medical Model, the Root Cause Medical Model, and the *"Ask 'Why' Until You Can't Ask 'Why' Anymore"* Model of true health care. Because of you, *The Shift* is on!

David Seaman DC, MS, is another pioneering hero in this important field. He beautifully explains the biochemistry of inflammation in his text, <u>The Deflame Diet</u> (Shadow Panther Press, 2016). Dr. Seaman explains:

Beside hormones, there are many other categories of biochemicals, such as eicosanoids (eee-kose-anoids), cyotokines, growth factors, and adhesion molecules, all of which have normal levels that are desirable. Most of these chemicals are either anti-inflammatory and associated with health, or pro-inflammatory and associated with disease. Imbalance occurs with all biochemicals discussed thus far when we eat a pro-inflammatory diet. In other words, the body produces an excess of pro-inflammatory eicosanoids, cytokines, growth factors, and adhesion molecules when we eat too much refined sugar, refined grains, refined omega-6 seed oils, and trans fats.[48]

As a result, this production of too many pro-inflammatory biochemicals can lead to chronic, uncontrolled inflammation, which is, as we have seen, a great destroyer of complete health.

In December 2012, I attended Dr. Roizen's Integrative Medicine Conference in Las Vegas. The meeting focus was on brain health, dementia and Alzheimer's. As I recall, there were only two dentists in an audience of several hundred physicians: myself and my dear friend **Dr. Michael Schuster** (a true pioneer in age-reversing dentistry, and a highly revered mentor/coach to many dental professionals). One of the keynote speakers was **Marwan Sabbagh, MD**, a geriatric neurologist, dementia specialist, and research director. He described modifiable risk factors to prevent Alzheimer's, with an emphasis on reducing inflammation.

He linked the following to Alzheimer's:
- Hypertension
- Elevated cholesterol
- Diabetes (with its elevated insulin levels and associated metabolic syndrome)
- Obesity (especially during midlife)
- Deficiency of vitamin B9 (also known as folic acid or folate)
- Heart disease and high homocysteine levels

During his presentation, Dr. Sabbagh also introduced his recently published book entitled, <u>The Alzheimer's Prevention Cookbook</u> (Ten Speed Press, 2012).

"But what exactly does diabetes have to do with Alzheimer's disease? The answer, scientists are discovering, seems to be a great deal. Links between abnormal insulin regulation or insulin resistance, both precursors of type 2 diabetes, and a person's risk of Alzheimer's disease have been borne out in numerous epidemiologic and clinical studies.

In cases of type 2 diabetes, the body makes plenty of insulin (the hormone responsible for getting sugar into cells) but the cells stop using insulin, so glucose (blood sugar) accumulates outside of cells instead of being transported into them. This leads to a state of chronic inflammation.

The brain needs a near-constant supply of glucose to keep it going, and insulin is a key player in providing it. Insulin is also responsible for regulating much of the activity within the brain cells themselves, as well as conveying signals from one neuron to the next. Because it's constantly transported across the blood-brain barrier, the levels of insulin found in the rest of the body tend to correlate with the levels found in the brain. It follows that when insulin and glucose metabolism are impaired, cognitive function likewise suffers.

> One study has indicated that up to 43% of dementia cases could be attributed to diabetes, stroke or a combination of the two. Another study found that patients with borderline diabetes aged seventy-five or older had a 77% increased risk of developing Alzheimer's compared to patients who had normal blood-sugar levels…The exponentially increasing prevalence of type 2 diabetes worldwide could mean that more and more people are also at risk for Alzheimer's. And a root cause of both these conditions is chronic inflammation…
>
> …By eating the right foods and keeping our weight down, we'll be protecting our bodies from diabetes and our brains from degeneration."
>
> Dr. Marwan Sabbagh and Beau MacMillan
> <u>The Alzheimer's Prevention Cookbook:</u>
> <u>Recipes to Boost Brain Health</u>

Inflammation/Infection:
History: *Signs & Symptoms*
7. Chronic Pain/Stress

Infection/Inflammation		
Caries/Toothaches	–	+
Bleeding Gums	–	+
Oral Sores	–	+
Tobacco/Toxins	–	+
High Blood Pressure	–	+
Pro-inflammatory Diet	–	+
Chronic Pain/Stress	–	+

Pain is very often synonymous with inflammation. Dr. Seaman describes the biochemistry of dietary-induced systemic inflammation by showing:

* Refined sugars, refined carbohydrates and refined seed oils represent 60% of the calories in the typical western diet.
* These are all pro-inflammatory. Once inside a cell, an inflammatory response is stimulated (NF-kB), which generates the expression of inflammatory mediators (IL-1, IL-6, TNF, MMP, VEGF, PLA-2, COX, LOX, PGE-2, LTB-4).
* When these inflammatory mediators become active outside the cell, there is a rise in C-reactive protein (CRP) from the liver, indicative of a systemic inflammation response.

* Sensory C neurons are also stimulated, resulting in the experience of diffuse chronic pain.

Dr. Seaman often lectures on nutritional inflammation to chiropractic societies. He begins his lectures by asking several questions.

- *First Question:* "*How many of you, as chiropractors, see patients with* **chronic pain**?"

  Every hand naturally goes up. They see patients with back pain, neck pain, muscle pain, joint pain, and more. We would expect the same response from a group of physical therapists, massage therapists, or orthopedic surgeons.

- *Second Question:* "*How many of you see patients with* **chronic inflammation**?"

  The response is very limited. Most doctors have focused on pain and pain management but have not thought about inflammation as a potential driver of the pain experience. Dr. Seaman will then state that essentially all chronic pain patients have a component of systemic inflammation. He will then ask one final question.

- *Third Question: "What do you think is the number one cause of systemic inflammation that causes patients to experience chronic pain?"*

  To a puzzled audience, he answers, "A pro-inflammatory diet and nutritional deficiencies."

I'm quite confident that Dr. Esselstyn would agree…as would Dr. Roizen…as would Dr. Masley…as would many other authoritative MDs, DOs, PhDs, DCs and researchers around the world.

"Every single disease or condition of metabolic syndrome is driven by fructose, including hypertension, through increases in uric acid; high triglycerides and insulin resistance, through synthesis of fat in the liver; diabetes, via increased liver glucose production combined with insulin resistance; accelerated aging, due to damage to lipids and protein; likely cancer, due to DNA damage, high insulin levels, and the fact that some cancers seem to use fructose preferentially for energy; and likely dementia, through insulin resistance in the brain."

Robert H. Lustig, MD, MSL
<u>Fat Chance: Beating the Odds Against Sugar, Processed Food, Obesity, and Disease</u>

I suspect that there are many vaguely understood disorders in which the primary unknown, underlying cause is inflammation. Consider Fibromyalgia and Chronic Fatigue Syndrome for example. Both include generalized soreness of muscles and joints, with no known origins, despite years of research. The prescribed therapy is gentle exercise and anti-inflammatory medications. Recently, fibromyalgia has been associated with vitamin D deficiency (nutritional deficiency inflammation) and sleep apnea (elevated stress hormones inflammation). These are lifestyle concerns, which drive inflammation, which drive pain and fatigue.

Or consider the many patients presenting daily with "TMD", or Temporomandibular Disorders. Their chief complaints often include sore muscles, sore joints, sore necks, fibromyalgia, and having to subside on *anti-inflammatory* meds. Why do anti-inflammatory meds help? That's right – because the problem involves inflammation.

Along with a very detailed evaluation of the health of the temporomandibular joints, the dental occlusion, the cervical spine, and breathing/airway/sleep concerns, the IDM Checklist will guide us through evaluating all possible sources of systemic inflammation that may produce pain.

We must always keep in mind that TMJoint osteoarthritis is an inflammatory disease, in which inflammatory mediators play a significant role.

In 2012, the Osteoarthritis Research Society International published the following statement:

> *Osteoarthritis (OA) has long been considered a "wear and tear" disease leading to loss of cartilage. OA used to be considered the sole consequence of any process leading to increased pressure on one particular joint or fragility of cartilage matrix. Progress in molecular biology in the 1990s has profoundly modified this paradigm. The discovery that many soluble mediators such as cytokines or prostaglandins can increase the production of matrix metalloproteinases by chondrocytes led to the first steps of an "inflammatory" theory. However, it took a decade before synovitis was accepted as a critical feature of OA, and some studies are now opening the way to consider the condition a driver of the OA process. Recent experimental data have shown that subchondral bone may have a substantial role in the OA process, as a mechanical damper, as well as a source of inflammatory mediators implicated in the OA pain process and in the degradation of the deep layer of cartilage. Thus, initially considered cartilage*

driven, OA is a much more complex disease with inflammatory mediators released by cartilage, bone and synovium. Low-grade inflammation induced by the metabolic syndrome, innate immunity and 'inflamm-aging' are some of the more recent arguments in favor of the inflammatory theory of OA.[49]

The lesson is to always consider inflammation as a significant factor of pain.

Dr. Seaman is a dear friend and mentor of mine. One day, as we were discussing systemic inflammation, he contrasted how to recognize someone with lots of inflammation as opposed to little inflammation.

A person with a lot of systemic inflammation, he said, is the one who goes to the fitness club (finally!), does a gentle half-hour work out, with very light weights, plus a short time on the treadmill walking, and the next day can barely get out of bed due to soreness!

In contrast, consider a person with very little systemic inflammation, who is accidentally scratched on the arm superficially, but deeply enough to draw blood. They will feel very little pain and will heal quickly. Theoretically, this makes sense.

Exactly three days after our conversation, I saw a dear patient of mine in the office who was a very strict vegan; she raises vegetables at home in her organic garden and is a big fan of Dr. Esselstyn. Four months earlier she had lost a tooth due to fracture, and a dental implant was placed by our surgeon. As we were taking final impressions for an implant crown, I asked her how the surgery had gone for her. She said surprisingly well. She had been given a prescription for a pain reliever the day of the surgery, but she had forgotten to fill it on the way home. When the anesthetic wore off, she still had no pain, so she decided to wait until the next day to fill the prescription. To her surprise, she slept well that night, with no pain the next morning. She never took any pain relievers and was very comfortable. Seven days later, she returned to the surgeon's office for suture removal and to check healing of the incision site. The surgeon told her he was amazed. He said he had never seen anyone heal so quickly and that he could barely see an incision line. She had no idea why she had responded and healed so well.

With my 72 hours of Seaman insight into systemic inflammation, I was able to very professionally respond and say, "You know why you had no pain and healed so quickly, don't you? It's because of your anti-inflammatory diet and lifestyle. You have no inflammation in your body and therefore your pain threshold is very high and your healing is very rapid." She was very impressed with my knowledge —and so was I!

Inflammation/Infection:
History: *Signs & Symptoms*
8. Diabetes

Infection/Inflammation		
Caries/Toothaches	−	+
Bleeding Gums	−	+
Oral Sores	−	+
Tobacco/Toxins	−	+
High Blood Pressure	−	+
Pro-inflammatory Diet	−	+
Chronic Pain/Stress	−	+
Diabetes	−	+

I'll never forget hearing Dr. Roizen speaking about diabetes at the Cleveland Clinic 2012 AAOSH Conference, describing it this way: **"Diabetes is like having shards of glass scraping the walls of your arteries all day long."**

With this in mind, it's safe to say that uncontrolled diabetes is one the most severe sources of destructive inflammation in every organ and cell of the body. It is virtually impossible to live a healthy life with uncontrolled diabetes.

But there is good news. Joel Fuhrman, MD, in his book, <u>The End of Diabetes</u> (Harper One 2013), reports

Type 2 diabetics can become non-diabetic, achieving complete wellness and even excellent health. They can become diabetes-free for life. In my twenty years of clinical experience with this program, I have experienced that more than 90% of type 2 diabetics who follow this diet and exercise lifestyle are able to discontinue insulin within the first month.[50]

Dr. Fuhrman also explains that 90% of diabetics in the U.S. are Type 2.[51] He further explains that this form of diabetes occurs most often in people who are overweight and do not exercise sufficiently.

The number of diabetics in the U.S. has skyrocketed in the last 25 years, paralleling the rise in the number of people who are overweight. Type 2 diabetes almost never occurs in people who are healthy eaters, exercise regularly, and have a low body fat percentage. It is a disease that was almost nonexistent in prior centuries, when food was not so abundant and when high-calorie, low-nutrient food was not available.

Inflammation/Infection: History: *Signs & Symptoms*
9. Gastric Reflux or Gastroesophageal Reflux Disease (GERD)

Infection/Inflammation		
Caries/Toothaches	−	+
Bleeding Gums	−	+
Oral Sores	−	+
Tobacco/Toxins	−	+
High Blood Pressure	−	+
Pro-inflammatory Diet	−	+
Chronic Pain/Stress	−	+
Diabetes	−	+
Gastric Reflux	−	+

Gastric reflux has recently become a common disorder in the Western world, affecting millions of people. 60% of the adult population in the U.S. will experience some type of gastroesophageal reflux disease (GERD) within a 12 month period. Less than 15% will be screened. 20-30% will have weekly symptoms.

This is an epidemic disease of Western diet and airway complications. It is estimated that as many as 30 million people suffer from sleep apnea in the United States. Sleep physicians report that the vast majority of their patients also have gastric reflux. There appears to be a direct relationship.

There are two separate explanations for the most common causes of gastric reflux:

1. Sleep Apnea/GERD interaction

Like two sides of the same coin, there is an interaction between these two disorders. One explanation is that obstructive sleep apnea is caused by a blockage of the posterior throat and airway, lasting ten seconds or longer per apneic event. During these events, when there is an effort to breathe, a negative pressure is created from the abdomen, and the acids from the stomach may come up the esophagus, into the throat, mouth, and nasal airway, as well as into the primary bronchioles of the lungs. Therefore, in this case, we would take the following view:
- ➤ Cause = Negative pressure from sleep apnea
- ➤ Effect = Gastric reflux

On the flip side, another explanation is that stomach acids come up the esophagus during the night, causing both airway inflammation and swelling. They might also cause vocal cord spasms, thereby producing sleep apnea. With this perspective, we would consider the cause/effect relationship to be:
- ➤ Cause = Gastric reflux inflammation and vocal cord spasms

➤ Effect = Sleep apnea

2. Acidic Diet

Jamie Koufman, MD, FACS, has a different explanation for gastric reflux, or acid reflux as she describes it. Dr. Koufman is a leading clinician, researcher and educator in the field of laryngology and the voice for more than 25 years, practicing in New York City. In her books, <u>Dropping Acid: The Reflux Diet Cookbook & Cure</u> (2010) and <u>Dr. Koufman's Acid Reflux Diet</u> (2015), she describes it as a Western disease of an acidic diet and digestive enzymes. Dr. Koufman explains that when stomach acids, bile and the digestive enzyme pepsin enter the esophagus and airway, very negative things can happen, especially when coupled with an acidic diet.

Pepsin is the primary digestive enzyme for protein in the diet, residing in the stomach. When food is swallowed and moves down to the stomach, stomach acids activate pepsin to digest proteins. When pepsin moves into the airway tissues and attaches to the walls, the ingestion of acidic foods and beverages (such as acidic sodas, sports drinks, canned foods preserved at a lower pH, and naturally acidic foods) can activate the enzymatic activity of pepsin even in the absence of protein. In 2010, the average 12-to-29 year old American consumed 160 gallons of acidified soft drinks, nearly a half-gallon per day. Pepsin molecules and acids can cause irritation of the esophagus walls, inflammation of the esophagus, Barrett's Esophagus, and are associated with esophageal cancer.

Dr. Koufman states: *"Reflux-related diseases affect at least half of Americans. Since the 1970's, the prevalence of reflux disease has increased 400%, and reflux-caused esophageal cancer has increased more than 850%; in terms of incidence, it has become America's fastest growing cancer."*

According to Dr. Koufman, the most common symptoms of acid reflux (by percentage) include:

Symptom of acid reflux	%
1. Post-nasal drip	15%
2. Chronic throat clearing	14%
3. "Lump in the throat" sensation	14%
4. Hoarseness	12%
5. Sore throat	11%
6. Heartburn	10%
7. Chronic cough	9%
8. Difficulty swallowing	8%
9. Choking episodes	7%

Some people who have acid reflux do not notice having any of the above symptoms. Therefore, they are classified as having **"silent reflux"**.

In all of these cases, the earliest signs of the destructive effects of acid reflux will often be seen in the mouth. Bio-corrosive wear on the teeth will be observed as cupping out on the occlusal and incisal surfaces and as smooth wear on root surfaces. Additionally, irritation to soft tissues in the mouth may create swelling in the posterior throat and on the tongue.

We will address gastric reflux as a disorder that involves both issues of airway-related sleep apnea/obstruction and an acidic diet. We will note that in both the case of sleep apnea and of gastric reflux, **weight loss** is often therapeutic in reversing the disorder.

Inflammation/Infection:
History: *Signs & Symptoms*
10. Physical Inactivity

Infection/Inflammation		
Caries/Toothaches	−	+
Bleeding Gums	−	+
Oral Sores	−	+
Tobacco/Toxins	−	+
High Blood Pressure	−	+
Pro-inflammatory Diet	−	+
Chronic Pain/Stress	−	+
Diabetes	−	+
Gastric Reflux	−	+
Physical Inactivity	−	+

Physical inactivity is also associated with systemic inflammation. Naomi Hamburg, MD, MS, and her research cohort from Boston University School of Medicine, studied healthy volunteers who remained bedridden for five days. The findings reported contained the following conclusions:

> *In summary, we observed the concurrent development of insulin resistance, microvascular dysfunction, dyslipidemia, and increased blood pressure following a short period of bed rest in healthy volunteers. There is a growing epidemic of diseases associated with physical inactivity and insulin resistance including obesity, the metabolic syndrome, and diabetes mellitus. Our data are consistent with the hypothesis that insulin resistance has deleterious effects on the vasculature or that common pathophysiological mechanisms account for both effects of bed rest. Our study suggests that the vasculature is highly sensitive to the metabolic changes associated with physical inactivity.*[52]

Many other studies also demonstrate the deleterious effects of physical inactivity and its relationship to systemic inflammation.

Clearly, infection and inflammation are key concerns when implementing the IDM Model of dental and medical practice. It is important to thoroughly screen (both in written form and in verbal interviews) for the presence of the issues addressed so far under **History: Signs & Symptoms.**

> Once a thorough written and verbal **History: *Signs & Symptoms*** is completed, proceed to **Evaluation: *Clinical Signs*** and then to **Screening & Testing.**

6. INFLAMMATION & INFECTION – EVALUATION/SCREENING & TESTING

Now we are prepared to move on to **Evaluation**: *Clinical Signs*.

Inflammation/Infection:
Evaluation: *Clinical Signs*
* **Visual inspection**
* **Periodontal Probing**
* **Oral Lesions**
* **Lymph Nodes**
* **Swollen Tonsils**

	–	+
Visual Inspection		
Periodontal Probing		
Oral Lesions		
Lymph Nodes		
Swollen Tonsils		

Visual inspection for signs of inflammation and infection is something very familiar to dental professionals. ***Moving from the outside in,*** we begin with external palpation of **muscles** and **lymph nodes**. Are any masses noted, especially unilateral enlargements of nodes or soreness to palpation?

Next, moving to the lips and intraoral tissues, are any **oral lesions** noted? If so, related/follow-up questions would include:
—Does the patient have any active herpetic lesions, or a history of them, and/or lesions of any other kind?

—Has the lesion appeared acutely in the last 7-14 days?
—Does it appear to be healing (vs enlarging) since first appearing?
—Does the lesion appear raised, discolored, or have an indurated appearance?
—Does the lesion warrant a biopsy?
—Do the lips look dry or chapped?
—Could this be related to mouth-breathing?

Next, do the **periodontal tissues** look inflamed, swollen, or discolored? Does **periodontal probing** produce bleeding? Are pockets greater than 3 mm present? Are the gums sore and tender upon probing?

Next, are the tonsilar tissues present? Are the **tonsils swollen**? Does the back of the **throat or tongue** look swollen or inflamed, as might occur with **gastric reflux** or **chronic mouth breathing**?

Are there any lesions in the cheeks, on the tongue or adjacent to teeth? Are there any **fistula tracts** adjacent to any root surfaces?

A thorough **History:** *Signs & Symptoms* and **Evaluation:** *Clinical Signs*, with positive indicators for possible issues of inflammation/infection, will then trigger the need for specific **Screening & Testing**.

Inflammation/Infection: Screening & Testing
1. Radiographic Imaging

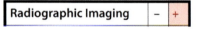

Radiographic imaging is needed to evaluate for caries, periodontal and periapical infections, and any bony pathology. A **full mouth radiographic series** provides a critical view of several things, including:
- interproximal tooth surfaces where hidden decay may reside
- periapical root pathology
- periodontal bone loss
- bony lesions
- broken root tips
- impacted third molars
- the status of implant positions and osseointegration

Depending on the screening status of the temporomandibular joints and airway, further testing may warrant specialized imaging using **CBCT** or **MRI**.

Inflammation & Infection: Screening & Testing
2. HbA1c (Blood Sugar)

Radiographic Imaging	−	+
Hb A1c Testing	−	+

HbA1c testing measures what percentage of a patient's hemoglobin (**Hb**) – a protein in red blood cells that carries oxygen – is coated with sugar ("glycated"). A higher A1C level correlates directly with poor blood sugar control – and a higher risk of pre-diabetes or diabetes.

The following details are helpful when considering testing for HbA1c:
- HbA1c can be determined in a dental office after gathering a blood sample through a simple finger-stick. Results are available within 7 minutes, and the cost of testing is very reasonable.
- Scoring is as follows:[53]

Normal	Below 5.7%
Prediabetes	5.7% to 6.4%
Diabetes	6.5% or above

Indications for HbA1c testing include periodontal inflammation, weight gain, a history of family heart disease, strokes, diabetes, periodontal disease, or obesity.

A highly-respected colleague and dear friend, Susan Maples, DDS, conducted a HbA1c pilot study of 500 random patients, in her private practice in Holt, Michigan. 20% were found to have elevated blood sugar levels representing either pre-diabetes or diabetes. This is a very significant finding, demonstrating the high percentage of people in our nation who are unaware they may have dangerously high blood sugar levels. Screening is so important!

Inflammation & Infection: Screening & Testing
3. Salivary Testing

Radiographic Imaging	−	+
Hb A1c Testing	−	+
Salivary Testing	−	+

The importance of oral pathogens in causing both localized infections and inflammation and their significant role in influencing other systemic effects is clearly understood. It is possible to

determine the levels of 11 key oral pathogens, utilizing salivary samples for testing. Sample collection can be as simple as the following:
- The patient swishes a saline solution in the mouth for 20 seconds and then spits a **salivary sample** into a collection tube.
- The samples are sent to a laboratory for analysis and a full report including diagnosis and treatment recommendations, based on the latest research.
- The report is typically received within one week.

Oral pathogen samples can also be collected using a second method, involving **paper points** which are placed in 5-6 periodontal sites under the gum for 20 seconds. These paper points are then placed in a collection tube which is sent to the laboratory for analysis.

> **For more science and guidelines regarding regarding oral pathogens and salivary testing, please refer to Dr. Thomas Nabor's outstanding chapter in the Appendix.**

Inflammation & Infection:
Screening & Testing
4. Oral Cancer Screening

	-	+
Radiographic Imaging		
Hb A1c Testing		
Salivary Testing		
Oral Cancer Screen		

As oral physicians, dentists should carefully assess every patient routinely for oral cancer. There are a number of excellent methods for close examination. One such method utilizes a blue light that is emitted into the oral cavity, resulting in a green fluorescence of normal, healthy tissue and a darker appearance of any abnormal tissue. The dental professional can visualize the contrast with special glasses. Other systems utilize dye contrasts.

Oral cancers can be caused by over-usage of tobacco and alcohol, which are both carcinogenic. Sun exposure can cause lip cancers. The sexually-transmitted virus HPV (Human Papilloma Virus) is rapidly becoming the most common cause of oral cancer in the United States. A weakened immune system also increases the susceptibility to oral cancers.

Inflammation & Infection: Screening & Testing
4. Koufman Reflux Symptom Index (RSI) Quiz

	–	+
Radiographic Imaging		
Hb A1c Testing		
Salivary Testing		
Oral Cancer Screening		
Reflux Symptoms Index (RSI)		

Jamie Koufman, MD, FACS, has developed a written screening tool for gastric reflux.[54] This tool is recommended to be used with <u>every patient</u> both to screen and to educate about the signs and symptoms of gastric reflux.

Koufman Reflux Symptom Index Quiz (RSI)

Within the last MONTH, how did the following problems affect you? 0 = No Problem 5 = Severe Problem

	0	1	2	3	4	5
Hoarseness or a problem with your voice						
Clearing your throat						
Excess throat mucous or postnasal drip						
Difficulty swallowing food, liquids, or pills						
Coughing after you ate or after lying down						
Breathing difficulties or choking episodes						
Troublesome or annoying cough						
Sensations of something sticking in your throat or a lump in your throat						
Heartburn, chest pain, indigestion, or stomach acid coming up						

Your RSI is

A score of 15 or more means that you have a 90% chance of having reflux, especially airway reflux.

* * *

Following the Integrative Dental Medicine Checklist, we can work through a thorough examination including:
1. **History: Signs & Symptoms**
2. **Evaluation: Clinical Signs**
3. **Screening & Testing**

in order to then determine a **DIFFERENTIAL CONCLUSION**.

> This information would provide the foundation to show that the patient presents either **NEGATIVE** or **POSITIVE** for Local and/or Systemic Inflammation/Infection.
> If **POSITIVE**, the next step would be to proceed to the **TREATMENT** portion of the IDM Checklist.
> **The focus now turns to putting out the *fire of inflammation*.**

7. INFLAMMATION & INFECTION – TREATMENT

A **DIFFERENTIAL CONCLUSION,** from following the IDM Checklist History, Evaluation, Screening & Testing, has determined that the patient presents **POSITIVE** for Oral and/or Systemic Inflammation/Infection. We will next proceed to the **TREATMENT** portion of the IDM Checklist, where the focus now turns to **putting out the fire of** *inflammation*.

Remembering Our Mission:

*To educate each patient we serve about the multiple facets of oral and systemic inflammation.

*To empower them to move toward a life of complete health, through counseling and supporting an anti-inflammatory lifestyle.

Let's explore the multiple facets of addressing oral and systemic inflammation and how exactly we can educate patients to empower each one to pursue a life of complete health.

Inflammation & Infection: Treatment
1. Eliminate Dental Caries

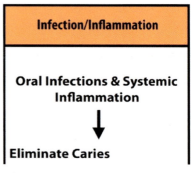

Dental caries results because the body loses a battle between the **pathologic factors** and the **protective factors** that are simultaneously active on and around the teeth.

John Featherstone, MSc, PhD, serves as Professor of Preventive and Restorative Dental Sciences at the University of California, San Francisco (UCSF) and Dean of the School of Dentistry. He is credited with pioneering a system for Caries Management by Risk Assessment (CAMBRA®), that has been implemented widely. He describes the occurrence of dental caries as follows:

> *The eventual outcome of dental caries is determined by the dynamic balance between* **pathological factors** *that lead to demineralization and* **protective factors** *that lead to remineralization.* **Pathological factors include acidogenic bacteria, inhibition of salivary function, and frequency of ingestion of fermentable carbohydrates. Protective factors include salivary flow, numerous salivary components, antibacterials (both natural and applied), fluoride from extrinsic sources, and selected dietary components.** *Intervention in the caries process can occur at any stage, either naturally or by the insertion of some procedure or treatment. Dental caries covers the continuum from the first atomic level of demineralization, through the initial enamel or root lesion, through dentinal involvement, to eventual cavitation. The dynamic balance between demineralization and remineralization determines the end result.* ***The disease is reversible, if detected early enough.***[55]

The reversible nature of this disease provides an incredible opportunity for practitioners to have a profound impact on their patients' oral health.

The CAMBRA® model of care is based on clinical scientific studies of thousands of patients of every age and is now considered to be the foundation of care in the future. It is a system that is both caries **preventative** and tooth-structure **proactive**, via the following strategies:

Caries Preventative
- Reduce cariogenic bacteria
- Reduce the ingestion of fermentable carbohydrates

Tooth-Structure Proactive
- Improve salivary function & flow
- Antibacterials
- Fluoride
- Dietary support

The CAMBRA® Caries Risk Assessment (CRA) Tool has now been used for over 14 years with remarkable findings and outcomes of treatment applications. Specific protocols are implemented for patients in the distinct risk categories of "low", "moderate", "high" and "extreme". Additionally, Dr. Featherstone's 2018 summary of this landmark work is extremely helpful:

> *This validated risk prediction tool has been updated with time and is now routinely used at UCSF and in other settings worldwide as part of normal clinical practice. The CAMBRA-CRA tool for 0 to 5-yr-olds has demonstrated similar predictive validity and is in routine use.* ***The addition of chemical therapy (antibacterial plus fluoride) to the traditional restorative treatment plan, based on caries risk status, has been shown to reduce the caries increment by about 20% to 38% in high-caries-risk adult patients. The chemical therapy used for high-risk patients is a combination of daily antibacterial therapy (0.12% w/v chlorhexidine gluconate mouth rinse) and twice-daily high-concentration fluoride toothpaste (5,000 ppm F), both for home use.*** *These outcomes assessments provide the evidence to use these CRA tools with confidence. Caries can be managed by adding chemical therapy, based on the assessed caries risk level, coupled with necessary restorative procedures.* ***For high- and extreme-risk patients, a combination of antibacterial and fluoride therapy is necessary. The fluoride therapy must be supplemented by antibacterial therapy to reduce the bacterial challenge, modify the biofilm, and provide prevention rather than continued caries progression.***[56]

Based on the CAMBRA® Model, products are now available on the market to optimally manage caries risk and prevention. The following is a description from one such company which produces a rinse and gel:

- **Rinse...** is designed to treat the cariogenic plaque biofilm, reduce the overpopulation of cariogenic bacteria, and neutralize oral pH.
- **Gel...** a low abrasion tooth gel that combines the proven anti-caries benefits of 1.1% neutral sodium fluoride with bioavailable nano hydroxyapatite crystallites, xylitol, and unique pH+ technology.

When an adult patient has no history of decay, tooth loss or periodontal disease, in almost all cases you can be confident that they eat a very healthy diet, low in refined sugars and refined carbohydrates. That is the goal for every patient, to establish and maintain optimum oral and systemic health, and to live free of caries. For patients for whom this is not yet a reality, a great place to begin is to suggest a sugar substitute that is both sweet and anti-cariogenic. Xylitol is the answer!

Xylitol

Xylitol is a natural sugar that has wonderful anti-cariogenic properties. It dramatically reduces dental caries, because:
- Xylitol raises the pH in the mouth. This decreases the presence of cariogenic bacteria, which proliferate in a low pH environment. An alkaline environment promotes oral health.
- Xylitol affects cariogenic bacteria's ability to produce acid.
- Xylitol disrupts the communication between bacteria so they stop producing the polysaccharide matrix that binds the biofilm on teeth.
- Xylitol significantly reduces the cariogenic bacterial population.

Xylitol comes in several forms, including granules, liquid, mints, candies and gum. Kids love it, and so do their healthy, cavity-free teeth. I would definitely recommend giving it a try!

Other potential strategies for the management of dental caries have been recently receiving attention. One that appears to be very effective is the combination of silver nitrate and fluoride.

Silver Nitrate + Fluoride

In 2018, Dr. Sherry Gao and cohort at the University of Hong Kong reported the following regarding silver nitrate and fluoride: *"studies have suggested that a combined application of silver nitrate solution followed by sodium fluoride varnish can be used to arrest dental caries. The treatment protocol is simple, non-invasive, painless, and low-cost. It can be a promising strategy for treating dental caries among young children, elderly populations, and people with special needs."* They added that *"as there are limited studies in the literature about this treatment, more randomized clinical trials should be conducted to provide stronger evidence for using silver nitrate solution followed by sodium fluoride varnish."*[57]

This is a promising strategy to further research and implement, as appropriate, in patients needing extra help in the management of their caries.

> For more science and guidelines regarding clinical implementation of caries management, please refer to Dr. Kim Kutsch's outstanding chapter in the Appendix.

Inflammation & Infection: Treatment
2. Periodontal Protocol

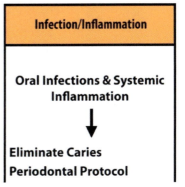

The principles that apply to the understanding and management of dental caries can be similarly applied to addressing periodontal disease. The objectives here are to prevent and eliminate the destructive effects of acid-producing oral pathogens both locally and systemically, to raise the pH in the environment, and to stabilize (and even reverse) the loss of bone and soft tissue attachment around the teeth.

There are many effective methods that can be implemented to achieve these objectives. If a desired goal is to identify specific pathogens that are active at elevated levels, then the use of **salivary testing** or paper-point sub-gingival samples can be conducted.

The results are used for **specific targeting of oral pathogens**, as directed by specific protocols that accompany the lab report. These may include local debridement, root planing and curettage (RP&C), antimicrobial rinses, and specific systemic antibiotics for 7-10 days. (Whenever a systemic antibiotic is used, an oral and systemic probiotic should be given as well. Antibiotics destroy the oral and gut flora and can themselves create a microbiome imbalance. Probiotics repopulate the oral cavity and gut with healthy new populations.) Retesting of the saliva is recommended after several weeks, in order to assess therapeutic outcomes.

Another approach is to use multiple means to reduce inflammation and infection both locally and systemically, while using **generalized targeting of oral pathogens**. Some of the possible therapeutic strategies include:

- **Root Planing and Curettage** (RP&C)
- **Laser Curettage**
- **Antimicrobial Rinses**
- **Trays for Antimicrobial Gel Delivery**
    - Specialized trays, designed to create a 360 degree gasket-like effect at the gingival margins of each tooth, delivering a specific formulation of hydrogen peroxide, have been scientifically proven to create a powerful oxygenating and anti-bacterial "hyperbaric oxygen chamber" that can destroy harmful periodontal pathogens and regenerate a healthy periodontal environment with long-term daily use. The wonderful advantage of such a system is the targeted destruction of subgingival anaerobic bacteria, the avoidance of problematic systemic antibiotic therapy, and the patient's ability to proactively treat or prevent periodontal disease, in most cases, with a simple home technique. Localized antibiotic applications, in a liquid droplet form, can be utilized inside the trays for tooth-specific delivery.[58]
- **Oral Probiotics**
    - Oral probiotics are live bacteria that are identical to the beneficial microorganisms found naturally in your mouth. The addition of oral probiotics to an oral care regimen can restore the natural balance of beneficial bacteria, which can be depleted by diet, stress, medication, illness or other factors.
    - Dr. Tom Hillman and Dr. Sig Socransky researched this subject for many years at the Forsyth Institute and found that the oral bacteria *Streptococcus oralis*, *Streptococcus uberis*, and *Streptococcus rattus* produce

hydrogen peroxide that positively influences the oral microbiome, thereby positively affecting caries and periodontal disease. They developed an oral tablet that is dissolved in the mouth to release billions of these probiotics. The image is one of sending in the good troops (probiotic bacteria) to crowd out the bad (pathogenic bacteria).
- o Excellent results have been reported regarding the efficacy of oral probiotics.[59]
- **Irrigation Systems** (utilizing water and/or antimicrobial agents)
- **Specialized Toothpastes**
- **Electric/Sonic Toothbrush**
- **Sugar-free Diet**
- **Ozone Therapy**

> **Please refer to specific guidelines for ozone therapy, provided by Dr. Rachaele Carver's outstanding summary chapter in the Appendix.**

- **Periodontal Surgery**

This list only represents some of the treatment options currently available for the management and treatment of periodontal disease.

> **For detailed information on the diagnosis and management of oral pathogens, please refer to Dr. Thomas Nabor's valuable information provided in the Appendix.**

Inflammation & Infection: Treatment
3. Treat or Extract Abscessed Teeth

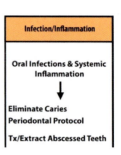

Abscessed Teeth typically have one of four primary etiologies:
1. Periodontal infection
2. Periapical infection
3. Fractured Root
4. Combination of #1-3

All of these problems represent both local and systemic sources of bacterial infection and inflammation.

The IDM model recognizes that dental caries, periodontal disease and abscessed teeth must be addressed. Bleeding and swollen gums, periodontal pocketing, radiographic changes, unresolved healing at the apex of teeth with previous endodontic therapy, remaining root tips, and fistulas are all significant concerns, even in the absence of pain. These findings should be addressed as immediate needs, regardless of the presence of symptoms.

Inflammation & Infection: Treatment
4. Counsel an Anti-inflammatory Diet

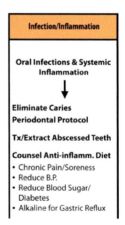

As we have previously discussed, **inflammation** is the chief cause of most chronic health concerns. **Inflammation plays a significant role in many dental concerns** such as periodontal disease, sore muscles, sore temporomandibular joints, breathing and sleep concerns that can affect nasal congestion, chronic mouth breathing, dry mouth, and even malocclusions.

It stands to reason that we must address every possible connection with inflammation in order to achieve optimal therapeutic results. As such, we must seek to leave no "stone" of inflammation unturned. Why would we not take every logical course of action, in order to empower those we serve in their journey toward complete health?

> **"ARE DENTISTS EXPECTED TO GIVE DIETARY GUIDANCE?**
> An emphatic 'yes' is the answer to this question on the responsibility of the dentist for providing dietary guidance. Of all the professional people in the healing arts, dentists are perhaps in one of the best positions to inform the public with respect to food and nutrition. They have regular contact with their patients over longer and sometimes more frequent periods than even the family physician. They, like the physician, develop a patient rapport and are recipients of a respect and confidence which makes for receptiveness on the part of the patient with respect to advice on health matters. For these several reasons, recognized knowledgeable experts, educators and scientists in medicine and nutrition are strongly recommending and even urging dentists to counsel their patients on proper diets."
>
> Abraham E. Nizel, DMD, MS, FACD
> <u>The Science of Nutrition and its Application in Clinical Dentistry</u>

In our efforts to achieve these goals, we must progress to the next step in the IDM checklist: counseling an anti-inflammatory diet. **Nutrition** has been a subject of much interest in dentistry for many years. In fact, the very first health practitioner to write about the role between diet, dental disease and physical degeneration was himself a dentist, Dr. Weston Price. In 1939, he wrote a pioneering book entitled, <u>Nutrition and Physical Degeneration</u>. Addressing nutrition still remains as an extremely helpful best practice to assist patients seeking complete health.

Dr. Peter Dawson is well-known as a giant in our field. He has long recognized the importance of counseling patients regarding their dietary choices. When I joined his dental practice in 1982, we still had paper charts with handwritten notes. I recall reviewing his charts and seeing "New Patient" and "Hygiene" entries going back to 1960, recording and monitoring the patient's sugar consumption. In his textbook, <u>Evaluation, Diagnosis, and Treatment of Occlusal Problems</u> (1974), he wrote in Chapter 1:

> *Those who believe nutrition is unrelated to either general health or dental disease should try this experiment. They*

should ask the next ten patients who have severe, active periodontal destruction what they ate for breakfast that day. Almost all will report that they do not eat breakfast. Further questioning will almost always reveal an unbalanced diet, high in refined carbohydrate intake and low in protein. The results of this questionnaire should be compared with the answers received from patients who have maintained exceptional health of their mouths. The results may be surprising. It will be obvious that poor nutrition is a potent contributing factor to accelerated deterioration of the oral tissues. Good nutrition is apparently important in deterring premature aging of the dentition.[60]

Based on both established findings and current research, it is clear that nutrition is important to properly manage the health of teeth and periodontal tissues; to build strong bone and gums; and to reduce blood sugar levels.

Nutrition is also important in the management of TMD, chronic pain and soreness. It is important in the management of allergies, airway, breathing and sleep disorders. Additionally, it is a key factor in supporting an alkaline environment in the airway, in order to reduce the dangerous effects of gastric reflux.

Good nutrition can provide the fuel and building blocks needed for growth, energy, regeneration, recovery and healing of damaged tissues throughout the body. Contrastingly, it has been scientifically proven that poor nutrition can be a major factor in systemic inflammation, periodontal disease, dental decay, sore muscles, sore joints, and osteoarthritis.

The basics of a healthy dental diet are not complicated. Three recommendations to get started are:
1. **Eat whole foods, 90% of the time – Fruits, Vegetables, Clean/Lean Protein, and a small amount of <u>Whole Grains</u>, remembering:**
    - God made everything on earth good for man to eat – fruits, vegetables, fish, birds and land animals.
    - All the chemistry for health is built into the whole foods we grow and raise.
    - Eating foods in their whole state is best; most of the time the more we alter a food, the more we detract from its inherent good chemistry.
    - Don't add hormones or antibiotics.
    - Don't use cheap refined grain foods to feed poultry or beef.

- Don't spray plants with pesticides.
- Don't refine or bleach the nutrition out of grains and rice.
- Don't refine seed and vegetable oils.
- Don't fry foods.
- Don't use preservatives, which have no nutritional value.
- Read labels and avoid ingesting chemicals you can't pronounce, such as the preservative "tert-butylhydroquinone" (TBHQ)!
- Beware of the 56 different names for sugars hidden in packaged foods, such as barley malt, brown rice syrup, corn syrup, corn syrup solids, dextrin, dextrose, diastatic malt, ethyl maltol, etc…it's all just SUGAR, and you don't want it!
- Beware of High Fructose Corn Syrup (HFCS); it can hide in so many foods and it acts like a poison in our bodies (many countries have banned its use).
- Beware of food coloring, which is very unhealthy.
- For healthy teeth and gums, remember that we need protein, calcium, phosphorous, zinc, antioxidants, folate, iron, omega-3, vitamin A, Bs, C, D3, and K2 (see next section for more information).
- Remember that eating well 90% of the time allows you 10% to enjoy a treat or a craving! When you intentionally want to indulge in, say, a pizza, enjoy it — and don't feel guilty!

2. **Take high quality supplements (such as a multivitamin, Omega-3, Vitamin A, D3, and K2) and/or eat foods rich in the following:**
    - Vitamin A: 700 mcg for women, 900 mcg for men
    Best sources: Liver & Fish Oils, Milk/Cheese, Eggs, Tomatoes, Green Leafy Vegetables, Fruits, Supplements
    - Vitamin D3: 400-800 IU/day
    Best sources: Sunlight, Cod Liver Oil, Bacon, Wild Salmon, Oysters, Caviar, Egg Yolks, Shrimp, Supplements
    - Vitamin K2: 50-1,000 mcg
    Best Sources: Leafy Green Vegetables (such as kale), fermented soy and dairy, scallions, brussels sprouts, prunes, cucumbers, broccoli, asparagus, supplements

3. **Read Dr. Steven Lin's exceptional book:** *The Dental Diet, the Surprising Link Between Your Teeth, Real Food, and Life-Changing Natural Health* **(Amazon 2017).**

> "Food is medicine.
>
> Food has the power to heal us. It is the most potent tool we have to help prevent and treat many of our chronic diseases – including diabetes and obesity. Truly, what you put on your fork dictates whether you are sick or well, slim or fat, depleted or energized.
>
> How does food do all this? Through the groundbreaking science known as *nutrigenomics*. The molecules in your food do much more than provide fuel for your body. They provide instructions that tell every cell in your body what to do every moment. More than 95% of chronic illness is not related to your genes, but to what those genes are exposed to in your lifetime.
> We call that the *exposome*.
>
> The exposome is the sum of everything you eat, breathe, drink, think and feel, plus the toxins in our environment and even the 100 trillion bacteria that live inside your gut. This is good news because it means that you have almost complete control over your health. And the most important thing you do every single day to interact with your genes is eat.
>
> ***Food is medicine. It is the most powerful tool we have to combat chronic disease.***"
>
> Mark Hyman, MD
> The Daniel Plan: 40 Days to a Healthier Life
> By Rick Warren, DMin, Daniel Amen, MD, and Mark Hyman, MD

Nutrition can become a very important and exciting subject in your life and in the lives of your dental patients. Additionally, incorporating dietary counseling is a wonderful way to demonstrate your commitment to your patients' complete health. When I became convinced that we should include nutritional counseling in our dental practice, I searched our community for a nutritional expert for advice on how to get started. The name I was given was

Isabelle Simon. A top expert in the Tampa/St. Petersburg area, Isabelle is a Board Certified Clinical Nutritionist, Holistic Health Practitioner & Wellness Consultant. When we met together to discuss possible collaboration, we both became very excited about the potential for bringing the subject of nutrition into the dental office setting. It became clear that it would be a natural fit. When I asked if she knew of anyone qualified to work with our patients, she responded with, "Well, I'm available on Fridays." A wonderful professional partnership was forged that day – one that has benefited the lives of many of my patients.

Isabelle's Mission Statement for her consulting services is as follows: *"Good health is a CHOICE, not a chance! My mission is simple: give my clients and students the wellness education, tools and resources they need to become the pro-actors of their vibrant health rather than the victims of their poor health. I encourage you to make small, sustainable, realistic behavioral and nutritional changes, adopting a healthier lifestyle, not just for a day, a week or a month, but for life!"*

I couldn't agree more, Isabelle…your mission beautifully describes the mission of *The Shift!*

I believe there are many similar like-minded professional partnerships waiting to happen – when we, as complete health practitioners, seek them out. Dental professionals who chose to practice the IDM model should consider the benefits of finding a highly-qualified nutritionist willing to partner with them in providing the best care possible for their patients. Some practices utilize a nutritionist who can "remote in", via online video conference, from any location, at any time that is most convenient for the patient.

Inflammation & Infection Treatment
5. Counsel an Anti-inflammatory Lifestyle

Even beyond the foods we eat, what we are promoting is an *anti-inflammatory life-style*. As we have discussed, it's important to remember that systemic inflammation can come from several sources, including:
- Oral Pathogens
- A Pro-inflammatory Diet
- Physical Inactivity
- Stress

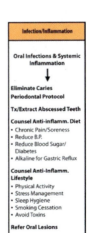

- Poor Sleep
- Smoking
- Toxins

Avoiding each of these as much as possible is important in order to establish and maintain a healthy lifestyle.

So far we have described the strategy for addressing the first two: (1) **creating a healthy oral environment** and (2) **counseling proper dietary goals**. Next we will address how we can advise patients regarding these **remaining key lifestyle concerns**.

Physical Inactivity

Kenneth Cooper, MD, is the founder of the renowned Cooper Clinic in Dallas, Texas. He is known as the "father of aerobics", a pioneer promoting the relationship between exercise and overall health. He has written more than 30 books on the subject in the last 37 years. Dr. Cooper was the keynote speaker for the American Academy for Oral Systemic Health (AAOSH) in 2016. He reported on the extensive work that he and his colleagues have done, studying a range of patients, clients, professional and Olympic athletes, middle-aged men and women, and retirees. He summarized his work in very simple terms: **simple physical activity, such as fast-walking 30 minutes per day, 6 days a week, will provide 90% of the cardiovascular benefits of exercise.** This means we can go to the gym and work out two hours a day, or we can train and run half marathons and more, but according to one of the world's leading authorities, doing so will only provide an increase of 10% of additional benefit to heart health than would be obtained through walking briskly 30 minutes a day, 6 days a week! This is great news, as this goal is something that almost everyone can achieve.

This is exciting in a world where most people cringe at the word "exercise". To many, it represents a commitment of time, discipline and pain which they agree is important but which most feel they can't achieve, and therefore they don't even try. Many people end up joining a local fitness club out of guilt, but they never darken its door. We call them fitness club "sponsors". Due to the negative connotations that the word "exercise" elicits for most people, I tend not to use it anymore; when counseling others, I instead refer only to "physical activity". It is very important to understand and promote the truth that everyone needs physical activity. I encourage even my sedentary elderly patients to get out and take a walk, a mere 15 minutes from home and then 15 minutes back home, 6 days a week.

My personal physician and integrative health authority, Dr. Steven Masley, also emphasizes the benefits of maintaining muscle mass and strength. It is often the loss of muscle that ultimately causes systems' failure in the elderly and a subsequent decline in their quality of life. Therefore, when possible, it is very important to include strength training with daily physical activity. For further information on this and many other related subjects, I highly recommend Dr. Masley's books <u>Ten Years Younger</u>, <u>The 30-Day Heart Tune Up</u>, <u>Smart Fat</u>, and <u>The Better Brain Solution</u>."

Stress

While there are many potential sources of systemic inflammation that can significantly compromise your health, one of the most dangerous of all is *STRESS*!! A very poor diet, obesity, diabetes, alcohol and cigarettes can ruin your health over many years, but stress can kill you much faster! This is not an exaggeration!

Stress in the mind and body can produce a dysregulation of the involuntary nervous system (sympathetic nervous system activation), whereby stress hormones, such as cortisol and adrenaline, are continuously being released from the adrenal glands into the bloodstream, with very dangerous consequences. The result is that the body's emergency "fight or flight" response system remains activated and on high alert 24/7.

If someone has a life-altering event that creates traumatic loss, fear, anxiety, or depression that remains unresolved, it can cause stress hormones to chronically flow throughout the body, creating effects such as insulin resistance, hormonal imbalances, cardiac arrhythmia, and even sudden death. This represents systemic inflammation at its worst.

Many feel that we live in the most mentally, emotionally and physically stressful era in history. Cell phones, emails, texts, financial pressures, politics, terrorism, road rage, fast food diets, physical inactivity and TMD have created a culture of exhaustion. This is not healthy!

Recognizing the importance of addressing stress in our lives is the first step to stress relief. The second step is to develop a daily plan to reduce stress and the constant production and release of stress hormones, which interfere with the body's normal functions. The plan does not have to be complicated, but it should be purposeful. Even 20 minutes a day of conscious stress management can make a tremendous difference. Fortunately, the solutions can be obvious and simple.

Here are some suggestions:
- 20 minutes of daily **aerobic activity and stretching**
- 20 minutes of **Scripture reading, prayer and meditation**
- 20 minutes using **Apps** to reduce Sympathetic activity/"Fight or Flight" mode and to increase Parasympathetic activity/a "Rest & Digest" state (one such app that can be downloaded on your mobile device is **AddressStress**).
- 20 minutes of walking on the beach or in a park, especially with a dog or friend
- 20 minutes in a hot bubble bath with Andrea Bocelli music!
- 20 minute massage by someone with great hands!

Be intentional and just "let it go"…on purpose, each and every day from now on! Release stress and embrace faith, love, joy, gratitude, grace, beauty, sunshine, rain, singing, whistling, smiling, laughing, and relationships!

Manage STRESS *each day* as if your life depended on it, because it does!

Sleep Hygiene

We spend almost one third of our lives resting in bed, hopefully sleeping most of that time. Many very important things happen in our bodies during sleep. Not only do we physically rest, but many critical restorative biologic functions are very active during sleep.

During sleep, growth hormones are released; the brain sorts, files and organizes information received during the day; memory and learning functions are very active; mood states are regulated; and tissues are repaired — to name a few things! It used to be thought that sleep was not that important; in college and graduate school programs, it was almost a badge of honor to say, "I pulled an all-nighter last night". Many of you will remember hearing the old saying, "No one ever died from lack of sleep". This is flat out wrong!

The National Sleep Foundation currently recommends the following general sleep guidelines:[61]

Toddlers (1-2 years old)	12-15 hours/day
Preschoolers (3-5 years old)	10-13 hours/day
School-aged (6-13 years old)	9-11 hours/day
Teenagers (14-17 years old)	8-10 hours/day
Young Adults (18-25 years old)	7-9 hours/day
Adults (26-64 years old)	7-9 hours/day
Older Adults (> 64 years old)	7-8 hours/day

When presented with this information, many people will quickly recognize that they are not meeting these recommendations. This is not a small matter.

Beyond the hours per day allotted for sleep, there are many factors that affect a person's sleep quality and quantity, including:
- Airway/breathing disorders, such as UARS and sleep apnea
- Anxiety and Stress
- Sleep disorders
- Hormonal dysregulation
- Exposure to light at night, affecting the body's Circadian rhythm
- Physical inactivity
- Pain in muscles and joints
- Obesity
- Medications, alcohol and drugs

A shortened/disrupted night's sleep can be very disruptive to our health and is a major source of *STRESS*. Therefore, educating patients on the importance of sleep is central in managing systemic inflammation. We will further explore this subject in great detail in the following chapters, but the underlying principle of the importance of adequate, restful sleep is paramount for dental practitioners following the IDM model to grasp.

Smoking Cessation

Smoking and chewing tobacco create inflammation in cells throughout the body. They can cause COPD, emphysema, asthma, heart disease, strokes, diabetes, poor healing, negative reproductive effects in women, premature/low birth-weight babies, blindness/cataracts/macular degeneration, lung cancer, and at least ten other cancers including cervical, colon, liver, stomach, colorectal and pancreatic. For the sake of reducing oral and systemic inflammation and to improve their overall quality of life, every smoker should be counseled to seek help, as needed, for smoking cessation. Some dental offices have implemented very effective in-house programs toward this goal. For other offices, patients can be directed toward a wide variety of clinics and/or services, available in almost every community, that specialize in smoking cessation.

Avoid Toxins

Isabelle Simon, our sage nutritionist, has stated, **"The number one toxin is not smoking; it's the food we eat."** Additives, preservatives, refined sugars/carbohydrates/vegetable & seed oils, BPA, trans fats, hormones, antibiotics, PAHs, food coloring, and frying all serve as toxins endangering complete health. This reality is at the heart of the recommendation to "eat clean".

We are commonly exposed to multiple toxins that are harmful and of which we must be aware. Some of the most dangerous are **heavy metals such as mercury and lead**. Mercury levels have increased in fish, both in fresh and salt water. It is recommended to limit the intake of large-mouth fish, such as tuna, bass, and catfish. Checking mercury levels during routine physicals is wise. Additionally, lead exposure may be elevated in older homes with lead painted walls. **Heavy metal toxicity can produce systemic inflammation and neurologic symptoms.**

Additionally, the following guidelines regarding **pesticides are very helpful:**
- Be aware that pesticides, especially those used in lawn care, may produce signs of systemic inflammation.
- Particle pollution, especially from dust, mold, fungus, and fuel emissions, is an important subject. Systemic inflammation is commonly exacerbated by dirty air particles found in our homes, resulting from pollution within the home and from close contact to fuel emissions.
- Air conditioning ducts can develop dust, mold and fungus, which can create systemic inflammation for the inhabitants who breathe them. Additionally, animal dander can produce allergic reactions. Changing A/C filters monthly and keeping pets out of bed can go a long way toward avoiding these problems.
- Close contact with fuel emissions, such as from a lawn mower or leaf blower, can produce systemic inflammation.

Therefore, it is advisable to use electric lawn equipment to eliminate fuel emissions.

* * *

Identifying sources of inflammation and infection throughout the body, and appropriately addressing these concerns, play a major role in the journey towards complete health. Dentistry has a unique opportunity to provide awareness, screening, testing, and practical solutions for many of these concerns. The Integrative Dental Medicine Model of care is founded upon the role that dentists and dental teams can have as the **gatekeepers of systemic inflammation**.

8. INFLAMMATION & INFECTION: FREQUENTLY ASKED QUESTIONS

What have we learned so far? Before moving on to the next section, let's consider eight great questions that dental teams frequently ask regarding the IDM philosophy of care.

Question #1:
What's the real story of the "Oral-Systemic Connection"?

The real story is that *the mouth is the gateway into the whole body*. Through the oral cavity passes life and health or sickness and accelerated aging. We will continue to explore this subject together in detail throughout the chapters of this book.

As an example, there are estimated to be over 700 varieties of oral bacteria in the mouth; most of these are symbiotic, promoting healthy digestion and immune system function. There are, however, a dozen or so currently identified bacteria that can be very harmful if they are heavily concentrated in the occlusal grooves or interproximals of teeth, creating an acidic, toxic environment in the periodontal sulcus. In addition to the harm caused by localized infections, when these pathogenic bacteria penetrate the gingival soft tissue and bone, entering the bloodstream, they are associated with systemic infection and inflammation. Inflammation is the body's way of resolving infections and insults through the immune system's response. Unfortunately, if the source of infection and insult becomes chronic, the body's immune system weakens; this results in illness, disease, and chronic pain. Medical authorities today (whether their focus is diabetes, cardiovascular disease, dementia, sleep apnea or cancers) all emphasize the critical role of inflammation in the disease process. That's why *periodontal disease is a very big deal to overall health.* Scientific studies are exposing the harmful effects of oral pathogens in cardiovascular disease, certain cancers, pregnancy complications, and several chronic illnesses.

As we continue to progress through the message of *The Shift*, we will further dive into other oral-systemic connections that significantly contribute to a state of wellness or of inflammation and illness. These connections come through the food we put in our mouths, toxins we inhale through our mouths, and chronic mouth breathing due to airway obstructions occurring both during waking hours and sleep.

We also recognize there is a "systemic-oral connection" as well. In the oral cavity, we see signs of systemic inflammation such as pregnancy gingivitis and diabetes. When there is poor circulation, hormonal changes, and/or compromised immune system function, the tissues in the mouth will change. ***The dental team is very likely to be the first health care provider to discover early signs of systemic compromise.***

Question #2:
Why would a dental team be interested in transitioning into an Integrative Dental Medicine style of practice?

Over the years, dentistry has progressed through several eras. Our profession's initial era was limited to extractions and dentures. As knowledge grew regarding the cause and management of periodontal disease, we moved into the era of preservation and restoration. In recent years, with an advancement in porcelain technology, we experienced another era, sometimes referred to as "the cosmetic revolution". Dentistry is now entering its next era — the Complete Health Era.

As previously mentioned, Michael Roizen, MD, is the prominent Medical Director of the Cleveland Clinic Wellness Institute. During his keynote address to the 2012 annual meeting of the American Academy for Oral and Systemic Health (AAOSH), he described a health care crisis in the United States that is escalating annually. This crisis is driven by poor Western diets (high in refined carbohydrates, refined oils, and fried foods); physical inactivity; high stress levels; high cholesterol; high blood pressure; high blood sugar levels; obesity; diabetes; and cardiovascular disease. He projected that health care costs will bankrupt our nation in the next several years – unless something changes. Due to insurance constraints, many physicians find themselves seeing 30-40 patients each day. Many are quick to point out that the average amount of time physicians are able to spend face-to-face with their patients is about 15 minutes every two years.

In a powerful keynote address, Dr. Roizen challenged his dental medicine colleagues to serve on the front lines in educating the public and turning the crisis around. He called upon us to take advantage of the reality that, in most cases, dental teams spend more quality time with patients than any other health care providers.

Dental teams are perfectly positioned to be the gatekeepers of systemic health. Through screening, testing, treatment, and referrals, not only can a dental team experience great internal, spiritual reward, but they can also build a wonderfully differentiated professional business model.

> **The Integrative Dental Medicine era will significantly elevate the status of dentistry in the larger medical community…and it offers an invitation to increased levels of excellence and service for those dental teams who join in its mission.**

Question #3:
Why am I not as healthy as I want to be?

Research shows that most health issues are related more to personal lifestyle practices than to genetic factors passed down from our parents. DNA studies show that the our regulatory DNA act like "switches" that turn "on" or "off" the genes which express disease.

- What are the factors that turn on these switches?
- How do we keep those switches turned off?
- How do we promote staying healthy for a lifetime?
- How do we become as healthy as we want to be?

The Cleveland Clinic Wellness Institute suggests five lifestyle practices that will best ensure optimal health long-term for each of us:

1. **Stress reduction,** through purposeful practices of prayer, meditation, and physical activity.
2. **Proper Nutrition** of complex carbohydrates through fruits and vegetables, clean and lean protein, healthy fats, and appropriate dietary supplements daily.
3. **Physical activity,** through exercising daily.
4. **No Smoking,** to prevent its inflammatory and carcinogenic damage systemically.
5. **Flossing Daily,** taking care of periodontal health and reducing systemic inflammation.

Additionally, weight gain is highly associated with most chronic health issues. Maintaining an ideal weight, through implementing the Cleveland Clinic recommendations, with a waist/hip ratio of 1:1 or less, is a very effective starting point to avoid metabolic syndrome, diabetes, cardiovascular disease, accelerated aging, sleep apnea, gastric reflux, heart attacks, strokes and dementia.

If you are not as healthy as you would like to be, a strong recommendation would be to focus on these 5 lifestyle practices, along with obtaining a complete physical examination with an Integrative Medicine Physician.

Question #4:
What are some ways to get healthier as a dental team?

Commit as a team to getting healthy together. Read books together that educate you on correct practices of stress reduction, proper nutrition/supplements, and physical activity. Enlist multiple members of the team (in addition to the dentist) to lead discussions on special topics of the group's interest. Go out to healthy restaurants together. Cook healthy meals together, shared at team meetings or in a home. Share healthy recipes. Invite an informed physician, nurse, nutritionist, personal trainer or health coach to speak to your team. Set team goals that relate to weight loss, fitness, and participation in a local charity walk-a-thon or run. Plan a special celebration for the whole team when the group's goals are achieved.

It is important to have fun together in the journey towards increased health in a loving, supportive, accountable culture, which you uniquely create together. Remember to talk with your patients about these activities and your personal commitment to getting healthy — that's where it all begins!

> "Foods that are high in fiber, which provide fuel to the gut bacteria, and reduced in refined sugars support a robust mélange of bacterial species, which helps maintain the integrity of the gut wall, keep blood sugar in check, reduce inflammation, and manufacture all those important substances and molecules critical for brain health and function. Moreover, there's a big difference between fats that fuel inflammation and fats that help control inflammation. Omega-6 fats dominate in the Western diet today; these are the pro-inflammatory fats found in many vegetable oils that have been linked to an increased risk for brain disorders as well as heart trouble. Omega-3 fats, on the other hand – such as the fats found in olive oil, fish, flaxseed, and wild grass-fed animals – boost brain function, help stamp out inflammation, and can actually counterbalance the detrimental effects of the omega-6 fats. Anthropological research reveals that our hunter-gatherer ancestors consumed omega-6 and omega-3 fats in a ratio of roughly 1:1. Today we consume an astronomical ten to twenty-five times more omega-6 fats than those ancestors did."
>
> David Perlmutter, MD
> Brain Maker: The Power of Gut Microbes to Heal and Protect Your Brain – for Life

Question #5:
In what ways are dental team members uniquely positioned to help guide patients toward complete health?

There are many ways to introduce, influence, and guide patients toward complete health. This process begins with our own personal commitment and enthusiasm for total wellness. Personal stories are always the most influential in helping others understand the need for change. Your commitment to total health and wellness should be a verbalized part of the office Vision and Mission Statements. It should be represented visually as well, reflected in the types of magazines in the reception area and books on shelves. New Patient Health History forms should include questions related to complete health, which can serve to open the door for meaningful conversations. An example could be as simple as "Do you take vitamins or supplements?" Experience has shown that about 50% of patients will check "No". When reviewing the health history with the patient, the dentist or clinical assistant can comment, "So I see you don't presently take any vitamins or supplements?" The most common response is, "No, should I?". The door is now open for a brief conversation; in our practice, this includes handing the patient a copy of Dr. Steven Masley's paperback book <u>Ten Years Younger</u>. This excellent guide covers the topics of nutrition, fitness, stress reduction, and includes a recommended total wellness program, all from a leading medical authority. (For more information, please see the interview with Dr. Masley provided in the next chapter.) Any patient with a significant health history of high blood pressure, high cholesterol/heart issues, high sugar levels/diabetes, or inflammatory disorders, among many others, would be a great person for whom to suggest some helpful resources.

Other ideas include enlisting hygienists and clinical assistants to help educate patients on the key topic of inflammation. Nutrition, weight management, stress management, and physical activity are all natural topics of conversation for hygienists and clinical assistants to engage in while with the patient. Additionally, practice newsletters can effectively introduce new health topics to your patients. Various screenings can be done as well. For example, the Epworth Sleepiness Scale or STOP-BANG questionnaire are simple, brief written tools that are helpful in uncovering patients who may have a sleep/airway problem, often related to sleep apnea.

Question #6:
How do dentists become distinguished in their communities as leaders in Integrative Dental Medicine?

A distinguished leader is someone whose vision for helping others inspires enthusiastic followers. What more inspiring vision could there be than creating a dental practice centered on helping people reach their maximum complete health goals? We lead by reaching out to our community with great information, practical support, and genuine compassion.

Our foundational commitment must be to learn **great information** through sources that can provide sound, scientific wellness principles. We as dentists must seek out trustworthy institutions, researchers, and clinicians to teach us transferable concepts aimed at helping our patients, family members, neighbors, and community achieve better health. In doing so, we can become passionate communicators of a healthful message within our circles of influence.

Our next commitment is to provide ***practical support*** to others. Everyone has read articles about periodontal disease, the oral-systemic connection, our poor Western diet, metabolic syndrome, the obesity epidemic, the benefits of exercise, the importance of reducing stress, the dangers of sleep apnea, and the link between smoking and cancer. Though all these concerns are real, many people will not take the steps toward positive lifestyle changes without help. That help is often hard to find. We can provide that necessary help to others as we become a practical resource for education and support. We as dentists can be the gatekeepers who screen for systemic inflammation. We can provide the information that motivates others to action. Furthermore, we can team up with other like-minded health professionals to create a practical support network for our patients. As dentists, we have a unique and exciting opportunity to make it easier for those we serve in our communities to get the help they need.

The overriding commitment supporting all the others is ***genuine compassion*** for those we serve. When we come alongside people, as their advocates for total wellness, treating them as we would a family member, they will sense our genuine care for them. It's a matter of continuing to gain and be worthy of their trust.

Every patient asks three questions when listening to our advice:
Does he/she really care about me?....................*Genuine compassion?*
Can I trust him/her?..*Practical support?*
Can he/she really help me?...................................*Great information?*

The Integrative Dental Medicine model will prove to be the most successful in helping dentists build well-deserved reputations as distinguished leaders in complete health.

> "Some of the findings, published in the most reputable scientific journals, show that:
>
> ➤ Dietary change can enable diabetic patients to go off their medication.
> ➤ Heart disease can be reversed with diet alone.
> ➤ Breast cancer is related to levels of female hormones in the blood, which are determined by the food we eat.
> ➤ Antioxidants, found in fruits and vegetables, are linked to better mental performance in old age.
> ➤ Kidney stones can be prevented by a healthy diet.
> ➤ Type 1 diabetes, one of the most devastating diseases that can befall a child, is convincingly linked to infant feeding practices.
>
> These findings demonstrate that a good diet is the most powerful weapon we have against disease and sickness. An understanding of this scientific evidence is not only important for improving health; it also has profound implications for our entire society."
>
> T. Colin Campbell, PhD, and Thomas M. Campbell II, MD
> <u>The China Study: Startling Implications for Diet, Weight Loss and Long-term Health</u>

Question #7:
How will a new identity and mix of services enhance the success of my practice?

Success should always be defined first and foremost as it relates to helping others. As a dental team, our most significant identity is found in being *problem solvers*. Whether the problem originates with a poor bite, clenching and grinding, temporomandibular joint (TMJ) pain, periodontal infection/inflammation or an unsightly smile, our clinical identity and success is best measured by our ability to help solve the problems of our patients. This new service mix is not a paradigm shift to an all new identity but instead serves as a *paradigm expansion*, broadening our ability to help others.

The emphasis of Integrative Dental Medicine will bring a new identity to your practice. Patients will appreciate and be impressed by your unique effort to solve more problems and provide more valuable services than other dental teams. Patients who experience significant positive changes in their lives will soon share their excitement with others in the community. Word will spread as patients share with those they know about how you have helped them, and you will attract new patients who are interested in a more comprehensive dental experience.

Your success will also be reflected on the business side as well. In the physician's office, the majority of income is generated through examinations, consultations, testing, treatment, re-testing, and follow-up consultations. In the conventional dental office, we are accustomed to being reimbursed primarily for services physically performed by the dentist, such as prepping the tooth for an MO inlay. With this increased knowledge base and enhanced practice model, the service mix can now expand to include diagnostic and preventative services and new types of interventional care – all of which will benefit your patients. Many of these services can be performed by team members. There will be a multiplicative effect in overall practice production that will be reflected in a significant increase in net income – as well as increased health and quality of life of your patients. You will find that the definition of "success" grows to include spiritual/emotional rewards, a well-deserved reputation within your community, and the financial rewards that rightfully compensates your efforts to launch your patients toward a new world of health they might not have otherwise known.

Question #8:
What is the future role of the dental team as a co-diagnostician in primary care?

The dental team will become increasingly involved in primary care. The focus will be to serve as gatekeepers of systemic inflammation and complete health. It has been said, "where there is smoke, there is fire". We must add, *"where there is inflammation, there is fire"*...and that *"fire"* is what the dental team will continually monitor through tracking signs of inflammation. As discussed, inflammation has several sources of *"fire"*, including oral pathogens; airway obstructions; toxins/smoking; a pro-inflammatory diet; lack of physical activity; and stress. These are the primary fires that the *dental team fire fighters* will battle to extinguish, working side-by-side with other fire-fighting health professional colleagues.

It is helpful to review a few examples of how this plays out. As we have noted, one major source of systemic inflammation comes from the *"fire"* caused by oral pathogens. Scientific studies are enlightening us to understand that bacteria from the mouth can invade the bloodstream, penetrate the arterial endothelial lining, and establish bacterial colonies of *"fire"* within arterial plaque. Concentrated levels of oral bacteria have been identified in blood thrombi (clots) of heart attack victims. **As physicians recognize that patients with atherosclerosis likely also have oral pathogen infections (fires), dental teams will be asked to assist with both co-diagnosis and treatment.**

Upper Airway Resistance Syndrome (UARS) and Obstructive Sleep Apnea (OSA) are significant sources of *"fire"* leading to systemic inflammation and are associated with high blood pressure, cardiac arrhythmias, elevated stress hormones, insulin resistant diabetes, obesity, sleep, weight and emotional dysregulation, and gastric reflux. The dental team is ideally positioned to screen for obstructions that occur in the back of the oral cavity, through a thorough health history, clinical examination, and the use of screening tools, such as home sleep monitors. This primary care role can work very well when combined with the expertise of a board-certified sleep physician, neurologist, allergist, internist, otolaryngologist, oral-myofunctional therapist, and medical sleep laboratory.

Another area of great significance involves the expanded use of saliva testing. Saliva testing can identify *"fire"* markers related to the endocrine system, the immune system, inflammatory and infectious processes, and several types of cancer, including oral, breast, prostate and pancreatic.

Quoting J. Max Goodson, DDS, PhD, Clinical Professor of Oral Medicine, Infection, and Immunity at the Harvard School of Dental Medicine, "saliva is likely to provide us with an overall health monitoring tool that can lead to better overall wellness and help fight the biggest health issues of our lifetime – obesity and type 2 diabetes." Furthermore Goodson's research reveals that clues found in the saliva may be the key to improved quality of life for patients not only with metabolic disorders but also with heart disease, kidney disease, concussions and Alzheimer's disease. As we have seen time and time again, **the mouth is the gateway to learning more about human health and disease.**

An additional simple test with great promise for systemic *"fire"*-fighters is oral swabbing. The following quote from the Harvard Gazette is most compelling:

> *Eyes may be a window to the soul, but Donna Mager, DMD (Forsythe Institute, Harvard Dental School), prefers looking into a mouth. She sees it as a mirror that reflects the body's health. It can reveal evidence for diabetes, measles, leukemia, syphilis, AIDS, bulimia, irritable bowel syndrome, heartburn, and other maladies. Obviously, oral cancer shows itself here, and she thinks it can be identified in its earliest stages by the communities of bacteria living in and on the mouth lining, tongue, and throat.*[62]

The exciting future role of the dental team will be as gatekeepers, *"fire"*-fighters, and co-diagnosticians, promoting the primary care of whole body concerns, manifested through the oral cavity.

"Since the 1960s, artificial food, hazardous chemicals, trans fats, high-fructose corn syrup, hybridized and genetically modified foods, toxic preservatives and other additives have caused the most prevalent and preventable disease of our time. The unhealthy American diet is responsible for epidemics of obesity, diabetes, heart disease, osteoporosis, asthma, sleep apnea, acid reflux, and esophageal cancer.

Reflux-related diseases affect at least half of Americans. Since the 1970's, the prevalence of reflux disease has increased 400 percent, and reflux-caused esophageal cancer has increased more than 850 percent; in terms of incidence, it has become America's fastest growing cancer.

In just 40 years, the acid reflux epidemic has occurred despite more than $1.5 trillion spent on medical surveillance procedures, such as endoscopy, and widespread use of acid-suppressive medications, the most notable being proton pump inhibitors (PPIs). Although they seldom control reflux, we spend $15 billion a year on PPIs alone.

The impact of the Western diet is now global. and where the Western diet goes, a reflux epidemic follows. Interestingly, the rise in reflux diseases directly parallels the arc of soft drink consumption. However, while the relationship between sugary soft drinks and obesity and diabetes is in the news, another negative impact of soft drinks on our health is being ignored.

Acids — most commonly citric, phosphoric, and ascorbic, often just labeled as *vitamin C* — are the main preservatives in almost everything in a bottle or can. Today, fruit juices, vitamin waters, energy drinks, and soft drinks all have the same acidity as stomach acid, and this causes serious problems for all people with reflux. In fact, these products are the actual *cause* of reflux for many people."

Jamie Koufman, MD, FACS
<u>Dr. Koufman's Acid Reflux Diet</u>

9. A CONVERSATION WITH STEVEN MASLEY, MD

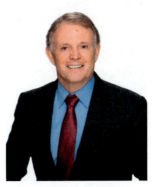

Steven Masley, MD is a highly respected researcher and clinician in Integrative and Functional Medicine. He served as the Medical Director at the world famous Pritikin Longevity Center in Miami, Florida. He presently directs the Masley Optimal Health Center, in St. Petersburg, Florida. Dr. Masley is well known across the United States for his nationally televised wellness programs on PBS. He has authored four books entitled Ten Years Younger, The 30 Day Heart Tune Up, Smart Fat, and The Better Brain Solution.

I feel very privileged that Steven is my personal physician, mentor and friend. We recently sat down together and had a personal conversation. I'd like to share that conversation with you. I know you will find it to be as valuable as I did.

* * *

Dr. Wilkerson: "Steven, it seems as if we are moving deeper into a greater and greater health crisis. Describe, as a wellness physician, what you see happening through the years with our country's health and with patients' health in general."

Dr. Masley: "Well, it's really a time of transformation because for years now, we have looked at people only with regard to what diseases they had and then treated them for those diseases – and we have never looked at them as a person. Whether you've got a cavity in your mouth or high blood pressure, we didn't think it was your lifestyle that was the key player. It was the disease that we needed to treat – like a bug that we had to fight. That worked fine if you had an accident and you had a trauma to "fix" – like a broken tooth or a broken arm. We fix that. However, it doesn't work well if your health is falling apart, and you have bad gums and bad arteries and a shrinking brain. The transformation that I think we've seen in recent years is that we are realizing we can make total health much better, on a large scale. We can transform, even rejuvenate, people. We can do so much more for them than sit back and deal with their acute symptoms and problems."

Dr. Wilkerson: "What do you think are the root causes of people not being well?"

Dr. Masley: "First of all, we eat a lot more junk; we've gone so far from eating real food to eating so much processed sugar and chemicals. What we eat today is nothing like what we ate 50 or 100 years ago – and certainly not thousands of years ago. Secondly, our food is so heavily processed that our nutrient levels are way down. We used to get a lot more nutrition from our food supply. We ate lean protein, vegetables, fruits and beans, and all of those had a very high density of nutrients. Thirdly, our fitness levels have significantly dropped. We're not nearly as fit. A fourth major root cause is stress. We're more stressed than we've ever been. It used to be that it got dark, and you went to bed in a cave. You might have had a little campfire if you were lucky. But now we're up 24/7. We've got all these personal gadgets, people communicating with us, calling, texting, and emailing us at 2:00 in the morning. It's endless. I think those are the four biggest factors that we see – more processed food, less nutritious food, less fitness and increased stress. Those have seriously impacted our energy, weight, mental sharpness, and accelerated our aging."

Dr. Wilkerson: "How do all these things relate to metabolic syndrome, as you described in your book, <u>Ten Years Younger</u>?"

Dr. Masley: "To a large degree, accelerated aging is a result of metabolic syndrome. It's a syndrome of your metabolism being out of whack. We don't burn calories well, so we gain weight. If our metabolism is out of whack, our blood sugar goes up, all our tissues are harmfully "sugar-coated", and we age faster. When our metabolism is out of whack, we are more inflamed; as a result our joints ache, we're more likely to clot, we're more likely to have a heart attack, and our tissues are breaking down. So accelerated aging results from your metabolism being out of balance – or, metabolic syndrome. For me, that's the greatest aging factor we see today. It affects a third of all adults. And more specifically, 50% of baby boomers have metabolic syndrome and accelerated aging – it's tragic."

Dr. Wilkerson: "What are some of the signs and symptoms that go along with metabolic syndrome over time?"

Dr. Masley: "One of the clearest signs of metabolic syndrome is an expanding waistline. Also your blood sugar's going up, so you're sugar-coating your proteins, and you're internally setting yourself on fire. Your cholesterol profile gets worse, HDL drops, the triglycerides go up, and there's a worsening of your cholesterol profile – so we grow a lot more plaque, even with the same cholesterol numbers. Because of that, our blood pressure goes up. Our arteries are sick; they're growing plaque; they're getting stiff, and so we have a rise in blood pressure and are even more inflamed. You can measure it with blood tests. You can actually see with some blood tests that our blood is more inflamed, our joints are more achy, our brain is shrinking, our arteries are growing plaque, and none of that sounds good."

Dr. Wilkerson: "No, it doesn't. We see it happening all around us. What do we do?"

Dr. Masley: "It's happening nationwide, on a massive scale. And it's time for us as medical professionals to stand up and stay, 'You've got to stop!' It's time to say, 'Enough!' We've got to stop looking at the acute thing – 'my tooth hurts,' 'my back hurts', 'I have a cold' – and get past that to say, 'You're slowly dying…what can we do to transform your life?' That's what we need to look at, beyond just the acute symptom."

Dr. Wilkerson: "As you examine patients, day in and day out, what percentage of your patients would you say are sick because of a self-inflicted lifestyle?"

Dr. Masley: "More than 80% of my patients, when I first see them, are grossly nutritionally deficient. And I see smart people – these are people working 40-60 hours a week. They're very professional; they know what to do in life. But they don't know how to meet their nutrient needs. They're misguided."

Dr. Wilkerson: "Do most people think they understand nutrition, and yet they really don't?"

Dr. Masley: "I'd say, of the 80% that are grossly nutritionally deficient, half likely know they are, and half think they are doing a pretty good job – until we evaluate their nutrient intake. Most of the people I see think they are fitter than they are. When we actually measure their fitness, they're like 'Holy moly, I thought I was in pretty good shape!'

Dr. Wilkerson: "What are the some of the things that some people eat that they think are just fine, but really they shouldn't be eating?"

Dr. Masley: "One of the biggest things is that we are eating way too much sugar – sugary drinks, sweetened soda and teas. Anything with flour counts as sugar as well, including whole wheat bread. When we look at flour, essentially we find that a bowl of flour and a bowl of sugar produce the same chemical response in your blood stream. That means that whole wheat bread, pasta, bagels, and cereal end up, essentially, being treated by your body the same way as sugar. You know, people are eating cereal thinking it's a good idea, but if it's ground into flour, it's raising their blood sugar and raising their metabolic syndrome. So I'd say that sugar is #1 – and #2 is hydrogenated fat. Most people know they should avoid it, but they don't realize that when they buy processed food or packaged restaurant food that they are basically eating embalming fluid. They don't read the label or check it out, so they are basically poisoning themselves and don't even realize it."

Dr. Wilkerson: "Why are those harmful things in these foods?"

Dr. Masley: "Well, I think they put sugar in processed foods because it's addicting. The way I see it, we have dealt with famine for thousands of years, and to fight it, as a survival mechanism, we learned that eating sweets tastes good because it helps you store calories and prevent famine. The problem is, most of us don't have to deal with famine anymore, and our genes haven't changed in the last 50-100 years. Sugar tastes pleasant and is addicting, so we don't even realize how dependent on sugar we have all become – and that when you eat sugar you can't really taste anything else. It's like having a shot of tequila and then trying to taste the difference between two pieces of fruit – you can't taste anything. Well, sugar has just about the same impact. It's amazing really. If that wasn't enough, we now have many toxins in our food. I'm not just talking about pesticides that are increasingly common; the linings of cans have a carcinogen called BPA, and most sandwich meats, hot dogs, and bacon have a toxin that kills brain cells – called 'nitrosamines.' Most processed foods have become toxic."

Dr. Wilkerson: "So now that we know what the problem is, would you say that we're getting sicker as a nation, as the years go by?"

Dr. Masley: "Absolutely. Every year that goes by, we see a worsening in American health."

Dr. Wilkerson: "What about children?"

Dr. Masley: "Well, I read about 20 medical journals per month, and I think the most important article in the last decade was the one in the New England Journal of Medicine showing that today's children are going to die at a younger age than ever before. So we are killing our children. There was an article published showing the average obese adolescent, aged 16-20, has the arterial plaque of someone in their 40's, and I couldn't believe that. So in our clinic, I checked 20 adolescents, aged 16-20, and measured their arterial plaque – and found that the average obese adolescent had the plaque of a 42-year-old. That's more than double their age! We are killing our children today with the lifestyle that we're offering to them, and it's time to change what we are doing. It's not just for us. It's going to be important for our children as well."

Dr. Wilkerson: "In your book, <u>The 30-Day Heart Tune Up</u>, you describe a medical plan for preventing and reversing heart disease. Can you tell us about it?"

Dr. Masley: "We tried to make it easy. I've tried some complicated things before, and people just aren't going to follow them. It has to be realistic. It has to include food they like, and it has to be something they could follow. We also looked at foods that you could add in. Our research was based on measuring arterial plaque in our clinic. We looked at hundreds of things that predict if someone's growing plaque at an accelerated rate or not. We could see things like sugar, and flour, and hydrogenated fat were really bad, but we also realized that there are some things that are awesome for health. It's so simple to add those things in. We realized that there were 5 key factors that helped you not grow plaque. Additionally, if you had plaque, we're now publishing data on what helps to reverse and shrink arterial plaque. The 5 key factors are:

#1. **Fiber** – not what's advertised in breakfast cereal, but what's in vegetables, fruits, beans and nuts.

#2. **Fitness** – your aerobic fitness. What matters is how fit you are. It doesn't matter how many minutes you work out, but it's how fit you are that matters.

#3. **Fish oil and Fish** – because those Omega 3's are very beneficial to heart health.

#4. **Food Nutrients** – everyone in the dental community needs to realize that there are some specific nutrients that are really good for our health, our bones, our tissues and our hearts, in particular vitamin K, vitamin D, and magnesium.

#5. **Body Fat** – because if your body fat is up, you're going to grow fat a lot faster. But here's the good news – if you add the fiber and increase your fitness, you almost always lose weight."

Dr. Wilkerson: "The Five F's. We can certainly remember Fiber, Fitness, Fish Oil & Fish, Food Nutrients, and Body Fat. You have recently completed writing <u>Smart Fat</u> and <u>The Better Brain Solution</u>. What's the main message of these books for our health?"

Dr. Masley: The book <u>Smart Fat</u> clarifies why we don't want to follow a low-fat diet, because healthy fats are good for us. However, we have to be selective about the fats we eat, because some fats are harmful, some are neutral, and many are clearly beneficial to our health. Healthy fats that we should eat often are avocados, olive oil, wild salmon, dark chocolate, and nuts. The book also identifies which fats can tolerate heat and which are destroyed by overcooking. The goal is to use the right fat at the right temperature, such as using extra virgin olive oil in a salad, while sautéing and cooking at medium-high heat with avocado oil.

The Better Brain Solution is based upon research from my clinic, showing that my average patient with the right information can improve their cognitive function by 25% and help prevent memory loss. The key to success is avoiding abnormal blood sugar levels and insulin resistance, plus eating more brain friendly foods, such as colorful vegetables, olive oil, fatty cold water fish, dark chocolate, spices and herbs like Italian herbs and curry spices, as well as tea. We also identified that increasing fitness, managing stress, and avoiding common toxins all complement a healthy diet, and doing these things together is far more effective in protecting the brain than just making a single change. It's amazing to think that going forward that we could prevent the majority of memory loss that we see today – and feel mentally sharper and more productive at the same time.

Dr. Wilkerson: "The Shift addresses Integrative Dental Medicine. As a physician, how do you see the dental profession making a difference?"

Dr. Masley: "The dental profession can make an enormous difference. It's a huge opportunity. People come into the dental office for their dental and oral health. The concept of dentists dealing with what occurs in the mouth, including what we eat, is so natural. It's a lot closer connection than they would consider a physician would address. So for the dental community to ask patients questions such as 'What do you eat?', 'What do you put in your mouth?', and 'Are you meeting your nutrient requirements?'…that's a huge opportunity. Also the average dental visit includes a lot more time with the practitioner than the average physician visit. And when you think about it, the 5 key nutrients we talked about could be addressed so easily. Asking 'Are you getting your fiber? Do you get your magnesium? Your potassium? Your vitamin D and vitamin K?' – those questions could be very easily addressed as a simple part of your dental evaluation. It wouldn't even have to be a part of each visit, but at least once a year there could be something related to how they are doing in these areas that are so important to their health. Let's address them as part of your dental evaluation. That would make a tremendous difference in people's lives."

Dr. Wilkerson: "Do you think that there is a growing community of people who care about total wellness among medical professionals? In other words, do you see physicians getting this? Do you think it's going to grow?"

Dr. Masley: "Presently, the community of medical professionals engaged in total wellness is way too small. People are getting it – the public is getting more interested, even ahead of the medical community. So whichever medical professionals get started, they are going to be way ahead in meeting the needs of the community and in taking this to the next step in transforming lives. This is a beautiful opportunity, and I'm rooting for whomever can get there first. I applaud you, Witt, for encouraging your colleagues to adopt an integrative philosophy of dental care."

Dr. Wilkerson: "Thanks, Steven. Is there anything else you would advise dental teams?"

Dr. Masley: "I think dental teams often don't realize the impact they have on their patients' cardiovascular health. If gums are inflamed, there is an increase in inflammatory markers, and an increase in carotid IMT (intima-media thickness) and arterial plaque growth. People grow more plaque in their arteries when their gums are inflamed, so dental care makes a big difference in reducing cardiovascular risk, and I don't think most people in the dental community realize that. Periodontal care has a much bigger impact than just the teeth. If we could get the dental team to look at the 5 factors – those that are associated with accelerated aging, accelerated arterial plaque growth and heart disease – and help people add the foods and the nutrients that would correct them, that would make a huge difference. The key point is, if you're focusing on improving your circulation and your heart health, it doesn't just help your heart. It's going to help improve your energy; you're going to be trimmer and fitter; you're going to have a better waistline; you'll increase weight control; and your brain speed improves. We have randomized trials showing that when you do these things, it increases brain speed and helps prevent memory loss. It's great for your romantic life; you feel better, and your overall function improves. It affects your entire quality of life. There's a theme I commonly hear when I see people. They ask me, 'What improvement can I get in just thirty days?' Well, in thirty days, you can sleep better; your energy level can be better; your romantic life can function better; and we can start taking people off their medicines – after thirty days! They are losing weight, and they feel awesome. Probably one of the most common comments I hear afterwards is, 'I forgot how great I could feel – I'd totally forgotten I could feel this good.' That is so gratifying to hear. It's not just that you're preventing heart disease, but that they feel great. So you can prevent heart disease – and, if you already have it, you can shrink it and reverse it and feel incredible at the same time. And that's the message that I think we need to spread."

Dr. Wilkerson: "Thank you, Steven! Working together, we will spread the message."

"Modern science shows that most common ailments in today's world are the result of nutritional ignorance. However, we can eat a diet rich in phytochemicals from a variety of natural plant foods that will afford us the ability to live a long and healthy life.

I always try to emphasize the benefits of nutritional excellence. With a truly healthy diet, you can not only expect a drop in blood pressure and cholesterol and a reversal of heart disease, but your headaches, constipation, indigestion and bad breath should all resolve. Eating for nutritional excellence enables people to reverse diabetes and to gradually lose their dependence on drugs. You can expect to reach a normal weight without counting calories and dieting, as well as achieve robust health and live a long life free of the fear of heart attacks and strokes.

Nutritional excellence, which involves eating plenty of vegetables, fruits, and beans, does not have to exclude all animal products, but it has to be very rich in high-nutrient plant foods (which should make up well over 80% of your caloric intake). No more than 10% of your total calories should come from animal foods."

Joel Fuhrman, MD
Eat To Live: The Amazing Nutrient-Rich Program for Fast and Sustained Weight Loss

Part III:
The Great Awakening
Airway, Breathing, and Sleep

10. "DENTISTRY'S GREAT AWAKENING"

Airway and breathing health can significantly affect dental and total health.

In the 1730-40s in America, a social movement, led by a Protestant Revivalist named Jonathan Edwards, created a fundamental *shift* within the culture that directly opened the door for the American Revolution against Great Britain. Using timeless Scriptural principles, Edwards spoke about human rights throughout New England. He proclaimed revolutionary principles such as the fact that people are created equal by their Maker and that taxation without fair representation is not right. He was also ahead of his time in speaking against slavery. One of Edward's biggest supporters was Benjamin Franklin, who often quoted him in his newspaper, the <u>Pennsylvania Gazette</u>. This societal *shift* has been described as "The Great Awakening."

Throughout the history of dentistry, there have been many important breakthroughs, such as:
- the breakthrough in understanding and treating periodontal disease;
- the breakthrough in understanding masticatory system dynamics between the joints, muscles and dental occlusion;
- the breakthrough in integrating dental implants with alveolar bone;
- the breakthrough in computer technology guiding all phases of orthodontic and prosthetic therapy.

It is the observation of many that we are currently experiencing another important breakthrough, one that will once again change dentistry forever: "Dentistry's Great Awakening".

"Dentistry's Great Awakening" refers to the sudden appreciation of the central role of a compromised airway in influencing breathing disruption, adverse craniofacial growth and development, dental malocclusions, sleep disturbances, TMD-like symptoms, cognitive impairment in all ages, autonomic dysregulation, and a general compromise in overall health.

In October 2017, the American Dental Association (ADA) released a policy statement addressing dentistry's role in diagnosing and managing sleep-related breathing disorders.[63] **The policy encourages dental professionals to screen their patients for Obstructive Sleep Apnea (OSA), Upper Airway Resistance Syndrome (UARS), and other breathing disorders. The ADA advocates working in collaboration with other trained medical colleagues and emphasizes the effectiveness of intra-oral appliance therapy for treating patients with mild to moderate OSA and CPAP-intolerant patients with severe OSA. With the endorsement of the ADA, screening and treating sleep-related breathing disorders has become the newest focus of Integrative Dental Medicine.**

Breathing is the most essential bodily function for survival. Every cell in the body depends on oxygen from the air we breathe to help metabolize the nutrients released from food for energy. Without oxygen, we can only survive for a matter of minutes. Air that enters the body through the nose is humidified and warmed as it swirls through the scroll-like turbinates. It passes over respiratory mucous membranes, which contain innumerable tiny hair-like cells designed to collect impurities, and it is sterilized by the powerful antimicrobial effects of nitric oxide, produced in the paranasal sinuses. Nitric oxide also dilates the nasal passages and airway and relaxes smooth muscle cells, resulting in bronchodilation and arterial vasodilation throughout the body.[64] [65] [66] [67]

In his book, <u>The Oxygen Advantage</u> (Amazon 2015), researcher and clinician Patrick McKeown, describes multiple physiologic advantages of nasal breathing, including:
- Increased red blood cell production, improving O_2 delivery to tissues
- Increased CO_2 in the blood, releasing more O_2 into tissues
- Controls hyperventilation

- Filtering of airborne pathogens
- Unblocks nasal congestion
- Improves overall breathing and lung function, including asthma
- Improves VO2 in the lungs, improving athletic performance

Breathing is a fascinating subject. A short lesson in the basic physiology of breathing helps us understand the goals of proper breathing.

Dr. Christian Bohr (1855-1911), a Danish physician, described the *Bohr Effect* in 1903. He explained that the affinity of hemoglobin in red blood cells to bind to oxygen is inversely proportional to both the acidity of the blood and the concentration of carbon dioxide. In other words, hemoglobin is the FedEx carrier of the package (oxygen), which is picked up in the distribution center (the lungs), carried along the highway (the bloodstream), and then delivered to homes (cells), all across the country (body). When the blood pH is lowered (becomes more acidic) – because carbon dioxide arrives, combines with water, and forms carbonic acid – hemoglobin releases the oxygen package to the cells. The Bohr Effect describes an equilibrium in the bloodstream. When carbon dioxide levels are low, oxygen remains bound to hemoglobin. When carbon dioxide levels are high, oxygen is delivered to the cells. Why is this important? This is all about healthy breathing.

We inhale oxygen from the air. We exhale carbon dioxide produced in the body. When breathing slowly and deliberately through the nose, the amount of carbon dioxide exhaled is low, the pH of the blood is more acidic, and more oxygen is delivered to cells in the brain, heart, muscles, and in fact every cell throughout the body. This is the goal. This is why yoga instructors emphasize breathing slowly and deliberately through the nose. You are promised better mental clarity and health. This is true, for physiologic reasons – better oxygen delivery. This will produce calming effects, reduced stress, and relaxation.

Why is it a popular home cure for hyperventilation to breathe into a paper bag? Exhaled air contains a high concentration of carbon dioxide. When exhaled air is collected in a paper bag and re-breathed, a higher level of carbon dioxide goes into the bloodstream, lowering the blood's pH, and more oxygen is delivered to the cells, which has a calming effect. This is the Bohr Effect in action.

Let's see if we understand the principle with a simple quiz. If you were about to run a 5K race in the next 5 minutes, what would be the best way to get prepared? I'm sure that, instinctively, many of us would take very deep breaths in and out through our mouths, trying to fill our lungs with oxygen. Dr. Bohr would disagree!

In reality, the best way to prepare would be to breathe very slowly through the nose for 30 seconds or so, hold your breath for 5-10 seconds, breathe slowly again through the nose 30 seconds, hold your breath for 5-10 seconds, and repeat for 5 minutes.

Why would this be the best way to prepare for the race? The Bohr Effect. Maintaining a higher level of carbon dioxide in the bloodstream, through less exhaling volume, delivers more oxygen to the cells you will use in the race.

In The Oxygen Advantage, Patrick McKeown reports that many athletes today are training with their mouths taped shut. This is a breathing training method, developed by Russian Physiologist Dr. Konstanin Buteyko. The *Buteyko Method* has been used extensively in the treatment of asthma. When respiratory problems are present, such as allergies, asthma, nasal congestion, and poor health, there is often a conversion to mouth breathing — which is shallow, from the chest rather than from the diaphragm, and is accompanied by a characteristic forward head posture and rolled shoulders. (This can be observed as one of the physical characteristics of those with Down's Syndrome – mouth open, head and tongue forward.)

Individuals with such characteristics demonstrate overbreathing, which is a form of pathologic breathing. The ideal goals for breathing are:
- primarily through the nose
- at a controlled, calm rate
- from the diaphragm and lungs
- with the shoulders back
- **nasodiaphragmatic breathing day and night**

Proper nasal breathing at night is important. Michael Fitzpatrick, MD, and his cohort at Queen's Medical Center, Ontario studied the effects of nasal vs. mouth breathing with healthy subjects, reporting: "Upper airway resistance during sleep and the propensity to obstructive sleep apnea are significantly lower while breathing nasally rather than orally. This mechanical advantage may explain the preponderance of nasal breathing during sleep in normal subjects."[68]

What are some of the factors involved in an airway becoming compromised?

Think of the airway as a "garden hose", from the tip of the nose to the lungs. It can be compromised by any change that obstructs the passageway, including a congenitally-deviated nasal septum; trauma at birth or following, producing nasal stenosis; turbinate hypertrophy from allergies, inflammation and infection; defective nasal wall collapse on inspiration; and sinusitis. When breathing through the nose, the lymphoid tissues of the adenoids (nasopharyngeal tonsils) and tonsils (palatine and lingual), act as secondary lines of defense against bacteria and viruses. Swelling of these tissues, due to hypertrophy from increased lymphocytic activity, inflammation and infection, can compromise the normal airway.

What are some of the possible influences of a compromised airway?

Nasal breathing provides all the benefits of the body's "air filtration system". When the nasal airway (upper airway) is compromised it can disrupt ideal physiologic breathing. Upper airway constrictions will often result in the conversion of nasal breathing to mouth breathing. Dr. Christian Guilleminault, a pioneering researcher in airway, breathing, and sleep disturbances, at Stanford University, first coined the term **"Upper Airway Resistance Syndrome" (U.A.R.S.)** to describe this breathing disorder.

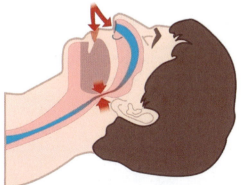

Figure[69]: Compromised airway and breathing compromises complete health. A structural and/or functional compromise can be present during both wakefulness and sleep.

Several consequences may follow chronic mouth breathing:
- In one highly referenced study, Dr. E.P. Harvold, at the University of Michigan Center for Human Growth and Development, did unique experiments with rhesus monkeys. He placed silicone nasal plugs in the experimental group, forcing conversion from nasal to mouth breathing. All of the experimental animals gradually acquired a long narrow facial appearance and dental occlusion compared to the controls.[70]
- Dr. James McNamara, also at the University of Michigan, later summarized their studies as follows: "Low tongue posture and dysfunctional swallowing patterns disrupt craniofacial-respiratory growth and development, resulting in narrow maxillary arches, longer faces, tongue thrusts and crowded malocclusions."[71] Additionally he states that "there is a relationship between upper airway obstructions and undesirable dental and craniofacial development. Significant improvements are seen when the obstructions are removed."[72]
- Furthermore, mouth breathing bypasses the nose, so that the tonsils and adenoids become the first line of defense against incoming bacteria, viruses, pollens, allergens, and pollutants. This "dirty air" can lead to inflammation, infection, and swelling of these lymphoid tissues, compromising the posterior airway in the back of the throat.
- Labored breathing symptoms related to Upper Airway Resistance Syndrome (UARS) are also associated with micro-arousals during sleep. UARS can produce classic "TMD"-like symptoms, such as chronic fatigue, non-refreshing sleep, disrupted sleep, bruxism, morning headaches, and daytime performance impairment.[73][74][75]
- Oxygen desaturations, related to Obstructive Sleep Apnea (OSA), can occur when a person's tongue and soft palate drop against the back wall of the throat. "Apnea" means the absence of breath, and it is defined as the cessation of breathing for 10 seconds or longer, an average of 5 or more times per hour, all night long, producing significant systemic repercussions. Many, if not most, sleep apneics are mouth breathers.
- Compromised airways and breathing disturbances are commonly associated with several extremely serious health

problems, which affect millions of undiagnosed (or misdiagnosed) people of all ages. For example:
- o **In children**, UARS and OSA are common, and their effects are frequently misdiagnosed as **ADHD**.[76]
- o **In young and middle aged adults**, UARS and OSA are common and frequently diagnosed coincident with **TMD**.[77]
- o **In middle aged adults**, OSA can take a toll on brain function, producing signs and symptoms of **dementia, poor concentration, difficulty with memory, decision making, depression and neurotransmitter dysregulation**.[78]
- OSA appears to activate both the systemic sympathetic/adrenomedullary and the HPA (hypothalamic-pituitary-adrenal) axis limbs of the ***STRESS* response system**. Nocturnal awakenings and micro-arousals are associated with chronic episodic cortisol release.[79]
- OSA is associated with obesity, insulin resistance/diabetes, systemic inflammation and a general compromise of overall health.[80]

Learning from History

Our understanding of the importance of airway and breathing in dentistry and medicine is rapidly *shifting*, but we have a rich history of research guiding our thinking. Let's review some invaluable lessons from the past.

Robert Ricketts, DDS, MS (1920-2003), was a prominent U.S. orthodontist and educator. He often made the statement, "respiration and mastication are inseparable." Breathing, biting, chewing, swallowing, and the nose, jaw, tongue, palate, and throat are all closely intermingled together.

What does an ideal respiratory/masticatory system look like? Let's describe it:
- The tongue is well-developed from birth, exercised by breastfeeding, not passive feeding (bottle), and the muscles of mastication are also very active from day one.
- When comfortably breathing through the nose, the mouth is typically closed.
- The tongue rests on the roof of the mouth when swallowing (approximately 1,200-2,400 times each day).

- The tongue is not functionally immobilized by a "tongue-tie", created by a short, thick lingual frenulum tethering it.
- The maxilla (upper jaw) develops broadly, due to tongue pressure upward and outward; additionally, the maxilla is not retruded, which could reduce the airway space in the throat.
- The upper teeth come in on a broad round arch, uncrowded, with enough room for the 3rd molars (wisdom teeth) to erupt and function as part of the normal dental occlusion.
- The mandible (lower arch) follows the dimensions of the upper arch and teeth and is also broad and rounded, uncrowded, and has room for the 3rd molars to fully erupt and function.
- The bite is straight, and the teeth fit together nicely.
- The cheekbones are high and well-developed by the influence of active muscles of mastication.
- The face is more square than long.
- The jaw muscles are well-developed.
- The chin is well-defined, strong, not retruded, and well-differentiated from the neck.
- The back of the throat is open when breathing and sleeping.
- The eyes are bright and appear well-rested, with no dark bags or swelling beneath them.

The above is a description of "normal". How many people do we see today who look normal? How many people have no crowded teeth with 3rd molars that are fully erupted and functioning? I'm confident the answer is less than 10%.

Now here's what's most interesting. Anthropologic studies show this is exactly what most people looked like — just a few hundred years ago. The worldwide studies of dental anthropologists have revealed significant insights. In 1939, Weston Price, DDS, wrote a book entitled <u>Nutritional and Physical Degeneration</u>, describing isolated indigenous tribes with primitive diets, who showed straight beautiful teeth, broad rounded dental arches, fully erupted and functioning 3rd molars, with some tooth wear but little decay.

More recently, Robert S. Corruccini, PhD, wrote <u>How Anthropology Informs The Orthodontic Diagnosis of Malocclusions</u> (1999), which details his studies of both museum skulls and living tribes. He reports that crooked smiles and bad teeth are a "malady of civilization", since the Industrial Revolution. In India, he discovered "village-dwelling Punjabi youth show significantly better dental occlusion and [levels of] respiratory allergy than their city-dwelling counterparts."

Allergies in the upper airway are a major source of congestion, U.A.R.S. and conversion to mouth breathing. There has been a significant rise in allergies in the modern world. For example, hunter-gathers of by-gone areas lived in small communities of 150 or less people. They were typically related and shared the same common genes. They frequently moved around with minimal interaction or contact with outsiders. They lived in an atmosphere of clean air, with no pollution, and with open spaces, lots of physical activity and sunshine. That all changed dramatically in the last several hundred years. We now live in very close quarters, under complex environmental conditions. These changes have produced many more allergens.

The other important factor highlighted by both Price and Corruccini is a significant change in **diet**. City-dwelling and the Industrial Revolution have led people to eat more **processed food**, rather than farmed and captured food sources. Processed food requires no chewing, no use of the masticatory muscles or tongue to break food down, and less stimulation of alveolar bone development. Here the old adage definitely applies – *use it or lose it!*

Disuse atrophy of the jaw system is a sign of modernization, and it shows in smaller maxillas, smaller nasal passages (superior side of the maxillary bone), smaller mandibles, smaller dental arches, more crowding of the teeth, less room for 3rd molars and the tongue in the mouth, and more airway problems in the back of the throat.

Jerome Rose, PhD, and Rick Roblee, DDS, MS, published an article in Compendium (2009) entitled "Origins of Dental Crowding and Malocclusions: An Anthropologic Perspective." Studying thousands of ancient museum skulls in the Nile Valley Region of Egypt, they identified a clear comparison between those from antiquity and today:

Hunter-Gatherers	Modern Industrial
similar skeletal bases	similar skeletal bases
massive masseter & pterygoid muscles	small masseter & pterygoid muscles
massive alveolar bone	smaller alveolar bone
straight teeth	crowded teeth
functioning 3rd molars	impacted 3rd molars

Conclusion: There is a clear connection between an industrial diet, dental crowding and malocclusion.

Let's do another comparison. This time let's compare the typical facial characteristics of a nasal breather vs. a mouth breather:

Nasal Breather	Mouth Breather
Good development of cheekbones	Poor development of cheekbones
Wider face	Narrower face
Straight teeth	Crowded teeth
Well-developed jaw(s)	Set back jaw(s)
Straight nose	Crooked nose
Alert eyes	Tired eyes
Good-sized airway	Smaller airway

Nasal vs. mouth breathing, allergies, soft diets, crowded dentitions, tongue crowding, blocked throats, enlarged tonsils, respiratory and sleep disturbances…these all tie together to expose airway and breathing as a top priority in Integrative Dental Medicine.

Dr. Tom Colquitt, illustrious Past-President of the American Academy of Restorative Dentistry (AARD), one of my personal heroes and dearest friends, said it best in his exhortation at the 2016 AARD Annual Session, *"Our new priorities, other than emergency care — the FIRST procedure performed by every dentist, for EVERY patient, of ANY AGE — should be a proper airway examination and evaluation of breathing function. The primary duty of every dentist is to promote proper nasodiaphragmatic breathing for every patient. The teeth are of secondary importance."*

Dentistry's Great Awakening!

In 2016, Dr. Suzanne Karan and Dr. Yehuda Ginosar wrote an editorial for the International Journal of Obstetric Anesthesia, entitled "Gestational Sleep Apnea: Have we been caught napping?" Borrowing from their theme of not missing the possibility of sleep apnea occurring during pregnancy, let us not get caught napping, but rather let's share in the "Great Awakening" – immersing ourselves in the strong body of evidence pointing out the central role of airway and breathing disorders in the comprehensive care of dental medicine, alongside the evaluation, diagnosis and treatment of systemic inflammation & infection and TMD & malocclusion disorders.

The "Great Awakening" is a critical piece of the Integrative Dental Medicine Model and the *shift* in our approach to empower our families, patients, and communities toward complete health.

Let's direct our attention to the Integrative Dental Medicine (IDM) Checklist to organize our discussion of Airway, Breathing & Sleep Disorders.

To do this, we will follow the IDM Checklist sequentially as follows:
1. **History:** Signs & Symptoms
2. **Evaluation:** Clinical Signs
3. **Screening & Testing**
4. **Treatment**

	Airway /Breathing Disorders			Airway /Breathing Disorders
History **Signs & Symptoms**	Mouth Breather	−	+	**Management & Resolution** ↓ **Nasal Breathing** • Buteyko Training • Mouth Taping **Oral Myofunctional Therapy** **Allergist-Allergy Testing** **E.N.T.-Airway Evaluation** **MANAGEMENT PROTOCOL** • Increase Vertical Airway • Increase Horizontal Airway • Sleep Position, Non-Supine • Weight Loss • Retest • Work with Sleep MD **RESOLUTION PROTOCOL** • Expand Oral Airway • Expand Upper Airway • Expand Posterior Airway • Release Tongue-Tie
	Snoring	−	+	
	Sleep Apnea	−	+	
	Daytime Sleepiness	−	+	
	Poor Sleep Quality	−	+	
	Nasal Congestion	−	+	
	Forward Head Posture	−	+	
	Tongue Tie	−	+	
	Chronic Cough	−	+	
	Deviated Septum	−	+	
Evaluation **Clinical signs**	Neck Circumference >16"	−	+	
	Mallampati Score >2	−	+	
	Scalloped Tongue	−	+	
	40% Tongue Restriction	−	+	
	Nasal Stenosis	−	+	
	Skeletal Profile		+	
Screening & Testing	Overnight Pulse Oximetry	−	+	
	Home Sleep Test	−	+	
	Heart Rate Variability(HRV)	−	+	
	Polysomnogram(PSG)	−	+	
Differential Conclusion	− Negative		+ Positive	

> "Airway obstruction, sleep-disordered breathing (SDB), obstructive sleep apnea (OSA), snoring, and other airway dysfunction such as mouth breathing affect us from cradle to grave. Silently and beneath the surface, the structure and function of your airway influences every aspect of your life, from birth and growth and development, to the early years and behavior and academic performance, on up to forgetfulness and fatigue in middle age, and early dementia in our elders. Open or obstructed airways affect sleep, inflammation levels, chronic disease, relationships, workplace performance and even how long we live and how we die. Given the far-reaching consequences of breathing disorders, it behooves all of us to do everything we can for our airways."
>
> Dr. Michael Gelb and Dr. Howard Hindin
> <u>GASP: Airway Health — The Hidden Path to Wellness</u>

11. Airway, Breathing & Sleep – History: Signs and Symptoms

Airway/Breathing/Sleep: History: *Signs & Symptoms*
1. Mouth Breather

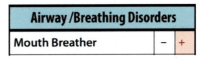

"The nose is for breathing, and the mouth is for eating."

Studying the research literature, plus good old common sense, supports this adage and shows us the important relationship between healthy breathing and a healthy body. There are two options for how air enters the body, through the nose or through the mouth. When entering through the nose, air is humidified and warmed as it swirls through the scroll-like turbinates. It passes over respiratory mucous membranes, which contain innumerable tiny hair-like cells to collect impurities, and is then sterilized by the powerful antimicrobial effects of nitric oxide, produced in the paranasal sinuses. This is very important for long-term health, as the air we breathe initially arrives in a very "dirty" state due to the outside environment.

To illustrate this, think of an air conditioning filter in the ceiling of a home. Living in Florida, our A/C runs almost every day of the year. It's recommended to change out the filter every month. Sometimes, I forget. When the filter remains for 45-60 days, it's disgusting, full of dirt and completely clogged. That's inside the house. Imagine what's in the air we breathe outside – bacteria, fungi, viruses, spores, pollutants, allergens, concrete dust, pollen…you get the picture. The nose is beautifully designed to collect, isolate, and destroy these invaders.

Nitric oxide is one of the great wonders of the human body. In fact, in 1998, three American pharmacologists, Dr. Robert Furchgott, Dr. Louis Ignarro, and Dr. Ferid Murad, were awarded the Nobel Prize in Science for their discoveries of how the body produces nitric oxide in the para-nasal sinuses, mediating the dilation of blood vessels throughout the body (healthy heart), helping to regulate blood pressure (healthy heart), battling infections (reducing infection and inflammation), preventing the formation of blood clots (healthy vascular system) and acting as a signal molecule in the nervous system.

When someone has chest pain (angina), they are typically prescribed a nitroglycerin tablet sublingually. How does it work? Nitric oxide is produced and the smooth muscles around the constricted heart vessels relax, providing relief.

Why are kale, swiss chard and arugula so popular for preventing and reversing heart disease? They are all very high on the nitric oxide index. Nitric oxide plays a powerful protective role against invading pathogens, but only when a person is breathing through his or her nose, where it is released.

Humans normally convert to mouth breathing when under high exertion, such as high intensity exercise. Under ideal circumstances, this should only be a temporary accommodation. Interestingly, we often associate mouth breathing with compromised health, and (most of the time) that is an accurate observation. Think of people suffering from colds, the flu, asthma, emphysema, or chronic illness, or consider the elderly and the handicapped. Mouth breathing is a sure sign of a struggle with proper breathing.

Mouth breathing has broad implications for abnormal craniofacial growth and development, dental malocclusions and compromised oral and systemic health. When mouth breathing, the tongue remains low in the mouth, failing to fill the palatal vault, which changes the normal "neutral zone" forces of the tongue outwardly against the maxillary bone and teeth (opposing the pressures of the cheeks and lips inwardly). Therefore, the maxillary vault will develop narrow and high, and the narrowed dental arch may be "V" or "Omega" shaped. If a forward tongue thrust is present, the anterior teeth will become separated, creating an anterior open bite. A cross-bite of the upper and lower teeth may be also present.

Some of the potential signs of mouth breathing include:
- Nasal congestion ("blocked" nose)
- Allergies (airborne, food)
- Poor asthma control
- Noisy, visible breathing
- Snoring
- Frequent night waking
- Frequent night trips to the bathroom – due to poor breathing related microarousals
- Dry mouth and/or dry, cracked lips
- Periodontal compromise – due to the loss of salivary pH buffering
- Dental decay
- Bad breath
- Night sweating
- Daytime fatigue
- Behavioral issues – in children
- Memory issues – in children and adults
- Forward head posture, shoulder roll
- Dental malocclusion

It is important to remember that mouth breathing problems often begin very early in life, and they can last a lifetime if not addressed.

Roger Price, BS, PharmD, an internationally-recognized pharmacologist, functional physiologist, and a brilliant personal mentor and friend, illustrates a common mouth breathing scenario in a child as follows: "Dairy causes an allergic response which makes the child mouth breathe. It is then the mouth breathing that causes:
- lack of filtration and cleansing of the air, allowing airborne bacteria to settle and flourish
- increase in volume of dirty air over the lymphoid tissue
- increase in inflammation and congestion as a result of over breathing
- lack of release of nitric oxide from the para-nasal sinuses preventing bacterial control and vasodilation
- diminution of diaphragmatic breathing leading to reduced lymph flow to the tonsils and adenoids to remove the toxins

Restoring nasal breathing is a MUST after eliminating the allergic triggers. Shut the mouth and get the diaphragm working again, and nature protects the system."[81]

In Summary:
- Breathing dysfunction can significantly affect both dental and complete health.
- Airway and breathing dysfunction can lead to cranio-facial-respiratory growth and development changes that are reflected in dental malocclusions.
- Mouth breathing is an issue that can negatively affect the body's health all day, every day.
- Breathing dirty air into the respiratory system is linked with swollen tonsils, nasal congestion, labored chest breathing, asthma, asthma-like symptoms, and sleep-related complications.
- Breathing dysfunction is both a daytime and nighttime concern.
- Therefore, it is important to always inquire about mouth breathing on the health history and during the initial patient interview.

Airway/Breathing/Sleep: History: *Signs & Symptoms*
Intro to Signs/Symptoms Related to Sleep

* **Snoring**
* **Sleep Apnea**
* **Daytime Sleepiness**
* **Poor Sleep Quality**

Airway/Breathing Disorders		
Mouth Breather	−	+
Snoring	−	+
Sleep Apnea	−	+
Daytime Sleepiness	−	+
Poor Sleep Quality	−	+

Sleep is a most fascinating and complex subject. Sleep represents about 36% of a person's life units of time. Compare the time we sleep with other major activities[82]:

Activity	Percentage
Sleep	36%
"Other activities"	19%
Work related	16%
Watching TV	11%
Housework	8%
Eating & drinking	5%
Socializing/communicating	3%
Sports, exercise, recreation	1%
Telephone calls, e-mail	1%

The Anatomy of Sleep consists of cycles of four basic types and stages: Stage 1 (light), Stage 2 (light/deeper), Stag 3 (deep) and REM (rapid eye movement). Stage 1-3 are considered NREM (non-REM) sleep, which represents about 75% of the night. Generally, each cycle during sleep (Stage 1 → 2 → 3 → REM → 1 and repeat) lasts about 90 minutes, with an average of 5 cycles per night, totaling an average of 7.5 sleep hours.

- **Stage 1:** begins the sleep cycle and is very light sleep; in this stage, you can be easily awakened.
- **Stage 2:** sleep is deeper; you are disengaged from the surroundings; body temperature drops; breathing and heart rate are regular.
- **Stage 3:** the deepest and most restorative sleep; blood pressure drops; breathing becomes slower; muscles are relaxed; blood supply to the muscles increases; tissue growth and repair occur; energy is restored; and hormones are released (such as growth hormone for development, including the development of muscles).
- **REM:** first occurs about 90 minutes after falling asleep, in short episodes, recurring about every 90 minutes, with episodes becoming longer later in the 7.5 hours. In this stage, the body muscles are essentially immobile and relaxed (except for eye movements); energy is provided to the brain and body; the brain is active and dreams occur; REM supports daytime performance.

> *"It is a common experience that a problem difficult at night is resolved in the morning after the committee of sleep has worked on it."*
> **– John Steinbeck**

Sleep helps us thrive by contributing to a healthy immune system. It can also balance our appetites by helping to regulate levels of the hormones ghrelin and leptin, which play a role in our feelings of hunger and fullness. When we're sleep deprived, we may feel the need to eat more, which can lead to weight gain.

REM is most active during the last 25% of sleep, which is early morning. Respiratory events in patients with Obstructive Sleep Apnea (OSA) are often more frequent and longer during REM sleep, with more profound oxygen desaturation than in any other sleep stage. OSA patients are more resistant to "fight or flight" arousals during REM sleep. The most dangerous time for those with OSA is the last 25% of their sleep. Many OSA patients have been prescribed CPAP at night. Frequently, these will be worn at bedtime and removed around 12:00 a.m., after getting up for the bathroom. The hours from 12:00-6:00 a.m. are when it is most important to wear the CPAP, due to REM sleep. Frequently, respiration-related heart attacks occur in bed between those hours. Now we know why someone can suffer a heart attack during a time that seems the least likely – while asleep at night.

> "…I had just read an article on the similarity of the timing of heart attacks and the most concentrated time for rapid eye movement (REM) sleep (the dreaming stage). Another scientific paper found that people with OSA [obstructive sleep apnea] are more likely to have heart attacks in the early morning hours (midnight to 6 A.M.), whereas people without OSA are more likely to suffer a heart attack after waking from 6 A.M. to 12 noon.
>
> I was reminded of my days during surgical internship, when an alarming number of otherwise healthy people undergoing routine operations had heart attacks during my early morning shifts. We know that for certain people predisposed to sleep-breathing disorders, sleep position can play a major role in the quality of sleep. What I realized was that there are some people who prefer to sleep only on their sides or their stomach. Some absolutely cannot sleep on their backs and must sleep in the latter positions in order to breathe properly. I concluded that what was happening in these situations was that being forced to sleep on their backs for the first time in decades after surgery or another medical procedure resulted in an inability to breathe properly. This, in turn, placed stress on the heart, increasing their risk of heart attack.
>
> The critical issue here is that it's during REM sleep that the muscles of the throat are most relaxed. If susceptible people are forced to sleep on their backs, they can no longer adjust in a hospital situation by changing their sleeping position. They are simply forced to sleep on their backs as best they can. This realization led to yet another sleepless night for me. The implications were enormous."
>
> Steven Y. Park, MD
> <u>Sleep, Interrupted: A Physician Reveals the #1 Reason Why So Many Of Us are Sick and Tired</u>

Circadian Rhythm and Sleep

"Circadian" comes from two Latin words: "circa" ("around") and "diem" ("day"); it refers to the 24-hour cycle of the body each day. It's our body clock telling us when to be awake (64% of the day) and when to it's time to sleep (36% of the day).

This is controlled by a magnificent system that relates directly to light. In the brain, behind the eyes, right above where the optic nerves crisscross, is a small nerve center called the suprachiasmatic nucleus. It's the body's internal clock. When morning light enters the eyes and travels through the pathways of the optic nerves, the suprachiasmatic nucleus stimulates hormonal changes and increases body temperature, because it's time to get moving. Many hours later, in the evening, the programmed clock stimulates the release of melatonin, the sleepiness hormone, and lowers the body temperature in preparation for going to sleep.

We can see how this worked perfectly for those living during early settler times of <u>Little House on the Prairie</u> – up with the sunrise and down soon after sunset. It works today as well, if we stay in sync with the Circadian Rhythm.

Sleep disorders are very common today for many reasons. The dramatic lifestyle changes that have occurred with the advent of electricity, TV, computers, hand held devices, and video games, have created **Circadian Rhythm Chaos (CRC)**, which carries significant consequences to complete health for both children and adults. This is a major health crisis in and of itself.

As *gatekeepers of systemic inflammation and gatekeepers of complete health,* we fight the battle of CRC, through educating and discussing sleep disorders with our patients.

Airway/Breathing/Sleep:
History: *Signs & Symptoms*
2. Snoring

"Laugh, and the whole world loves you; snore, and you sleep alone!"

Airway /Breathing Disorders		
Mouth Breather	–	+
Snoring	–	+

Snoring is thought of as a social disease, and indeed it is. It is estimated that 30-40% of couples sleep in separate bedrooms due to snoring… and it's not just men who snore. The Wisconsin Sleep Cohort Study found that **44%** of all men surveyed and **28%** of all women surveyed were habitual snorers, a total of almost 90 million

Americans. It is estimated that **10%** of children snore. Through surveys, it is estimated that the bed partner of a snorer loses almost one hour of sleep every night.

The American Academy of Otolaryngology – Head and Neck Surgery lists four major reasons people snore,[83] to which we will add comments:

- **"Poor muscle tone in the tongue and throat"**: This may reflect a mouth breather whose tongue is not properly sealed against the roof of the mouth. The jaw drops open at night. This can also relate to severe fatigue or sedatives such as alcohol depressing respiration, or supine sleep position (on the back).
- **"Excessive bulkiness of throat tissue"**: This may reflect mouth breathing; unfiltered air inflaming tonsilar tissue; retrusion (under-development) of the maxilla (upper jaw) which can cause the soft palate to constrict the throat and airway; inflammation from smoking and gastric reflux; or being overweight, reflected in greater soft tissue mass – similar to weight gain and an increased waistline.
- **"Long soft palate and/or uvula"**: This may reflect maxillary retrusion, which is an underdeveloped upper jaw.
- **"Obstructed nasal airways"**: This may reflect allergies; turbinate congestion; polyps; deviated septum; nasal growths and/or obstructions; or enlarged adenoids.

Reggie White (1961-2004), the highly respected National Football League Hall of Fame player, died at the age of 43 in his sleep from a heart attack associated with sleep apnea. His wife, Sara, who now speaks nationally to educate the public through the Reggie White Sleep Disorders Foundation, tells the all too common story: "I noticed that he snored, but it was something I accepted. I would just elbow him; so many wives know about the elbow!" What a sad and unnecessary tragedy for an American hero and his family.

Lessons from Snoring:
- Snoring is much more than a social disease.
- Snoring is an alarm, telling you something is wrong with your breathing.
- Snoring, in combination with mouth breathing during sleep, can increase systemic risks.

- Snoring is considered a sign of the presence of a circadian rhythm disorder.
- Snoring is a risk indicator for Sleep Apnea.

Chronic snoring is not an innocent occurrence. It most likely reflects a structural or functional problem in the airway. It is a sign of breathing pathology that should be evaluated.

Airway/Breathing/Sleep: History: *Signs & Symptoms*
3. Sleep Apnea

Airway/Breathing Disorders		
Mouth Breather	–	+
Snoring	–	+
Sleep Apnea	–	+

The Neurology of Sleep

During sleep, body functions are regulated by the involuntary nervous system, also known as the **Autonomic Nervous System (ANS)**, controlling unconscious activities and actions. The ANS has two main divisions: the **Sympathetic (SNS)** and the **Parasympathetic (PNS)**. The Parasympathetic is the primary division active during normal sleep. The **vagus nerve,** which is known as **Cranial Nerve X (10)** from the Central Nervous System (CNS), controls the PNS, influencing smooth muscles of the GI tract. Known as the "**Rest & Digest**" system, vagus nerve stimulation also influences important healthful organ activities during sleep, including those of the heart, bronchi, stomach, liver, pancreas, adrenal gland, small & large intestine, kidney, bladder, rectum and genitals.

During sleep, if oxygen levels drop in the bloodstream beyond a normal range, there is a stimulation from the CNS to quickly activate the emergency response system, the Sympathetic Nervous System (SNS). This is known as the **"Fight or Flight"** or "Quick Response Mobilization" System. The SNS sends out impulses to the adrenal gland which releases the three major stress hormones, **cortisol**, **adrenaline** and **norepinephrine**, into the bloodstream. These elevate the heart rate and blood pressure, increasing blood flow to improve diminished oxygen delivery throughout the body. This can also stimulate an **"arousal"** from one sleep stage to a lighter stage or even consciously waking up.

Acute fight or flight responses are very important whenever danger is perceived. **The problem with chronically disordered breathing is that it can lead to chronic stimulation of the fight or flight response, chronically high levels of stress hormones released into the bloodstream, chronic arousals, chronically** disordered sleep, and chronically distressed health… in many ways.

Let's follow the cascade that can begin with disordered breathing, leading to breathing disordered sleep, and then to distressed health:

- **Reduced Oxygen** levels due to disordered breathing (UARS, OSA, CSA, mouth breathing)
- **O_2 Saturation decreased** in the blood and decreased O_2 supply to the organs and cells
- **"Fight or Flight"** response of the Sympathetic Nervous System
- **Cortisol** release into the bloodstream
- **Heart Rate** increase
- **Blood Pressure** increase
- **Stress Hormone levels chronically elevated**
- **Cortisol affects insulin regulation** in the bloodstream
- Increased risk for developing insulin-resistant **Type 2 Diabetes**
- Cortisol influences dysregulation of the metabolic hormones Ghrelin (which affects satiety) and Leptin (which affects hunger), increasing the risk of **Obesity**
- **Gastric Reflux** risk increases due to airway obstruction/Sleep Apnea
- **Daytime Fatigue**
- **Poor Mental Sharpness** (Brain Fog)
- **Anxiety & Depression** due to poor sleep quality
- **Fibromyalgia** found in 45% of sleep apneics, associated with ANS dysregulation and an associated increase in body-wide inflammation
- **Chronic Fatigue Syndrome**
- **Restless Leg Syndrome** (Willis-Ekbom Disease)
- **Reduced Libido** due to Sympathetic hyperactivity, Parasympathetic hypoactivity
- Increased risk for **motor vehicle accidents** due to sleepiness
- **Dental wear due to Bruxism/Clenching** related to SNS hyperactivity and associated stress
- **Headaches** due to O_2 desaturation, SNS hyperactivity
- **Congestive Heart Failure and Heart Attack** increased risk
- **Stroke** risk
- **Organ Failure** risk
- **Death** risk

3 Types of Sleep Apnea

The results of sleep apnea are oxygen deprivation and the cascade of consequences just reviewed. The etiology is not as simple. Sleep Apnea has 3 primary etiologies:

> - **Obstructive Sleep Apnea (OSA):** caused by a blockage in back of the throat due to enlarged tissues filling the airway (often associated with being overweight) and/or the tongue and jaw dropping back during sleep, especially due to mouth breathing and sleeping on the back (supine)
> - **Central Sleep Apnea (CSA):** caused by a failure of the respiratory drive center in the brain, the medulla. This results in a lack of respiratory effort and disrupted breathing. Rather than an inability to pass air through a blocked airway found in OSA, CSA is due to the brain not directing the muscles to breathe. In CSA there is no effort to breathe. **CSA is often associated with severe illness**, such as congestive heart failure, and diseases of infection, tumors, neurologic disorders, strokes, cervical spine damage, increased narcotic use, severe obesity, and lower brain stem problems.
> - **Mixed Sleep Apnea (MSA)** is a combination of OSA and CSA, present in the same individual.

Untreated Obstructive Sleep Apnea is estimated to carry the following risks:
- 5.5X greater risk for **HYPERTENSION**
- 4X greater risk of **STROKE**
- 2.5X greater risk of developing **DIABETES**
- 2.5X greater risk of developing **CANCER**
- 1.3X greater risk of **HEART ATTACK**

The way to simplify the explanation of what happens with breathing disordered sleep is as follows:
- **When we sleep, oxygen levels should remain very high in our bloodstream.**
- **If breathing is labored or ceases periodically during sleep, the oxygen levels in the bloodstream can drop.**
- **A significant drop in oxygen levels can turn on the "Fight or Flight" alarm in the body, which causes stress hormones to be released into the bloodstream.**
- **This causes the heart rate to increase.**

- If this happens frequently during sleep, it creates stress and increases systemic inflammation in the whole body, which is the number one factor for atherosclerosis and accelerated aging.

Disordered breathing is a major health concern, that is both a daytime and nighttime problem.

Peter Litchfield, PhD, Director of the Behavioral Physiology Institute in Santa Fe, New Mexico, has shared the following:
- 10-25% of the U.S. population demonstrate dysfunctional breathing.
- 90% of pain problems demonstrate dysfunctional breathing.
- 60% of ambulance runs in New York City are associated with dysfunctional breathing.
- Over-breathing (reduced carbon dioxide in the blood) can reduce brain oxygen by 40% in a matter of several minutes (Bohr Effect).

Sleep Apnea is the most serious commonly undiagnosed medical concern that can be easily screened in every dental office.

Sleep Apnea Diagnosis

Strong indicators of Sleep Apnea can be noticed by a bed partner or observer. **Snoring** is most often present, but not always. During sleep, sleep apneics **stop breathing** for intervals of 10 seconds, and sometimes much longer. Sleep apneics have been observed ceasing to breathe for as long as 2 minutes! During sleep, sleep apneics will often **struggle to breathe, gasp, grimace, grind their teeth, try to swallow,** or show **sudden body movements**. Any of these observations are good reasons to pursue a professional evaluation.

Screening:
* **Written screening tools** can help evaluate the degree of apparent severity of the breathing related sleep disorder. Several are found online including:
* **Epworth Sleepiness Scale** (good for all ages)
* **STOP-BANG** (best for middle-aged adults)
* **Apps** – Various downloaded apps can be used on smartphones for overnight self-assessments, including snoring and risk for sleep apnea.

* **Professional screening** – overnight data can be gathered at home, using:
  - **High Resolution Pulse Oximetry (HRPO)**
  - **Heart Rate Variability (HRV)**

Testing:
Testing will measure the specifics of sleep activity such as: heart rate, Apnea-Hypopnea Index (AHI), oxygen saturation, sleep position, and respiratory effort.
* **Professional testing:** overnight data is gathered using:
  - **Home Sleep Testing (HST)** through the dental or medical office
  - **Polysomnogram (PSG)** in a sleep laboratory

We will discuss the details of these different professional screening and testing tools in the next section.

Lessons to Remember:
* **Sleep disturbances, such as Upper Airway Resistance syndrome (UARS) and sleep apnea (OSA, CSA, MSA), stimulate a parasympathetic/sympathetic dysregulation that is very stressful to the body.**
* **Sleep apnea can be a source of chronic inflammation that can break down the body.**
* **Sleep apnea is a very common, life-threatening disorder. It affects nearly 25% of adults between the ages 30 & 70, and 2-4% of children…yet <u>less than 15% have been screened</u>!**
* **Sleep Apnea is found in every age and size person.**

Airway/Breathing/Sleep:
History: *Signs & Symptoms*
<u>4. Daytime Sleepiness and/or Poor Sleep Quality</u>

Airway /Breathing Disorders		
Mouth Breather	−	+
Snoring	−	+
Sleep Apnea	−	+
Daytime Sleepiness	−	+
Poor Sleep Quality	−	+

As we have seen, sleep is a most fascinating and complex subject. It is clear that daytime sleepiness and poor sleep quality can often be related to disordered breathing disturbances from airway issues.

Common observations regarding breathing-related sleep disturbances are the following:

—**Children**: snoring, gasping, restless sleep, kicking off the covers at night, head at the foot at the bed in the morning, bedwetting, tired in the morning, ADHD-like symptoms

—**Young Adults**: sore muscles, sore joints, A.M. headaches, TMD, chronically tired

—**Middle Age Adults**: frequent bathroom trips at night, sudden awakening, foggy thinking

—**Excessive Sleepiness (ES):** ES may result from neuronal injury caused by OSA. This injury of chronic oxygen deprivation (hypoxia), and the sleep fragmentation from multiple arousals, may impact the wakefulness part of the brain. In essence, studies report OSA-induced brain damage.[84][85]

There are multiple systemic and psychological reasons for poor sleep. Daytime sleepiness and poor sleep quality may have several possible etiologies:

The 3 Major Categories of Sleep Disturbances:

1. Disturbed Sleep, caused by:
* UARS
* Sleep Apnea
* REM Sleep Behavior Disorder
* Restless Leg Syndrome (Willis-Ekbom Disease)
* Periodic Limb Movement Disorder

2. Lack of Sleep, caused by:
* Insomnia

3. Excessive Sleep, caused by:
* Narcolepsy
* Cataplexy
* Sleep Paralysis
* Hypnagogic hallucinations

When discussing daytime sleepiness or poor sleep quality, remember that there are several possible explanations. The **Epworth Sleepiness Scale** (ESS) is a screening tool used widely in medicine to evaluate the degree of sleepiness during the day. This tool is helpful because many people deny daytime sleepiness due to being accustomed to it. The ESS asks questions related to sleepiness when in quiet situations, including: sitting and reading, watching TV, sitting in a movie theater or a meeting, as a passenger in a car for an hour without a break, in a car while stopped for a few minutes, lying down to rest in the afternoon, sitting and talking to someone and/or sitting quietly after lunch. If you're dozing off while reading this list, you may be sleep deprived!

Airway/Breathing/Sleep: History: *Signs & Symptoms*
5. Nasal Congestion

Airway /Breathing Disorders		
Mouth Breather	−	+
Snoring	−	+
Sleep Apnea	−	+
Daytime Sleepiness	−	+
Poor Sleep Quality	−	+
Nasal Congestion	−	+

Nasal congestion can have multiple etiologies including:
- Nasal Stenosis
- Sinus Infections
- Allergies – both food and environmental
- Septum Deviation
- Nasal Polyps
- Turbinate Enlargement
- Eustachian Tube Blockage

Integrative Dental Medicine practices will identify many patients with significant undiagnosed and untreated allergy-related and nasal/airway-related problems. Pediatric and adult otolaryngologists should be key members of the IDM team.

> "Itching, sneezing, and coughing during the night in allergic children may be relieved by clenching and grinding. In one study, investigators reported that the incidence of bruxing in allergic children is 60% whereas the incidence in nonallergic children is 20%. Marks postulated that allergic edema of the mucosa in the auditory tubes may lead to nocturnal bruxism. The mucosal swelling closes the auditory tube orifice at torus tubarius, which reduces the pressure in the middle ear by absorption of the trapped gases into the water of the vascular bed of the cavity lining. The dilator tubae and tensor veli palatini are attached to the fibrous anterior wall of the auditory tube. When they contract, their tension pulls the tube open. During sleep, these muscles scarcely function, but with decreased pressure stimulus in the middle ear, the patient bruxes to secrete saliva and swallows to open the auditory tube when the tensor veli palatini and dilator tubae contract. In these patients, bruxism has been eliminated or reduced significantly with appropriate treatment of allergies."
>
> Parker E. Mahan, DDS, PhD, and Charles C. Alling, III, DDS, MS
> <u>Facial Pain, 3rd Edition</u>

Airway/Breathing/Sleep:
History: *Signs & Symptoms*
6. Forward Head Posture

Airway/Breathing Disorders		
Mouth Breather	−	+
Snoring	−	+
Sleep Apnea	−	+
Daytime Sleepiness	−	+
Poor Sleep Quality	−	+
Nasal Congestion	−	+
Forward Head Posture	−	+

Forward head posture is closely associated with **Mouth Breathing Syndrome.** A Brazilian cohort reports that *"in the presence of a significant nasal obstruction, an effort occurs to overcome this resistance by increasing the work of accessory muscles of inspiration. Moreover, the forward head posture, common among mouth breathers, facilitates the air to enter the mouth which could lead to a deterioration of the pulmonary function. In the long run, the hyperactivity of the neck muscles may be associated with cervical changes that, as a result, can cause temporomandibular disorders (TMD) and spine cervical disorders."*[86]

In my clinical experience, it is very common for patients presenting with temporomandibular disorders (TMD) to report cervical neck issues. Many of these patients have histories involving whiplash-type injuries due to motor vehicle accidents, blows to the head, and falls. Many have internal derangements in the temporomandibular joints. They will report forward head posturing in an effort to gain some relief from pain. Other symptomatic patients are unaware of any history of trauma.

In these cases, questions should be asked about allergies, breathing and sleep concerns such as snoring, mouth breathing, and shallow breathing from the chest. It is common to receive affirmative feedback regarding these issues.

Airway/Breathing/Sleep:
History: *Signs & Symptoms*
7. Tongue Tie

Airway/Breathing Disorders		
Mouth Breather	-	+
Snoring	-	+
Sleep Apnea	-	+
Daytime Sleepiness	-	+
Poor Sleep Quality	-	+
Nasal Congestion	-	+
Forward Head Posture	-	+
Tongue Tie	-	+

Dr. Christian Guilleminault reports from his 2016 study at Stanford Sleep Center: *"A short lingual frenulum has been associated with difficulties in sucking, swallowing and speech. The oral dysfunction induced by a short lingual frenulum can lead to oral-facial dysmorphosis, which decreases the size of upper airway support. Such progressive change increases the risk of upper airway collapsibility during sleep."* [87]

A narrow palate, due to failure of the tongue to fill the maxillary vault, leads to a narrow nasal passage on the superior side of the maxilla, resulting in difficulty breathing through the nose at night. Dr. Guilleminault reports:

> When considering results of several of our investigations performed in children a pattern emerges: a dysfunction early in life involving abnormal nasal breathing, sucking and masticating leads to progressive dysmorphoses favoring increased collapsibility of the upper airway during sleep, which worsens with aging and leads to the development of SDB (sleep disordered breathing) over time up to adulthood.[88]

It is important to understand that tongue-tie in newborns can affect their breathing for a lifetime and increase their risk for UARS and OSA.

Additionally, Drs. Guilleminault and Huang report from their 2015 study:

We systematically investigated the presence of a short frenulum in children born full-term and referred for suspicion of OSA and performed a retrospective investigation of all pediatric cases seen during an 18-month period. Out of 150 successively seen children diagnosed with OSA, 42% had a short frenulum. The presence of the short frenulum was associated with abnormal development of the oral cavity including the presence of a high and narrow palatal vault...[89]

There is a strong correlation between a shortened lingual frenulum and tongue-tie, affecting both child and adult cranio-facial-respiratory development and breathing related sleep disorders.

This is a growing topic of great interest in Integrative Dental Medicine. **The International Affiliation of Tongue-tie Professionals (IATP)** is an organization focused on training medical doctors, dentists, chiropractors, osteopaths, IBCLCs (International Board Certified Lactation Consultants), speech-language pathologists, myofunctional therapists and other health professionals interested in this field of study.

Airway/Breathing/Sleep:
History: *Signs & Symptoms*
8. Chronic Cough

Airway/Breathing Disorders		
Mouth Breather	−	+
Snoring	−	+
Sleep Apnea	−	+
Daytime Sleepiness	−	+
Poor Sleep Quality	−	+
Nasal Congestion	−	+
Forward Head Posture	−	+
Tongue Tie	−	+
Chronic Cough	−	+

Chronic cough is included on the IDM Checklist under "Airway/Breathing Disorders" because of the common relationship between breathing disorders and **Gastric Reflux**. We discussed the signs and symptoms of Gastric Reflux under Inflammation & Infection.

There is a very significant second-most common cause for a chronic cough to keep in mind as an oral physician: **HPV (Human Papilloma Virus).** HPV is sexually transmitted. In the past, oropharyngeal cancers were mostly linked to smoking or alcohol abuse. Today, oropharyngeal cancers related to smoking and alcohol are on the decline while those caused by HPV are rising dramatically. Some experts predict that HPV-caused mouth and throat cancers will become more common than cervical cancer by 2020. There is currently a HPV vaccine available.

In a recent conversation with a local pathologist, I was told that there has been a significant upswing in middle aged men, with chief complaints of chronic sore throats, who are being diagnosed with HPV. Whenever a chronic sore throat is present, HPV testing is recommended. It is now possible to perform salivary testing for HPV in a dental office.

Airway/Breathing/Sleep:
History: *Signs & Symptoms*
9. Deviated Septum

Airway /Breathing Disorders		
Mouth Breather	–	+
Snoring	–	+
Sleep Apnea	–	+
Daytime Sleepiness	–	+
Poor Sleep Quality	–	+
Nasal Congestion	–	+
Forward Head Posture	–	+
Tongue Tie	–	+
Chronic Cough	–	+
Deviated Septum	–	+

The nasal septum is the separating partition between the two nostrils that is made up of both bone and cartilage. It can be deformed from birth with a curve to one side, or it can be damaged through injury and scarring.

The deviation can alter airflow through the nostril, affecting breathing through the nose. A deviated septum can be visually seen upon examination.

Once a thorough written and verbal **History:** *Signs & Symptoms* is completed, proceed to **Evaluation:** *Clinical Signs* and then to **Screening & Testing.**

"The philosophy of effortless breathing is echoed by authentic teachers of Indian yoga and traditional Chinese medicine. I use the word *authentic* in order to differentiate practitioners who have a deep knowledge of breathing and how it affects physiology from those who don't. Unlike many modern Western teachers of yoga, who instruct students to breathe hard in order to remove toxins from the body, authentic teachers know that when it comes to breathing, less is more. The traditional Chinese philosophy…succinctly describes ideal breathing as 'so smooth that the fine hairs within the nostrils remain motionless.' True health…occurs when breathing is quiet, effortless, soft, through the nose, abdominal, rhythmic, and gently paused on the exhale. This is how human beings naturally breathed until modern life changed everything."

Patrick McKeown
<u>The Oxygen Advantage</u>

12. AIRWAY/BREATHING/SLEEP – EVALUATION/SCREENING & TESTING

Now that a thorough History of Signs and Symptoms related to airway, breathing, and sleep has been obtained, the next appropriate step is to begin evaluating for Clinical Signs.

Airway/Breathing/Sleep:
Evaluation: *Clinical Signs*
1. Neck Circumference that is > 16" for Women or > 17" for Men

| Neck Circumference >16" | – | + |

It has been demonstrated through several studies that enlarged necks are associated with increased soft tissue volume in the throat area.[90] Neck size can be associated with being overweight, the same as with waist size. Enlarged neck size is to Upper Airway Resistance Syndrome (UARS) and possibly Obstructive Sleep Apnea (OSA) as waist size is to metabolic syndrome and possibly diabetes.

Measuring a neck size that exceeds 16" for women and 17" for men correlates with a very high probability of the presence of an airway and breathing obstruction.

**Airway/Breathing/Sleep:
Evaluation:** *Clinical Signs*
2. Mallampati Score >2

Neck Circumference >16"	–	+
Mallampati Score >2	–	+

The Mallampati Score[91] involves a visual assessment of the distance from the tongue base to the roof of the mouth – and, therefore, the amount of space for an adequate airway. The score is assessed by asking the patient, in a sitting posture, to open the mouth and protrude the tongue as much as possible, rating in 4 classes.

- Class 1: Soft palate, uvula, fauces, pillars fully visible.
- Class 2: Soft palate, uvula, fauces visible.
- Class 3: Soft palate, base of uvula visible.
- Class 4: Only hard palate visible.

A higher Mallampati score is a predictor for risk of OSA and can be a helpful screening tool during the clinical examination. However, its role in predicting the severity of OSA remains doubtful and needs further study.[92]

It is very common to identify patients with a Mallampati 3 or 4 who have significant airway challenges. There are occasions when patients present with a high Mallampati Score in the absence of airway obstruction. It should also be noted that some individuals with a Mallampati 1 or 2 may have airway compromise for other reasons.

**Airway/Breathing/Sleep:
Evaluation:** *Clinical Signs*
3. Scalloped Tongue

Neck Circumference >16"	–	+
Mallampati Score >2	–	+
Scalloped Tongue	–	+

When the size of the dental arches are narrower than the space required for the tongue, the tongue will overlap the lower teeth and indentations into the sides of the tongue will be made by the upper back teeth when the mouth is closed. This creates a "scalloped" appearance to the borders of the tongue on visual inspection.

The analogy is to consider that the dental arches are like a garage, and that the tongue is like a car parked in the garage. If the dental arch (garage) is built for a Mini-Cooper, but the tongue (car) is a Mini-Van, there will not be enough room to park it. The tongue (car), in fact, may have to back out of the garage into the alley, which is the throat and airway. Now the alley's blocked!

The presence of tongue scalloping has shown a high correlation for abnormal AHI (Apnea-Hypopnea Index) and nocturnal oxygen desaturation. The presence and severity of tongue scalloping has also shown a positive correlation with increasing Mallampati. In high-risk patients, tongue scalloping has been found to be predictive of sleep pathology. A Southern Illinois University study reports that

> [the] presence of tongue scalloping was 71% specific for abnormal sleep efficiency (<85%), 70% specific for abnormal AHI (>5), and 86% specific for nocturnal desaturation >4% below baseline. Presence of tongue scalloping also showed PPV of 67% for abnormal AHI, 89% for apnea or hypopnea, and 89% for nocturnal desaturation. Presence and severity of tongue scalloping showed positive correlation with increasing Mallampati and modified Mallampati airway classification. Conclusion: In high-risk patients we found tongue scalloping to be predictive of sleep pathology. Tongue scalloping was also associated with pathologic polysomnography data and abnormal Mallampati grades. We feel the finding of tongue scalloping is a useful clinical indicator of sleep pathology and that its presence should prompt the physician to inquire about snoring history.[93]

Tongue scalloping is a useful clinical indicator that should lead to further evaluation and/or discussion with the patient about the possibility of sleep pathology.

Airway/Breathing/Sleep:
Evaluation: *Clinical Signs*
4. 40% Tongue Restriction (Tongue-tie/Ankyloglossia)

A normal range of free tongue movement is greater than 16 mm.[94] Ankyloglossia can be classified into 4 classes based on Kotlow's assessment, as follows:

	-	+
Neck Circumference >16"		
Mallampati Score >2		
Scalloped Tongue		
40% Tongue Restriction		

    Class I: Mild ankyloglossia: 12 to 16 mm,
    Class II: Moderate ankyloglossia: 8 to 11 mm,
    Class III: Severe ankyloglossia: 3 to 7 mm,
    Class IV: Complete ankyloglossia: Less than 3 mm.

Class III and IV tongue-tie category should be given special consideration because they severely restrict the tongue's movement. Restrictions include limitations of movement protrusively, laterally

and vertically.⁹⁵ One screening evaluation to examine for possible tongue-tie involves:
1. Have the patient open his/her mouth as wide as possible. Normal maximum opening is 40-50 mm.
2. While maximally open, raise the tip of the tongue, attempting to touch the soft tissue incisive papilla behind the upper central incisors. Successful touching represents "normal" tongue mobility. Tongue restrictions can be visualized as a percentage of movement from rest to full extension towards the incisive papilla.

A restriction of 40% or greater often has significant clinical implications.

Airway/Breathing/Sleep:
Evaluation: *Clinical Signs*
5. Nasal Stenosis/Blockage

Neck Circumference >16"	−	+
Mallampati Score >2	−	+
Scalloped Tongue	−	+
40% Tongue Restriction	−	+
Nasal Stenosis	−	+

A simple visual observation can be made by having the patient breathe in and out through the nose. Does the nostril on one or both sides collapse during nasal breathing?

This provides a visible indicator of nasal airway collapse or obstruction. It would be common for the patient with visible nasal stenosis to struggle with upper airway resistance (UAR) and default to mouth breathing.

Airway/Breathing/Sleep:
Evaluation: *Clinical Signs*
6. Skeletal Profile

Neck Circumference >16"	−	+
Mallampati Score >2	−	+
Scalloped Tongue	−	+
40% Tongue Restriction	−	+
Nasal Stenosis	−	+
Skeletal Profile		+

Maxillary and/or mandibular skeletal underdevelopment can compromise airway volume.⁹⁶ This is described as **Bimaxillary Retrusion or Maxillo-mandibular Retrusion.**

Arnett's True Vertical is a useful visual and photographic assessment for evaluating mandibular retrusion, maxillary retrusion, and bimaxillary (maxillo-mandibular) retrusion by observing the patient's profile, facing to the right. A line dropped vertically down from the nose-lip intersection (Sella Nasion or SN) relates ideally to the fully developed lower face when:
-Upper Lip = 2-5 mm in front of the line
-Lower Lip = 0-3 mm in front of the line
-Chin Point = -4-0 mm behind the line

Measurements less than these ranges can correlate with craniofacial, mid-face underdevelopment, with increased risk for airway compromise.[97]

> When a thorough review of **History: *Signs & Symptoms*** and **Evaluation: *Clinical Signs*** reveals positive indicators for a potential airway and breathing disturbance, then **Screening & Testing** are routinely indicted.

Personally Speaking ... "Twelve Suggestions"
By John B. Harrison, DDS, MSc

Dr. Harrison was my orthodontist in 1966! After 53 years in dentistry, my dear friend is still practicing full-time, learning, growing, educating, and changing young lives every day. It is with great pleasure that I share his recent newsletter with you.

* * *

"OK, I am not Moses, and this message is a Commandment from Mt. Sinai, but I am invested in a towering mountain of current knowledge that has converted my understanding of dentistry. I aspire to be a disciple of truth but must admit that truth is often the needle in the haystack, yet to be discovered, and other times we trip over it obviously in front of us. Fortunately for all of us, a few good men and women are digging and sifting the evidence of how the human being should work as the Lord intended. Remember there is a snake in the garden who would love to mess us up. So, I am a learning student who wants to pass it forward.

First, admit we have a health problem in every village, town, city, and state. Statistics tell us our health is worse than it was in 1950 when most of our population was not even born and is declining at an alarming rate. I was born before WW2 and have never missed a day of school or missed a day of work in 53 years. I can say the same for my wife, Carolyn; we just don't get sick. What is going on here, and why? Can we ever get back to an earlier healthier time or are we headed for the second Plagues of Pharaoh?

Since Y2K (2000 AD), the health benefits of sound sleep have aroused my curiosity as the most important health remedy, surpassing nutrition and exercise as the "silver bullet", but others have influenced and convinced me to recognize that how our body works during the time we are awake determines how we sleep at night – an "aha" moment! Obvious and simple to understand. We don't have a sleep problem as much as an awake problem that affects our sleep at night. So, what are we doing all day? Breathing correctly or incorrectly. You breathe right, and you live right. It is a fundamental of health we have overlooked and don't understand…

To dentistry's credit, our expertise with the influences on the development of the anatomy of the face has proven irrefutably that breathing problems cause distortions and disruptions in overall health and physical development. The scary part is that it starts at or before birth and we all need to be aware of the harbinger of 'almost sick' before really sick.

What are the 12 signs or symptoms discovered by science that should be a wake-up call?

"Thou shall not:"
1. Mouth breathe.
2. Snore or audibly breathe.
3. Have enlarged tonsils or adenoids.
4. Be irritable and have mood swings.
5. Clench or grind your teeth.
6. Have a high narrow palate.
7. Have a tongue tie or low tongue posture.
8. Have a retruded lower jaw.
9. Have daytime fatigue.
10. Be hard to wake up.
11. Gasp for air during sleep.
12. Have a runny nose, ear infections or persistent allergies."

* * *

John, you are the best of the best, and I love you, man!

Airway/Breathing/Sleep:
Screening & Testing
1. Written Screening Forms

*Epworth Sleepiness Scale
*STOP-BANG

Written screening forms are useful tools to screen both a general population as well as individual patients. There are more than ten different written screening forms commonly used in different medical centers in the U.S. The two most commonly used are:

1. **Epworth Sleepiness Scale** (ESS)
Poor quality of sleep produces daytime sleepiness, especially at specific times and in specific circumstances. The ESS evaluates 8 of those times and circumstances, with the respondent rating their sleepiness from 0-3. The responses are totaled and Average Sleep Propensity (ASP) is determined. This correlates very well with quality and quantity of sleep, which may be related to UARS or OSA.

To learn more about the ESS or obtain the license to use the study, visit their website at http://epworthsleepinessscale.com/.[98]

2. **STOP-BANG**
The **S**noring, **T**iredness, **O**bserved apnea, high B**P**, **B**MI, **A**ge, **N**eck circumference, and male **G**ender (**STOP-BANG**) questionnaire is a reliable, concise, and easy-to-use screening tool. It consists of 8 "YES" or "NO" items related to the clinical features of sleep apnea. The total score ranges from 0 to 8. Patients can be classified for OSA risk based on their respective scores. The sensitivity of STOP-Bang score ≥ 3 to detect moderate to severe OSA (apnea-hypopnea index [AHI] > 15) and severe OSA (AHI > 30) is 93% and 100%, respectively. Patients with a STOP-BANG score of 0-2 can be classified as low risk for moderate to severe OSA, whereas those with a score of 3-4 can be classified as intermediate risk for moderate to severe OSA, and those with a score of 5-8 can be classified as high risk for moderate to severe OSA..[99]

NOTE: The STOP-BANG questionnaire is more useful for middle-aged patients.

Airway/Breathing/Sleep: Screening & Testing

Overnight Pulse Oximetry — +

2. Overnight High Resolution Pulse Oximetry (HRPO)

Overnight HRPO monitors two significant factors that relate to healthy or dysfunctional breathing:

- ➢ **Oxygen Saturation (SO2)** is the fraction of oxygen-saturated hemoglobin relative to total hemoglobin (unsaturated + saturated) in the blood. The human body requires and regulates a very precise and specific balance of oxygen in the blood. Normal blood oxygen levels in humans are considered to be 95-100%. **If the level is below 90%, it is considered low (hypoxemia).** If SO2 falls below 90% for a patient in a medical facility, they are typically administered oxygen. Blood oxygen levels below 80% may compromise organ function, such as in the brain and heart. Continued low oxygen levels may lead to respiratory or cardiac arrest.[100]

- ➢ **Pulse Rate:** During non-REM sleep, the pulse rate tends to slow down 14-24 beats per minute compared to wakefulness. The average heart rate range during all 3 stages of non-REM sleep is between 60-100. Some individuals may have a normally slower or faster heart rate range. Non-REM represents roughly 75% of the time during sleep. REM sleep includes periods of dreaming and increased heart rate, with more variability. Dreaming is very active during REM sleep. The relative muscle paralysis present during REM prevents acting out some of the more exciting dreams. REM is often concentrated in the last few hours of sleep. HRPO can screen for disordered breathing during sleep by observing the recorded "delta" of both SO2 and Pulse Rate. Delta involves the difference between high and low values. **Large swings in both SO2 and Pulse Rate over short intervals, on multiple occasions throughout sleep, may indicate a breathing disorder.** Precise interpretation is often difficult.[101]

Airway/Breathing/Sleep: Screening & Testing
3. Home Sleep Testing (HST)

Overnight Pulse Oximetry	–	+
Home Sleep Test	–	+

Home sleep testing has become a standard for evaluation and diagnosis of sleep disorders in recent years. Though less information is gathered relative to polysomnography (PSG) studies, the accuracy appears comparable.[102]

Most home testing recorders can track **time of the test period**, but not sleep time, which requires EEG signals. They also gather data about:
- **Oxygen saturation**
- **Pulse rate**
- **Sleep position**
- **Apnea & Hypopnea episodes (AHI)**
- **Snoring**
- **Chest effort**
- **Respiratory Event Index (REI)**, a new term adopted by the American Academy of Sleep Medicine to designate results from testing when true sleep time is not measured.

Additionally, there is a lot of other data that even such 'simple' tests can provide regarding a patient's sleep.

NOTE: Dentists are not qualified or licensed to diagnose sleep apnea. HST should be interpreted by a Board Certified Sleep Physician. Many HST manufacturers provide an interpretation service. Dentists are the ideal health professionals to screen patients and gather studies for potential airway, breathing and sleep disorders. When HST reveals significant signs of breathing dysfunction and elevated AHI, referral for an overnight laboratory PSG will analyze important additional information such as EEG and CSA. The results may significantly alter the treatment plan.

> Please see the recently released ADA Policy Statement on "The Role of Dentistry in the Treatment of Sleep-Related Breathing Disorders" (2017) in the Appendix for further information.

**Airway/Breathing/Sleep:
Screening & Testing
4. Heart Rate Variability (HRV)**

Overnight Pulse Oximetry	−	+
Home Sleep Test	−	+
Heart Rate Variability(HRV)	−	+

There is activity in the heart between heart beats. HRV is the physiological phenomenon of variation in the time interval between heartbeats. It is measured by the variation in the beat-to-beat interval.

This activity can vary according to several influences including the Parasympathetic (Rest & Digest, PSNS) and Sympathetic (Fight or Flight, SNS) divisions of the Autonomic Nervous System. It can be monitored using a simple portable device that measures HRV. Here's the take home:

- **Decreased PSNS activity or increased SNS activity will result in reduced HRV.**
- **Reduced HRV is a sign of increased *STRESS***

Frederic Roche, MD, PhD, and cohort in Lyon, France studied the effectiveness of using HRV for screening for OSA. They concluded that *"Time-domain analysis of HR variability, used as the only criterion, could thus represent an efficient tool in OSAS diagnosis with a sensitivity of 90%. The ease of use and interpretation are also of interest because of the high prevalence of the disease in the general population and the need for repeated control."*[103]

In conclusion, HRV provides an inexpensive and accurate method for dentists to evaluate potential OSA and stress levels related to the sympathetic nervous system.

**Airway/Breathing/Sleep:
Screening & Testing
5. Polysomnogram (PSG)**

Overnight Pulse Oximetry	−	+
Home Sleep Test	−	+
Heart Rate Variability(HRV)	−	+
Polysomnogram(PSG)	−	+

A PSG is performed in a professional sleep laboratory. It is considered the "Gold Standard" of definitive testing because of the many channels of body functions that are monitored. In addition to monitoring **oxygen saturation, pulse rate, sleep position, Apnea & Hypopnea Index (AHI), snoring,** and **chest effort,** PSG's also include **Respiratory Event Index (REI),** including **brain activity**

(EEG), eye movements **(EOG)**, muscle activity/skeletal muscle activation **(EMG)**, and **heart rhythm (ECG)**, during sleep.

Polysomnography is used to diagnose, or rule out, many types of sleep disorders other than sleep apnea, including **narcolepsy, idiopathic hypersomnia, periodic limb movement disorder (PLMD), REM behavior disorder**, and **parasomnias**.

The proper protocol in the medical management of health concerns is a thorough history, thorough clinical evaluation, and thorough diagnosis. If an airway, breathing and sleep disorder is unclear, use every resource to get an accurate and complete diagnosis. That may require an overnight PSG. **When in doubt, go find out!**

* * *

Following a thorough evaluation including:
1. **History: Signs & Symptoms**
2. **Evaluation: Clinical Signs**
3. **Screening & Testing**

This information gathered should be adequate to produce a **DIFFERENTIAL CONCLUSION.**

This information allows the practitioner to determine that the patient presents either
NEGATIVE or **POSITIVE** for Airway and Breathing Disorders.
If **POSITIVE**, proceed to the **TREATMENT** portion of the IDM Checklist.
The focus now turns to re-establishing a healthy airway, healthy breathing, and complete health.

> "Chronic pain and sleep disturbances are significant global health concerns. Each of these common problems has been independently linked to decreased quality of life, increased psychiatric and medical morbidity, and disability. An estimated 50% to 88% of chronic pain patients exhibit sleep disturbance, and when these conditions co-occur, their deleterious effects may be compounded, if not magnified.
>
> Temporomandibular disorders (TMD) are pain disorders that have been associated with significant sleep disturbance. TMDs, characterized by episodic, masticatory muscle and/or joint pain, are the most common chronic orofacial pain conditions. The estimated prevalence of TMDs in the general population is approximately 12%. While the pathophysiology of TMDs is poorly understood, the syndrome is often classified by the presence and degree of assumed masticatory muscle pathology, articular disc dysfunction, temporomandibular joint (TMJ) arthritis, and/or TMJ pain (arthritides). As in most chronic pain syndromes, poor sleep is a ubiquitous complaint among patients with TMDs; recent data suggest that up to 77% of orofacial pain patients report reduced quality and quantity of sleep."
>
> <u>Sleep Medicine for Dentists: A Practical Overview</u>
> Edited by Gilles J. Lavigne, DMD, MSc, PhD, FRCD(C),
> Peter A. Cistulli, MBBS, PhD, MBA, FRACP
> and Michael T. Smith, PhD, CBSM

13. AIRWAY, BREATHING & SLEEP – TREATMENT

A **DIFFERENTIAL CONCLUSION,** from utilizing the IDM Checklist History, Evaluation, Screening & Testing, has determined that the patient presents **POSITIVE** for Airway, Breathing and Sleep Disorder. We will next proceed to the **TREATMENT** portion of the IDM Checklist, where the focus now turns to re-establishing a healthy airway, healthy breathing, and complete health.

Remembering Our Mission:

* To educate each patient we serve about the multiple facets of a healthy airway, breathing, sleep and complete health.

* To empower them toward complete health, through counseling and supporting a healthy airway, healthy breathing and restorative sleep.

Let's explore these multiple facets of Airway, Breathing and Sleep, and how we can educate to empower each patient toward complete health.

Airway/Breathing/Sleep:
Treatment
1. A Strategic Plan

The great American architect Louis Sullivan (1856-1924) stated, *"Whether it be the sweeping eagle in his flight, or the open apple-blossom, the toiling work-horse, the blithe swan, the branching oak, the winding stream at its base, the drifting clouds, over all the coursing sun...form ever follows function, and this is the law. Where function does not change, form does not change."*

Form follows function in the masticatory system as well. The healthy form of the cranio-facial-respiratory complex follows healthy, functioning nasal airways and breathing. When unhealthy, dysfunctional blocked or congested airways lead to dysfunctional breathing patterns, tongue posturing, swallowing and sleep patterns, then the natural result that follows is deformation of the craniofacial-respiratory-dental occlusion complex.

As form follows function,
so deformation follows dysfunction.

DIAGNOSE THEN TREAT
A thorough evaluation of the complete masticatory system, including the temporomandibular joints, is critical to derive an accurate diagnosis and treatment plan related to potential airway, breathing and sleep concerns. The diagnosis of dysfunctional airways, breathing and sleep should lead us to anticipate possible craniofacial and dental occlusal deformation, depending on the severity of the problem. We must also clearly understand that **deformation can also precede dysfunction.** Deformation due to internal derangement of the temporomandibular joints ("TMJoints") can affect the airway and influence dysfunctional breathing, as well as distortions of the cranio-facial-dental occlusion complex.

As deformation follows dysfunction,
so dysfunction follows deformation.

We will discuss the implications of this statement as it relates to the TMJoints in further detail in the next section: TMD & Occlusion Disorders. Regarding issues of airway, breathing, and sleep, we must ask: when both dysfunction and deformation are diagnosed, what is the preferred treatment plan of action? Whenever possible, the preferred plan would be to correct <u>both</u> the dysfunction and the deformation.

Clinically speaking, treatment can be divided into two plans: Management and Resolution. In some cases sequencing may include "Phase 1" Management and "Phase 2" Resolution.

Management is working with the existing condition through reversible measures. An example would be the treatment of Type 2 Diabetes. We know this disease is primarily created by dysfunctional eating, blood sugar dysregulation, and inflammation. It can lead to significant body organ and weight deformation. One treatment plan is to chemically "manage" the disease with diabetic medications. The disease is still present but is hopefully being controlled much better than with no intervention.

Breathing disorders that affect sleep, especially if sleep apnea is diagnosed, are "managed" using CPAP and oral appliances. The dysfunctional airway and breathing are still present, but hopefully the oxygen and cortisol levels and heart rate are controlled much better than with no intervention. If a diagnosis of severe sleep apnea is made, then it is very important that proper ventilation during sleep be reestablished ASAP!

Resolution is working out a plan to correct the dysfunctional breathing and the deformational changes, with the goal of reversing the condition. In the case of Type 2 Diabetes, the treatment plan would be to implement an anti-inflammatory diet (eliminating sugar, refined carbohydrates, refined seed oils, and processed foods), increase exercise, stop smoking, control stress, and reduce weight in order to normalize blood sugar levels and reestablish healthy organ functions. As we discussed earlier, studies by Joel Fuhrman, MD, and others, reveal it is possible to reverse diabetes in 90% of cases. Dr. Esselstyn has done this with heart disease at the Cleveland Clinic.

Our preferred plan for airway, breathing, and sleep dysfunction and/or deformation is to stabilize or reverse it whenever possible.

Airway/Breathing/Sleep:
Treatment
2. Examples of Airway, Breathing and Sleep – *Management* **and** *Resolution*

Let's discuss Airway, Breathing and Sleep *Management* and *Resolution* through several example scenarios. The plan for addressing these disorders depends on the diagnosis.

Using the **IDM: 7 Key Questions**, let's consider various clinical scenarios.

Scenario #1:
The patient's chief complaint is SNORING. Nasal breathing is unobstructed and the patient reports no other dental or systemic concerns. A thorough clinical examination is performed with the following conclusions:

IDM: 7 Key Questions
*Does the **OCCLUSION** appear unstable? …**NO**
*Does the patient **BRUX**? …**NO**
*Does the patient have **SORE MUSCLES**? …**NO**
*Are there signs of **TMJ CHANGE**? …**NO**
*Could there be an **AIRWAY PROBLEM**? …**YES**
  ➢ Snoring is a sign of airway compromise that often accompanies underlying concerns of UARS or OSA. Further screening is indicated in this case.
  ➢ One option is the overnight use of portable High Resolution Pulse Oximetry (HRPO), which can determine if there are large delta changes in heart rate and oxygen desaturations. It is a screening tool but is non-specific for UARS and OSA.
  ➢ A second option is to use a portable Heart Rate Variability (HRV) monitor to assess overnight levels of stress related to sympathetic nervous system "fight or flight" stimulation.
  ➢ A third option is the overnight use a portable Home Sleep Test (HST). This test is more specific for both UARS and OSA. If the AHI > 5, the diagnosis of OSA should be made by a qualified physician reviewing the study.
*Are there signs of local or systemic **INFLAMMATION**? …**NO**
*Is there an **UNESTHETIC SMILE** concern? …**NO**

In this case, let's assume the sleep screening demonstrates no significant blood oxygen desaturations and a calm heart response. We will not have uncovered the true cause of what may be described as "simple snoring".

Based on the examination findings and what we've learned about airway and breathing, a question comes to mind: would the snoring improve or cease if the mouth were held closed all night, promoting physiologically preferred nasal breathing with better filtration and nitric oxide release into the upper airway?

Management Strategy (Phase 1): Patrick McKeown (The Oxygen Advantage, published by HarperCollins Publishers, 2015) reports working with his patients' sleep breathing by holding the mouth closed, using light **Paper Tape** (3M Micropore Tape) across the lips to prevent the mouth from falling open during sleep. In chapter 3, he reports,

> *Over the years, I have introduced this taping method to thousands of people with incredible results. Unless you breathe calmly through your nose at night, you have no idea what it feels like to have a great night's sleep. Taping the mouth at night is a simple but very effective technique, and while it may sound a little strange, it is well worth getting used to. Continue to wear the tape until you have managed to change to breathing through your nose at night. How long this takes will vary from person to person, but in general wearing the tape for a period of around three months is sufficient to restore nasal breathing during sleep.*

A good alternative to mouth taping is a **"stop snoring strap"** which keeps the lower jaw closed at night.

Nasal dilation during sleep, using **external breathing strips** or **nostril cones**, can be therapeutic as well. **Sleep position** and snoring are often related, especially sleeping on the back (supine). **Body pillows** can be used to wrap around the body and position the patient onto his/her side. There are a variety of sleep positioning aids available. Counsel the patient **not to drink alcohol** for several hours before going to bed, as alcohol is a CNS depressant and can impede restful sleep.

Resolution Strategy (Phase 2): Chronic snoring is often associated with weight gain, and many who previously snored report they ceased snoring after they lost weight. Therefore, in many cases losing weight can be a very effective way to stop snoring.

Enlarged tissues of the nasal and posterior throat airway may interfere with adequate passage of air and produce snoring. This may be related to allergies or damaged tissues. Allergist and ENT intervention may be appropriate. Maxillary and mandibular retrusion will provide inadequate room for the tongue – the garage may be too small for the car. Expansion of the dental arches orthodontically, along with oral-myofunctional therapy for proper breathing and tongue positioning, may eliminate the snoring.

Scenario #2:

The patient's chief complaint is **SNORING, SORE MUSCLES, A.M. HEADACHES and DAYTIME FATIGUE.** A thorough clinical examination is performed with the following conclusions:

IDM: 7 Key Questions

*Does the **OCCLUSION** appear unstable? ...**NO**
> The teeth showed no signs of wear, mobility, or drifting of position. The seated joints (in C.R.) and the fully seated bite (in maximum intercuspation position, or M.I.P.) are in harmony, with exclusive front teeth contact in all excursions (demonstrating anterior guidance).

*Does the patient **BRUX**? ...**YES**
> No wear due to grinding is observed on the teeth, but enlarged masseter and temporalis muscles are consistent with chronic clenching. Is this related to an airway problem?

*Does the patient have **SORE MUSCLES**? ...**YES**
> The patient reports tender clenching muscles, temporalis A.M. headaches 3-4 times per week, along with daily neck soreness. Could this be related to an airway problem? The patient also reports fibromyalgia-like generalized muscle fatigue.

*Are there signs of **TMJ CHANGE**? ...**NO**
> The jaw moved freely in all excursions within a normal range (ROM). The joints were comfortable to finger palpation and to orthopedic load testing, using Dawson's bilateral manipulation technique (described in the TMD/Occlusion section). Doppler auscultation was normal.

*Could there be an **AIRWAY PROBLEM**? ...**YES**
> A seasonal history of allergies is reported by the patient.

> High Resolution Pulse Oximetry (HRPO) overnight reports a high delta/variable in heart rate and oxygen desaturation.
>
> <u>*OR*</u>
>
> > Heart Rate Variability (HRV) reports high sympathetic stress levels.
> > A subsequent Home Sleep Test (HST) reports an AHI = 2 (normal <5) and a RERA =12 (Respiratory Effort Related Arousal is mildly elevated, most likely due to difficulty breathing). The patient doesn't stop breathing often, but breathing is challenged, producing a sympathetic (SNS) response.
> > Mallampati 1 (no maxillary retrusion or soft palatal tissue obstructing the airway).
> > Nasal breathing is possible without difficulty, but when inhaling through the nose, the left nostril collapses (nasal stenosis).

*Are there signs of local or systemic **INFLAMMATION**? ...**YES**

> The patient is lean, with a BMI (Body Mass Index) of 20 (BMI = body weight divided by the square of height). A BMI of < 18.5 is considered to be underweight, >24 is overweight, and >30 is obese. The patient's diet consists primarily of fast foods, with a high intake of refined carbs, including 4-5 diet colas daily.
> Physical activity is minimal due to soreness after strenuous exercise.

*Is there an **UNESTHETIC SMILE** concern? ...**NO**

Diagnosis:
- **UARS** – increased breathing effort, but no significant cessation of breathing.
- **Inflammation** – due to UARS, poor diet, seasonal allergies, possible fibromyalgia, and lack of physical activity

Dr. Christian Guilleminault coined the term "Upper Airway Resistance Syndrome" (UARS)[104]. In one of his Stanford University research projects, he studied younger, thin people with severe fatigue and poor sleep, but without any significant obstructive sleep apnea. He found from PSGs that they still had multiple partial to total breathing obstructions, which weren't severe enough to be called apneas (low AHIs) but which led to arousals from deep sleep to light sleep (high RERAs).[105]

The 30 subjects in the study were ages 22.8 +/- 1.8. All 30 were diagnosed with UARS and reported **chronic fatigue**; 28 reported **non-refreshing sleep**; 26 reported **disrupted nocturnal sleep**; 17 reported **morning headache**; and 29 reported **daytime performance impairment**.[106] These are complaints expressed by many patients who would be described in dentistry as "classic TMD" patients.

In this case, the "TMD" appears to be due to airway restriction, elevated breathing effort, oxygen deprivation, sympathetic dysregulation (fight or flight), and systemic inflammation.

Management: The immediate need is to open the airway all night. Consider:
1. Promote nasal breathing during sleep through **mouth taping**.
2. Open the vertical dimension of the dental occlusion (VDO), and position the mandible in a slightly forward posture, in order to create more room for the tongue and open the posterior airway (back of the throat). Trial oral appliances (MyTap) are available that accomplish both of the above and which can be fabricated chair-side within minutes. These can be adjusted for comfort by the patient. Additionally, as stated in the previous example, it is important to promote **nasal dilation** during sleep, and using **external breathing strips** or **nostril cones** can be therapeutic. **Sleep position** and snoring are often related, especially sleeping on the back (supine). **Body pillows** can be used to wrap around the body and position the patient onto his/her side. There are a variety of sleep positioning aids available. Counsel the patient **not to drink alcohol** for several hours before going to bed, as alcohol is a CNS depressant and can impede restful sleep.
3. Allergy testing and treatment

Resolution:
1. Evaluation with an ENT for left nasal stenosis treatment
2. Counsel an **anti-inflammatory diet** and **physical activity**
3. **Vitamin D3 supplement** – which has been found to be deficient in many patients with sleep apnea and fibromyalgia

4. **DHA/Fish Oil supplement** – which has been found to be deficient in many patients with sleep apnea due to oxidative stress
5. **Antioxidant supplements** – **Vitamin A, C, E** to combat the oxidative stress related to chronic sleep apnea[107]

Scenario #3:

The patient's chief complaint is SNORING, SORE MUSCLES, A.M. HEADACHES and DAYTIME FATIGUE. A thorough clinical examination is performed with the following conclusions:

IDM: 7 Key Questions
*Does the **OCCLUSION** appear unstable? …**NO**
*Does the patient **BRUX**? …**YES**
*Does the patient have **SORE MUSCLES**? …**YES**
*Are there signs of **TMJ CHANGE**? …**NO**
*Could there be an **AIRWAY PROBLEM**? …**YES**
*Are there signs of local or systemic **INFLAMMATION**? …**YES**
*Is there an **UNESTHETIC SMILE** concern? …**NO**

Evaluation:

- High Resolution Pulse Oximetry (**HRPO**) overnight reports a **high delta/variable in heart rate and oxygen desaturation**

  or

- Heart Rate Variability (**HRV**) reports **high sympathetic stress levels**

- A subsequent Home Sleep Test (**HST**) reports an **AHI = 12** and a **RERA = 10**

- No wear on the teeth, but **enlarged Masseter and Temporalis** Muscles

- **Mallampati 3** and **enlarged tonsils**

- **Nasal stenosis on one side**, some **stuffiness** most of the time

- **Allergies** seasonally; uses nasal sprays frequently

Diagnosis:
- This appears to be mild Sleep Apnea (AHI 5-15), but it will require a diagnosis by a **Sleep Physician.** Many HST companies have Board Certified Sleep Physicians available to interpret HSTs. When the AHI is in a **MILD** to **MODERATE** category, it is appropriate to obtain a remote diagnosis and interpretation from one of them. If the AHI is in the **SEVERE** category, it would be more appropriate to refer them for treatment by a Board Certified Sleep Physician. When the diagnosis is confirmed, the Physician will prescribe treatment options for the patient. These are typically CPAP, Oral Appliance and, if applicable, weight loss.
- **Allergist referral is needed** for testing
- **ENT referral** is needed for evaluation of nasal stenosis and enlarged tonsils

Management:

    Sleep Appliances for OSA should more correctly be described as **Breathing Appliances.** They are used during sleep, but their function is to manage breathing. They are typically fabricated in a forward mandibular position for the purpose of moving the mandible and tongue forward to open or dilate the airway.

    Conventional fabrication of breathing appliances requires recording the initial mandibular starting position, with measuring instruments such as the **George** or **TAP Gauge**. Once the appliance is placed, it is monitored for comfort and efficacy. Most oral appliances are adjustable, which allows for "titration" of the appliance, moving the mandible forward over time, if required, to improve efficacy.

    A newer technology, ©*MATRx Titration System,* has been recently developed by John Remmers, MD. Dr. Remmers is a highly esteemed physiologist, pioneer and innovator in sleep medicine, having invented products ranging from portable diagnostic sleep monitors to auto-titrating CPAP devices and now MATRx©. The MATRx© Plus monitors apneas and hypopneas during the home or laboratory sleep study and uses fitted bite trays, electronic sensors, and bluetooth communication to reposition the mandible during the study, without awakening the patient.[108] This uniquely permits active evaluation of the efficacy of oral appliance therapy during the pre-treatment phase. It also determines and records the optimum or target position of the mandible to minimize the AHI. This information is communicated, along with CBCT and dental arch scanning, to guide the digital fabrication of oral breathing appliances at the pre-determined target position of the mandible. Dr. Remmers' studies have demonstrated that close to 75% of apneic patients can greatly benefit from the use of oral breathing appliances during sleep.

*Note: **Oral appliances can potentially alter the dental occlusion adversely.** Despite careful management, a risk factor of repositioning the mandible for several hours per day is the possibility of bite changes. "A.M. Aligners" should be used with every case to minimize these changes.

*Note: **Oral appliances can potentially aggravate TMD symptoms.** Most often the symptoms are related to sore muscle responses to extensive protrusive repositioning of the jaw in the initial nights of treatment. For example, let's say a patient's maximum protrusive mandibular movement is 10 mm and an appliance is placed that positions the mandible forward 80% or 8 mm. The patient reports soreness in front of the TM joints in the morning. If the appliances is titrated back to 50% or 5 mm, the patient will most often report relief. Any titration forward of that position will be made by slowly adjusting the appliance over several weeks in very small increments. Patients who have a TMD history should be instructed to remove the appliance if any discomfort is experienced and to report this to the dentist.

Additionally, as stated in the previous examples, it is important to promote **nasal dilation** during sleep, and using **external breathing strips** or **nostril cones** can be therapeutic. **Sleep position** and snoring are often related, especially sleeping on the back (supine). **Body pillows** can be used to wrap around the body and position the patient onto his/her side. There are a variety of sleep positions aids available. Counsel the patient **not to drink alcohol** for several hours before going to bed, as alcohol is a CNS depressant and can impede restful sleep.

Resolution:
　* **Lose weight**, if appropriate
　* Implement an **anti-inflammatory diet** and **exercise**
　* **Vitamin D3 supplement** – which has been found to be deficient in many patients with sleep apnea and fibromyalgia; a deficiency of Vitamin D3 can add to fatigue

* **DHA/Fish Oil supplement** – which has been found to be deficient in many patients with sleep apnea due to oxidative stress
* **Antioxidant supplements – Vitamin A, C and E** to combat the oxidative stress related to chronic sleep apnea
* **Allergy resolution**
* **ENT Surgery if needed for tonsils and nasal stenosis**
* **Re-evaluate HST to determine AHI improvement and possible discontinuation of the breathing appliance**

Scenario #4:
The patient's chief complaint is SNORING, SORE MUSCLES, HEADACHES, CLENCHING, and DAYTIME FATIGUE. A thorough clinical examination is performed with the following conclusions:

IDM: 7 Key Questions
*Does the **OCCLUSION** appear unstable? …**NO**
*Does the patient **BRUX**? …**YES**
*Does the patient have **SORE MUSCLES**? …**YES**
*Are there signs of **TMJ CHANGE**? …**NO**
*Could there be an **AIRWAY PROBLEM**? …**YES**
*Are there signs of local or systemic **INFLAMMATION**? …**YES**
*Is there an **UNESTHETIC SMILE** concern? …**NO**

Evaluation:

- The temporomandibular joints are healthy

- The dental occlusion is stable (CR = MIP, acceptable anterior guidance)

- **HRPO** or **HRV** report red flags for airway compromise and high stress levels

- **HST** reports AHI = 34 and RERA = 37

- **Narrow maxillary arch morphology**

- **Tongue scalloping**

- **Tongue-tie 50% restriction** (and affected maxillary arch size)

- **4 Biscuspid extraction** for ortho and **3rd molars removed**

- **Mallampati 4** (Maxillomandibular retrusion)

Diagnosis:
* This appears to be severe sleep apnea, but it will require a diagnosis by a **Sleep Physician. A referral is made.** There will be a Polysomnogram Study **(PSG)** needed to complete the diagnosis. Is this Obstructive Sleep Apnea (**OSA**), Central Sleep Apnea (**CSA**), Mixed Sleep Apnea (**MSA**), or **Cheyne-Stokes** respiration with central sleep apnea (**CSR-CSA**), which presents with congestive heart failure signs that can be related to sleep apnea? More diagnostic information is needed in this case.

Management:
*A **CPAP** will be prescribed due to the severe nature of the sleep apnea. If resolution steps are taken moving forward, a CPAP will be used until completion and reevaluation with another sleep study.

Resolution:
*Considering the signs of crowding of the airway by a tongue-tie, tongue scalloping, narrow maxillary arch, bicuspid extractions, Mallampati 4 and maxillary retrusion, this would be a case to evaluate for **orthodontic arch expansion**. In severe cases, **orthognathic surgery**, to expand and rotate the maxilla and mandible away from the airway, would be considered.
***Tongue-tie release** and **oral-myofunctional therapy** would be considered for better function and neutral zone stability.

NOTE: It is important to understand that all of the above therapies may or may not assure major improvement in the breathing dysfunction. Sleep apnea is a complex subject and responses to logical therapeutic options vary from patient to patient. That being said, many patients frequently demonstrate amazing improvement following these "resolution" procedures.

Airway/Breathing/Sleep:
Treatment
3. Summary of Management and Resolution

Management of Airway, Breathing and Sleep Disorders primarily consists of:
1. Improving daytime breathing
    a. **Buteyko Breathing Techniques** (see <u>The Oxygen Advantage</u> for further details)
    b. **Oral-myofunctional Therapy** to train in proper breathing, tongue posturing, swallowing, and muscle strengthening.
    c. **Allergy Testing and Therapy**
2. Improving nighttime breathing
    a. **Nasal breathing**
        i. Mouth taping, or a "stop snoring" strap.
        ii. Nasal dilation using external breathing strips or nostril cones.
        iii. Nasal decongestants
        iv. Sleep position changes, from supine onto the side.
    b. **Open the VDO (vertical dimension of occlusion) and anteriorly reposition the mandible** with an oral breathing appliance. This will improve the airway and breathing for many patients, but not for all. Predetermination of this outcome through testing methods, such as Dr. John Remmers' ©MATRx Plus Titration System, is ideal when available. Utilizing inexpensive trial appliances, such as the MyTap, is another way to evaluate outcomes overnight subjectively, through the patient's reported improvement of signs and symptoms, and objectively, through repeated home sleep studies.
    c. **Sleep Physician and Sleep Laboratory** referral and guidance as needed
3. Improving systemic health
    a. **Allergy Testing,** through referral.
    b. **ENT evaluation of upper and posterior airway,** through referral
    c. As we have discussed, **inflammation** plays a role in airway, breathing and sleep concerns. **Anti-**

inflammatory, anti-oxidant, and anti-stress strategies should begin immediately.

Resolution strategies of Airway, Breathing and Sleep Disorders primarily consists of:
1. **Expansion of the Upper Airway** through correcting sources of obstruction, disease and inflammation in the nose and nasopharynx.
2. **Expansion of the Posterior Airway** through correcting sources of obstruction, disease and inflammation in the throat.
3. **Expansion of the Oral Airway** through expanding the maxilla, mandible and dental arches.
4. **Tongue-tie release** to free the tongue to fill the maxillary vault, reestablish a more physiologically ideal neutral zone (the muscle balance between the tongue and cheeks/lips), and to allow for better function, including swallowing.
5. **Oral-myofunctional Therapy** to train the tongue in healthy function, including nasal breathing, palatal seal, swallowing patterns and tongue strengthening.
6. **Improving Complete Body Health** with an emphasis on the factors that are anti-inflammatory, anti-oxidant, and anti-stress.

NOTE: Resolution strategies are based on the goal of improving airway restrictions and breathing pathology. It is not possible to always predetermine the degree of improvement each patient will experience. We are very encouraged that the resolution strategies mentioned above have produced many dramatic, life-changing improvements for many patients.

In conclusion, we must always remember:
Complete health requires a healthy AIRWAY.
Complete health requires healthy BREATHING.
Complete health requires healthy RESTORATIVE SLEEP.

Airway /Breathing Disorders
Management & Resolution **Nasal Breathing** • Buteyko Training • Mouth Taping **Oral Myofunctional Therapy** **Allergist-Allergy Testing** **E.N.T.-Airway Evaluation** **MANAGEMENT PROTOCOL** • Increase Vertical Airway • Increase Horizontal Airway • Sleep Position, Non-Supine • Weight Loss • Retest • Work with Sleep MD **RESOLUTION PROTOCOL** • Expand Oral Airway • Expand Upper Airway • Expand Posterior Airway • Release Tongue-Tie

---

Remembering Our Mission:

*To educate each patient we serve about the multiple facets of a healthy airway, breathing, sleep and complete health.

*To empower them toward complete health, through counseling and supporting a healthy airway, healthy breathing and restorative sleep.

Full implementation of the Integrative Dental Medicine Model means committing to educate and empower each person served to pursue complete health, through healthy breathing…24 hours a day.

14: "TREATING AIRWAY AND BREATHING DISORDERS: A KEY FOCUS OF INTEGRATIVE DENTAL MEDICINE FOR PATIENTS OF ALL AGES" BY DEWITT C. WILKERSON, DMD

The following article was published in <u>Inside Dentistry</u> in February 2018. It is reproduced here, with permission, with the intent of providing a useful guide for both patients and practitioners.

* * *

ABSTRACT

Patients can develop airway and breathing disorders at any stage of life. Issues such as allergic reactions, chronic congestion, malocclusions, mouth breathing, improper tongue position or tongue-tie, and other age-related and associated risk factors must be treated to correct the source of obstruction and reestablish proper naso-diaphragmatic breathing. Other conditions with similar symptoms, such as TMD, must be considered during treatment planning in order to avoid complications during therapy. Among older patients, treatment for airway and breathing disorders not only restores proper breathing function, but can also reverse some of the damage seen in brain scans. Because an open airway and proper breathing are foundational to oral and systemic health, every patient treated, regardless of age, should be screened for disordered breathing.

* * *

Learning Objectives:
• Identify the risk factors and describe the screening process for airway and breathing disorders among children.
• Discuss the areas of focus and techniques involved in the treatment of children with airway and breathing disorders.
• Explain the issues involved in diagnosing and treating patients with both TMD and airway/breathing disorders.
• Discuss the risk factors and treatment considerations for middle-aged patients with airway and breathing disorders.

* * *

Dentistry continues to grow as a true medical specialty. In the 1970s, the primary focus was on dental occlusion and restorative dentistry. In the 1980s, the focus shifted to dental implants and the treatment of temporomandibular disorders (TMDs). In the 1990s, the new focus was on esthetics, cosmetics, and ceramic materials. Since 2000, dentistry's focus has concentrated on digital technology and is now moving toward Integrative Dental Medicine. Integrative Dental Medicine looks at the dental patient as a whole person and is concerned with issues such as diabetes, systemic inflammation, cardiovascular health, gastric reflux, toxins, stress factors, drug interactions, and other issues related to the convergence of oral and overall health. In addition to these concerns, addressing airway and breathing disorders, both during childhood and throughout life, will be a key focus of Integrative Dental Medicine moving forward.

An understanding of the critical role of airway obstructions and disordered breathing significantly influences proper treatment planning in dentistry. Manifestations may include signs and symptoms such as dental malocclusions, bruxism, tongue-tie, attention deficit, poor sleep, sleep apnea, daytime fatigue, TMD, and morning headaches. Every patient treated, regardless of age, should be assessed for the presence of potential airway problems. (Note: Dentists are not trained or qualified to diagnose obstructive sleep apnea; this diagnosis must be made by a medical doctor. Dentists should work under the guidance of a qualified physician when treatment planning such cases.)

Risk Factors and Treatment for Children

These concerns may start at a very young age – even at birth. Adenoid hypertrophy is the most common cause of nasopharyngeal obstruction in children, the most common cause of pediatric sleep-disordered breathing, and a potential etiologic cause of altered craniofacial growth, characterized by a long face, retrusive chin, and narrow maxilla.[1]

Roger Price, BS, PharmD, describes a common childhood scenario in which an allergic reaction to dairy products induces mouth breathing. "This mouth breathing results in a lack of filtration and cleansing of the air, allowing airborne bacteria to settle and flourish; an increase in the volume of dirty air over the lymphoid tissue; an increase in inflammation and congestion as a result of over breathing; a lack of release of NO from the sinuses, preventing bacterial control and vasodilation; and diminution of diaphragmatic breathing, which can lead to a reduced lymph flow to the tonsils and adenoids to remove the toxins," Price explains. "After eliminating the allergic triggers, restoring nasal breathing is a must."

Mouth breathing has also been associated with dental malocclusions in children.[2] Zicari and colleagues' analysis of 71, 6- to 12-year-old mouth breathing children revealed a 72.5% incidence of reduced transverse diameter of the maxilla and increased vertical dimension, a 32.5% incidence of crossbite, a 43.7% incidence of skeletal class II malocclusions, and a 90% incidence of atypical swallowing patterns. The results showed a strong correlation between oral breathing and malocclusions, which manifests as both dentoskeletal and functional alterations, leading to a dysfunctional malocclusive pattern. The study concludes that "this dysfunctional malocclusive pattern makes it clear that the association between oral breathing and dental malocclusions represents a self-perpetuating vicious circle in which it is difficult to establish if the primary alteration is respiratory or maxillofacial. Regardless, the problem needs to be addressed and solved through the close interaction of the pediatrician, otorhinolaryngologist, allergologist, and orthodontist."

Children can suffer from both obstructive and central sleep apnea. Approximately 10% of children snore and 2% to 4% of them have obstructive sleep apnea (OSA) (including babies, but especially those between 2 and 8 years old). Up to 40% may experience subtle breathing disturbances, including those related to upper airway resistance syndrome (UARS) with sympathetic nervous system "flight or fight" response and blood cortisol stress hormone surges. Signs and symptoms of sleep apnea among children can include insulin resistance, cardiac modulation, mood swings, cognitive dysfunction/attention deficit, and behavioral changes such as hyperactivity and poor impulse control. In addition, these children are at an increased risk of future cardiovascular disease, especially those with childhood obesity. Most children with sleep apnea are mouth breathers, and many of them snore.

Bruxism commonly accompanies airway obstructions in children. DiFrancesco and colleagues evaluated 69 consecutive children who presented to the Otolaryngology Department of the University of São Paulo Medical School for tonsil and adenoid removal.[3] Before surgery, the children's parents reported that 100% experienced sleep apnea, 45.6% engaged in bruxism, and 60.7% possessed dental malocclusions. Three months after surgery, none of the children presented with breathing problems, and 11.8% presented with bruxism. Because there was a significant improvement in bruxism after surgery, the study data suggests that there is a positive correlation between sleep-disordered breathing and bruxism. The researchers conclude that otolaryngologists must be aware that bruxism is associated with airway obstruction and consider it when evaluating tonsil and adenoid hyperplasia.

When screening children for breathing and airway disturbances, integrative orthodontist Barry Raphael, DMD, recommends that clinicians ask the following questions:

- Does the child have any sleep issues such as restlessness, bedwetting, frequent awakening, or snoring?
- Is the nose chronically obstructed or congested in any way?
- Are the lips apart at rest?
- Does the tongue rest on the palate and stay there during swallowing?
- Are the chest and shoulders moving during breathing instead of the diaphragm?
- Is the child's respiratory rate greater than 16 breaths per minute?
- Is the child holding his or her head in front of the shoulders to keep the airway open?

Treatment for children's sleep-disordered breathing involves correcting the sources of obstruction and reestablishing naso-diaphragmatic breathing. There are several areas of focus, including the following:

- Treatment of any food and environmental allergies that may be causing upper airway inflammation and obstruction.
- Ear, nose, and throat treatment of airway obstructions, including nasal stenosis, deviated septum, and enlarged adenoids and tonsils. It is always best to treat the potential causes of lymphoid infection and inflammation, such as allergies or mouth breathing, before considering removal of the tissues, which provide a valuable first line of defense against invading pathogens.
- Surgical removal of restrictive tongue frenum.
- Orthodontic expansion of the maxillary and mandibular dental arches.
- Orofacial myofunctional therapy to train proper tongue position and swallowing.
- Training in proper naso-diaphragmatic breathing, including breathing exercises such as the Buteyko method.

Pediatric dentist and anthropologist Kevin Boyd, DDS, MSc, has uncovered published papers from the University of Michigan's archived dental library collection that clearly show that physicians, orthodontists, and general dentists from the mid-19th through the early 20th century were keenly aware of a possible connection between pediatric nasorespiratory dysfunction, somatic and neurological/neurobehavioral growth deficits, and dental malocclusion in the primary/early mixed dentition. Moreover, these medical and dental professionals of yesteryear were collaboratively exploring how preventing or reversing early malocclusion might also prevent or reverse associated systemic and neurological problems.

An open airway and proper breathing are foundational to oral and systemic health. Screening all children for disordered breathing should be a top priority in every dental practice.

<u>Airway/Breathing Disroders and TMD</u>
Young adults often present to the dental office with signs and symptoms that are categorized under the "basket syndrome" TMD. Common manifestations of TMD include sore muscles of

mastication, bruxism (clenching and/or grinding), morning headaches, joint soreness, joint clicking/locking, restricted range of mandibular movement, dental malocclusions, cervical neck problems, poor sleep quality, and chronic fatigue.

One of the pioneers in sleep medicine, Christian Guilleminault, MD, studied young, thin men and women who were exhausted despite regularly sleeping 8 hours and having sleep study results in the "normal" range.[4] In his classic experiment, he placed thin pressure sensors inside each patient's esophagus and measured pressures during sleep. All of the subjects had multiple episodes of only partial obstruction; however, they exhibited severe respiratory efforts that led to significantly negative pressures in the esophagus. After multiple episodes of labored breathing, patients would awaken from deep to light sleep, which is called an "arousal" in sleep medicine. Although the apneas and hypopneas among these patients were minimal, they experienced severely fragmented sleep. Guilleminault coined the term "UARS" to describe this common phenomenon.

In another Guilleminault study involving 30 subjects age 21 to 24 who were diagnosed with UARS, all reported chronic fatigue, 28 reported non-refreshing sleep, 26 reported disrupted nocturnal sleep, 29 reported daytime performance impairment, and 17 reported morning headaches.[5]

These are common complaints expressed when interviewing patients diagnosed with TMD as well. UARS and TMD can have many similar symptoms. In practice, it is not unusual to find patients who are suffering from both disorders simultaneously. When determining the appropriate treatment plan, it is important to clarify the cause and effect relationships that are resulting in the patient's symptoms.

Some patients with both TMD and airway/breathing disorders may actually suffer negative effects from traditional TMD therapy. Yves Gagnon, DMD, and Giles Lavigne, DMD, MSc, PhD, conducted a pilot study involving 10 subjects who were previously diagnosed with snoring and sleep apnea through polysomnography.[6] Each subject was fitted with a maxillary occlusal splint (ie, nightguard). After one week of wearing the splint to sleep each night, the participants underwent a new overnight polysomnography, during which the splint was worn. The results indicated that, with the splint in the mouth, the apnea-hypopnea index increased by approximately 50% in half of the subjects and the total time snoring while asleep was increased by 40% overall.

When airway/breathing disorders are present, including UARS and OSA, it is important to avoid prescribing overnight intraoral splint therapy that may crowd the tongue or allow the mandible to drop back during sleep.

Screening all TMD patients for disordered breathing should be a top priority in every dental practice.

Considerations for Middle-Aged Patients

Another segment that frequently suffers from airway and breathing disorders is the population of middle-aged men and women. For these patients, poor sleep, frequent sleep arousals, daytime fatigue, foggy thinking, early memory loss, tired eyes, bruxism, and gastric reflux can indicate the presence of an airway or breathing disorder. Research conducted at UCLA by Paul Macey, PhD, concluded that sleep apnea can take a toll on brain function[7]. Due to neurotransmitter imbalances, sleep apnea can result in poor concentration, difficulty with memory and decision-making, depression, and stress. There are two key neurotransmitters involved: gamma-aminobutyric acid (GABA) and glutamate. The neurotransmitter GABA acts as a brake pedal in the brain, producing a calming mood and helping to make endorphins, whereas the neurotransmitter glutamate acts as an accelerator in the brain, increasing when the brain is in a state of stress. Chronic high levels of glutamate can be toxic to nerves and neurons.

Sleep apnea may result in low levels of GABA and high levels of glutamate that can essentially produce brain damage. This is indicated by signs of memory loss and foggy thinking and may appear to mimic the early signs of Alzheimer's disease. The good news is that effective therapy can often reverse the damage. After less than one year of continuous positive airway pressure (CPAP) therapy, reversals attributed to increased oxygenation have been seen in brain scans. Millions of middle-aged men and women across the United States suffer from this reversible form of memory loss and brain damage, and dental professionals are perfectly positioned to screen and intervene. As such, screening all mature adults who snore or are overly tired for disordered breathing should be a top priority in every dental practice.

Conclusion

In October 2017, the American Dental Association (ADA) released a policy statement addressing dentistry's role in sleep-related breathing disorders. The policy encourages dental professionals to screen their patients for OSA, UARS, and other breathing disorders; advocates working with medical colleagues; and emphasizes the effectiveness of intraoral appliance therapy for treating patients with mild to moderate OSA and CPAP-intolerant patients with severe OSA. With the endorsement of the ADA, screening for and treating sleep-related breathing disorders has indeed become the newest focus of Integrated Dental Medicine.

* * *

NOTE: This article references different types of intraoral appliances – some which are helpful in cases of sleep-related breathing disorders and some which are not. For further information regarding different types of intraoral appliances, please see the "T.M.D. and Occlusion Disorders – Treatment" chapter in the *Great Imposer* section.

* * *

References

1. Major MP, El-Hakim H, Witmans M, et al. Adenoid hypertrophy in pediatric sleep disordered breathing and craniofacial growth: the emerging role of dentistry. *J Dent Sleep Med.* 2017; 5(4):83-87.
2. Zicari AM, Albani F, Ntrekou P, et al. Oral breathing and dental malocclusions. *Eur J Paediatr Dent.* 2009; 10(2):59-64.
3. DiFrancesco rC, Junqueira PA, Trezza PM. Improvement of bruxism after T & A surgery. *Int J Pediatr Otorhinolaryngol.* 2004;68(4):441-445.
4. Guilleminault C, Stoohs R, Clerk A, et al.. A cause of excessive daytime sleepiness. The upper airway resistance syndrome. *Chest.* 1993;104(3): 781–787.
5. Guilleminault C, Lopes MC, Hagen CC, et al. The cyclic alternating pattern demonstrates increased sleep instability and correlates with fatigue and sleepiness in adults with upper airway resistance syndrome. *Sleep.* 2007;30(5): 641-647.
6. Gagnon Y, Mayer P, Morisson F, et al. Aggravation of respiration disturbances by the use of an occlusal splint in apneic patients: a pilot study. *Int J Prosthodont.* 2004;17(4):447-453.
7. Perry, L. Sleep apnea takes a toll on brain function Page. http://newsroom.ucla.edu/releases/sleep- apnea-takes-a-toll-on-brain-function. Updated February, 11, 2016. Accessed November 22, 2017.

15. *THE SHIFT*: A PEDIATRIC PERSPECTIVE BY KEVIN BOYD, DDS, MS

Kevin Boyd, DDS, MS is a world renowned pediatric dentist from Chicago, Illinois, and a very special friend of mine. He has helped thousands of children suffering from a variety of developmental, breathing, and dental occlusion disabilities.

I am not a pediatric dentist. I have learned a lot about children though in studying Integrative Dental Medicine. We have briefly mentioned several signs and symptoms of airway and breathing dysfunction that may occur very early in life, even before and during birth. These can have very significant effects on complete health, both in childhood and later as adults. We are constantly surprised to find out just how early *"when"* may turn out to be for many people.

As a result, for all of us, *The Shift* is a work in progress, for a lifetime. There is so much to learn from the past and to discover in the future, regarding complete health. We must commit to critical thinking, grounded in two important questions: *"why"* and *"when"*.

For example, as we consider cardiovascular disease, we now know that the rupturing of unstable atherosclerotic plaque can cause acute cardiovascular events. We call these events "heart attacks" and "strokes." *Why* does atherosclerotic plaque occur? *Why* is it unstable? *Why* does it rupture? We discussed several of the known *"why"* answers when studying "The Great Fire."

Another important question is *"when"* does atherosclerotic plaque form? Many of us assume that vascular disease is a disease of adulthood. Is that true?

A study was conducted after the Korean and Vietnam Wars. 111 victims of non-cardiac trauma (mean age of 26 +/- 6 years), killed in battle, underwent pathologic examination of their coronary arteries, to estimate the presence and severity of coronary atherosclerosis. Signs of coronary atherosclerosis were seen in 78.3% of the total study group, with > 50% narrowing in 20.7% and > 75% narrowing in 9%.[109]

We learn from this study that *when* atherosclerosis begins is much younger than we would think. Cardiovascular disease can begin at a very young age due to a pro-inflammatory lifestyle and other factors.

The same can be true for the issues of dysfunctional breathing and breathing disordered sleep and their applications in the treatment of children. Even for practitioners who do not routinely treat children, it is important to be aware of how these principles can affect pediatric patients.

It is beyond the scope of this text to detail the complete range of applications that can be made for pediatric dentistry regarding this subject. Even so, it is exciting to think of the many ways children can benefit from an expanded awareness of and implementation of these principles. Practitioners who have the ability to screen children for possible airway issues (even if they partner with/refer to a pediatric dentist, pediatrician, ENT, etc. for treatment) can do a world of good in a child's life even by identifying possible warning signs of potential issues.

Furthermore, general dentists can educate their adult patients with young children regarding questions which they can discuss with their child's doctors. For example, three areas that could be discussed are (1) the role of breastfeeding in promoting good jaw development and tongue function, (2) childhood allergies affecting breathing, and (3) on-going research regarding breathing disordered sleep, including sleep apnea, in even very young children and how it might be related to SIDS and other complications. Additionally, as has been referenced, many children struggle with behavioral issues that are often labeled as ADHD, with treatment options that mostly involve medication. However, in recent years, many families have found that children who were diagnosed with ADHD actually suffer primarily from nasal allergies, dysfunctional mouth breathing, and poor sleep quality due to labored, interrupted breathing and sympathetic nervous system "fight or flight" responses, which were stimulating stress hormone release into the bloodstream. Resolving these issues has enabled countless children to regain their health.

The Foundation For Airway Health has produced a 5 minute YouTube video, entitled <u>Finding Connor Deegan,</u> presenting a dramatic testimonial of one child's airway and breathing concerns. It is highly recommended viewing for every parent, teacher, and pediatric health care provider.

For more on how *The Shift* affects our approach to pediatric dentistry, I have asked Dr. Boyd to share some of his perspective on this topic. Thank you, Kevin, for your invaluable insights!

* * *

> "...To know even one life has breathed easier because you have lived. This is to have succeeded."
> Ralph Waldo Emerson

In order to become a more complete and accurately-informed *pioneer* when embarking upon what DeWitt Wilkerson refers to as *Dentistry's Next Frontier*, clinicians, educators and researchers from *all* dental disciplines will need to acquire additional in-depth knowledge about topics that might on first glance seem apparently unrelated to dentistry. In addition to their dental school experience and subsequent post-graduate training and continuing education efforts, which are essential, they will also need to pursue topics that weren't a part of their core curriculum in dental school and in their post-graduate specialty training programs. For instance, when I was learning orthodontic cephalometric analysis during my Pediatric Dentistry residency training at the University of Iowa in the mid-1980s, we were not taught that certain malocclusion traits (such as retrognathia, deep overbites, anterior open-bites, obtuse naso-labial angles and anterior or posterior cross-bites, etc.) were often co-morbid with sleep-related breathing disorders such as snoring and pediatric obstructive sleep apnea. Additionally, when I first heard that dental caries (or, decay) had not appreciably appeared in the human skeletal record until our predecessors had discovered how to control agriculture and produce cereal grains, I didn't believe it was true. (It *is* true, by the way.) Then I was presented with reports showing that the appearance of the most frequently observed human malocclusion

(HM) phenotypes (such as retrusive, narrow and vertically-growing jaws, etc.) is an even more recent phenomenon than is caries and that malocclusion seldom occurred prior to the Industrial Revolution some 200-300 years ago. Again, I didn't believe it could be true (it is, by the way) – for the simple reason that it hadn't been taught to me in dental school or during my residency training program.

Referencing Dr. Dawson, in order to become what he would qualify as a ***complete dentist***, or what is otherwise described by him as a "**Masticatory System Physician**", practitioners *must* be willing to explore and eventually embrace novel and scientifically-supported concepts that at first glance might seem unrelated or irrelevant to their previous dental educational experiences and clinical practices. To that aim, Dr. Wilkerson invited me to write a brief ***pediatric perspective*** on The Shift. I will attempt to present the reader with a compelling argument in support of the reality that most of the adult oral (and systemic) health maladies addressed in Integrative Dental Medicine often can have their pathophysiological seeds sewn in childhood, and perhaps in some instances, even before birth.

The Masticatory Mechanism as a survival apparatus

Abilities for vocal communication, optimal breathing, hearing, chewing/swallowing and smelling are all essential to our survival. Together with the **speech mechanism**, the **respiratory mechanism**, the **auditory mechanism** and the **olfactory mechanism,** the **masticatory mechanism** is a member of the **Mammalian Survival Mechanism Complex** that *all* share the craniofacial complex as an essential structural and functional component. From dentistry's primal origins (described in an ancient Sumerian text detailing the misery wrought by tooth decay emanating from "tooth worms"), its main focus had been directed towards solving problems associated with treatment and prevention of pain originating from within the *masticatory system*. However, over recent decades the dental profession has discovered a new role for itself primarily within, but not limited to, the domain of the *respiratory system*. In this text, Dr. Wilkerson has referred to the work of Jim McNamara, DDS, PhD, MS, a distinguished academic orthodontist from the University of Michigan's Center for Human Growth and Development. He has alluded to a biological *hybrid* connection between the respiratory and masticatory systems when describing how, in Dr McNamara's words, "low tongue posture and dysfunctional swallowing patterns disrupt **cranio-facial-respiratory** growth and development, resulting in narrow maxillary arches, longer faces, tongue thrusts and crowded malocclusions."

As both the medical and dental literature dating back as far as the mid-19th century have documented, physicians and dentists working collaboratively have long understood about the harmful effects of chronic mouth-breathing in childhood and the intimate connection between growth and development of the craniofacial and respiratory complexes. Accordingly, what modern dentistry has apparently *discovered* is actually more accurately described as a *rediscovery* concerning their *new* role within the connected realm of airway, sleep and oral hygiene.

Dentistry's *New* Frontier – A Rediscovery

In 1913, E.A. Bogue, DDS, MD, a New York orthodontist and physician who published a series of several articles under the title of "Orthodontia of the Deciduous Teeth", stated *"In 1871, while spreading an upper arch, I believe I separated the two halves of the upper maxilla, in securing the upper width, thereby also enlarging the nasal passages,"* which later led him to propose that *"the purpose of rapid spreading is to enlarge the nasal passage and permit the nasal septum to straighten, not to correct the irregularities of the teeth."* Furthermore he said that *"the correction of impending irregularities by means of the deciduous teeth, when the child is not more than five or six years of age, is the most important factor in modern orthodontia."* As radiography technology was not yet available to verify his findings, Dr. Bogue described his observation of palate 'spreading' as being a *belief* that had likely been based upon his knowledge of human anatomy combined with what he'd observed in the improved naso-respiratory competence of children whose palates he had *spread* under his watchful eye. Furthermore, what Bogue described as *"impending irregularities by means of the deciduous teeth"* was likely his own wording for what had been described by E.H. Angle in the late 19th century when arguing against those who contended that (1) there is no relationship between the mouth breather and deformed arches; and (2) there is no connection between the morphology of the deciduous arch and that of the subsequent permanent arch – to which Dr. Angle responded *"any class of deformity of the second set, can be found in the first dentition."*

Rapid maxillary expansion and other validated dentofacial orthopedic treatment regimens of maxillary and mandibular arch development in three planes of space are increasingly being utilized as primary interventions in the treatment of pediatric patients. They are also being used as augmentative strategies alongside other medical and surgical efforts aimed at preventing, reversing or controlling/mitigating myriad negative somatic and neurological health consequences associated with specific constrictive and retrusive malocclusion phenotypes of the craniofacial complex and other survival complexes. Impairments in speech, hearing, vision, sleep, respiration, olfaction, mastication, and TMJ function (and other medical/dental concerns equally important to *quality of life*) can be associated with retrusive and constrictive malocclusion phenotypes at *any* stage of a person's lifetime. Conversely, they can often be *mitigated* by appropriately timed and applied orthodontic and dentofacial orthopedic intervention strategies – especially when addressed in childhood. Therefore, it is becoming increasingly apparent that inaction will *not* be an option for any practitioner striving to be a *Complete Dentist* and *Masticatory System Physician*.

Even when a *Complete Dentist* might not be inclined to actually *treat* children in his or her clinical practice, merely asking an adult patient a few important questions about physically and behaviorally-related sleep/airway issues can be helpful in identifying children who could already have (or later be at risk for developing) a sleep-airway disorder. These children might be their own, or they might be a grandchild or great-grandchild or a niece or nephew. Opening the door for such conversations can have a vast impact on countless children's lives.

On a closing note, in an address read before the E.H. Angle Society of Orthodontia in 1933 and published in the journal *The Angle Orthodontist*, orthodontist L.G. Singleton, DDS, contended that *"it is from the human side of orthodontia that the urge rises to harken to the appeal of the pedodontist. These specialists feel that the orthodontist, who examines the teeth of children from three to five years of age and presents to the parents a picture of incipient malocclusion, is not rendering his full duty to society if he has nothing better to offer than recommendations of delay until the malocclusion becomes objectively apparent when procedures of a mechanical nature may be instituted to correct the defect. Parents and dentists, too, want to know what is the matter with the natural courses of growth and development in children. We criticize the dentist for standing by until the dental organs actually break down before measures are adopted for prevention, but we do not even suggest a remedy for incipient malocclusion nor intimate that some obscure involvement of the biological organization may be operating to defeat the normal course of physical welfare."* Dr. Singleton continued, *"Every orthodontist should have continual opportunity to examine the mouths of very young children and witness the appeal of mothers for a more hopeful outlook regarding the mouths of their progeny."* In summarizing his address, Dr. Singleton stated, *"If Dr. Angle were here today, I can imagine him saying that a sufficient number of appliances for making any form of tooth movement have been devised and are at our disposal. He might also state that malocclusion is being anticipated five or six years before it actually occurs, but he certainly would not advise us to sit down and wait until the defects become entirely objective, so that these appliances could be used."* In his conclusion Singleton emphatically proclaimed, *"The problems of growth and development in infancy and juvenility should be attacked with vigor. The appeal of the children's dentist should receive a response, and the anxiety of the mothers who present their children for infantile diagnosis should be satisfied. The orthodontist should be no more be excused from his responsibility to society in making a more thorough investigation of the etiology of incipient malocclusion than the dentist should be relieved of his efforts to prevent dental caries by means of dietetic or prophylactic measures."*

When the above comments by Dr. Singleton were made, it had not yet been established that specific regimens of orthodontic and dentofacial orthopedic interventional strategies could often confer tremendous therapeutic outcomes for young children afflicted with co-morbid malocclusion and systemic disease. Keeping this in mind, it is clear that, like Peter Dawson and his protégé DeWitt Wilkerson, Lawrence Singleton seems also to have been way *ahead of his time.*

Kevin L. Boyd, Pedodontist
Chicago

* * *

Kevin is a board-certified pediatric dentist practicing in Chicago. He is an attending instructor in the residency-training program in Pediatric Dentistry at Lurie Children's Hospital where he additionally serves as a dental consultant to the Sleep Medicine service. Also is also a teaching faculty member for the Dawson Academy.

Prior to completing his dental degree from Loyola University's Chicago College of Dentistry in 1986, he obtained an advanced degree (MSc) in Human Nutrition from Michigan State University where his research interests were focused on unhealthy eating, dental caries, obesity and diabetes. Kevin attended the University of Iowa for his post-graduate residency training where he received a Certificate in Pediatric Dentistry in 1988. Dr. Boyd has served on the teaching faculties of the University of Illinois College of Dentistry, the University of Michigan's College of Dentistry, the University of Chicago Hospital, Rush Presbyterian-St. Luke's Medical Center and Michael Reese Hospital as an attending clinical instructor.

He is currently completing pre-requisite course work in Biological Anthropology at Northeastern Illinois University in preparation for graduate study and research in the newly emerging discipline of Evolutionary Medicine. His clinical focus is centered upon prevention of oral and systemic disease through promotion of healthy breathing and eating; his primary research interest is in the area of infant/early childhood feeding practices and how they impact palatal-facial development, naso-respiratory competence and neuro-cognitive development. He is currently a visiting Scholar at U. Pennsylvania doing research in the areas of anthropology and orthodontics.

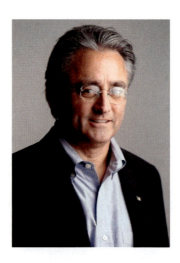

Part IV:
The Great Imposer
T.M.D. and Occlusion Disorders

16. T.M.D. & OCCLUSION DISORDERS AND INTEGRATIVE DENTAL MEDICINE

A Central Theme of Integrative Dental Medicine is TMD & Occlusion Disorders.

An "imposer" is one who intrudes on others, taking unfair advantage of them and misusing them. Since 1982, I've seen it happen over and over again, hundreds of times, in my clinical practice – weary patients coming to see us from near and far, who are hurting and discouraged. They arrive sore, tired, headachy, misunderstood and generally beaten up, both physically and emotionally by that *Great Imposer*, the one that we in dentistry and medicine call "TMD".

Who or what is this villainous imposer – TMD? **T**emporo-**M**andibular **D**isorder is a term that first received attention in the late 1970s. Anatomically, the hinge connection between the upper jaw (**T**emporal bone) and lower jaw (**M**andibular bone), right in front of the ear on both sides of the face, is called the **T**emporo-**M**andibular **J**oint (**T.M.J. or, "TMJoint"**). When the joint is uncomfortable or damaged, medically speaking, that represents a true "TMJ" problem. Through the years, the description has become much more vague. We frequently hear people describe themselves as a "TMJ patient", who present with chief complaints of clenching & grinding their teeth; bite problems; sore muscles of the jaw, neck, back, shoulders, face and forehead; headaches; earaches; vertigo; tinnitus; poor sleep; fibromyalgia; chronic fatigue syndrome; and poor concentration. Basically, any problem above the shoulders is often labeled by many, including doctors, as "TMD". It has become a basket term for many different problems in the head, face and neck.

"T.M.D." really describes a "syndrome", which is defined as a set of medical signs and symptoms that are correlated with each other. A syndrome is not specific to only one disease. Dr. Pete Dawson likes to point out during his lectures that saying you have "TMJ" is like saying you have a case of "elbow" or "stomach". You get the point! This is very important because it means **T.M.D. is a description, not a diagnosis**. A diagnosis is based on finding the specific source of the problem. A diagnosis explains *"WHY"* someone has TMD symptoms.

The bottom line is that we have a big problem. Millions of people are imposed upon by this Great Imposer, TMD. It is poorly understood by most doctors, poorly diagnosed by most, and most often empirically treated by trial and error. Sadly we see patients presenting with severely-damaged TMJoints who have been told that their TMD problem is primarily driven by psychological, hormonal, and emotional stress issues. Can you imagine telling someone with a torn ACL in their knee that their problem is mainly family stress and the cure is an anti-depressant prescription and counseling? That happens with TMD all the time! This needs to change.

The Integrative Dental Medicine model addresses TMD and Dental Occlusion as a major focus. For over 50 years, Dr. Pete Dawson's educational model, the "Concepts of Complete Dentistry," has strongly emphasized that dentists are the physicians of the masticatory system. TMD is primarily a masticatory system disorder. Dr. Dawson's textbook <u>Functional Occlusion: From TMJ to Smile Design</u> is the definitive resource on this subject.

TMD is primarily a problem of the TMJoints, dental occlusion (bite), muscles, CNS, airway and cervical region of the spine. To address these areas of focus, we will next direct our attention to the Integrative Dental Medicine (IDM) Checklist to organize our discussion of **TMD-Occlusion Disorders**.

Let's follow the IDM Checklist sequentially as follows:
1. **History:** Signs & Symptoms
2. **Evaluation:** Clinical Signs
3. **Screening & Testing**
4. **Treatment**

	TMD/Occlusion Disorders		
History *Signs & Symptoms*	Joint Discomfort	−	+
	Popping/Clicking	−	+
	Limited Opening	−	+
	Sore Muscles	−	+
	Nerve Pain	−	+
	Bruxism (Grind or Clench)	−	+
	Poor Bite	−	+
	Worn Teeth	−	+
	Tongue Thrust	−	+
	Crooked Teeth	−	+
Evaluation *Clinical signs*	ROM Atypical	−	+
	Muscle Palpation	−	+
	Joint Palpation	−	+
	TMJ Load Testing	−	+
	CR to MIP Slide	−	+
Screening & Testing	Doppler Auscultation	−	+
	Imaging (CBCT/MRI)	−	+
	Dawson Photo Series		
	Diagnostic Study Models		
	Dawson Wizard Analysis		
Differential Conclusion	**− Negative**	**+ Positive**	

TMD/Occlusion Disorders

Phase 1 / Phase 2

↓

Phase 1
- Appropriate Orthotic
- Anti-inflammatory Meds/Diet
- Physical Therapy prn
- C1/C2 Therapy prn
- Injection Therapy prn
- Surgical Referral prn

Phase 2
- Definitive Occlusal Therapy
- Post Tx Orthotic prn

> "The clinical management of the dentition comprises the major day-to-day duties of the practicing dentist. Management of the masticatory system, however, does not end with providing the presence, normal structural form, proper alignment, and harmonious occlusion of teeth. The dentition proper represents only the working ends of the apparatus, the tools by which mastication is accomplished, not the system itself.
>
> Prehension, incising, grinding, and swallowing foods are vital body functions. The same is true of respiration and speech, in which the oral structures participate importantly. The mechanisms of oral communication and orofacial expression make social intercourse pleasant and profitable. Chronologically, the oral cavity is the initial organ of sexual expression and throughout life never completely loses this emotional association. The mouth and orofacial structures constitute a region of unusual emotional significance that remains sensitive to threat and responsive to clinical management.
>
> The masticatory system is a complex one indeed. During the many patterns of action required for the preparation of food prior to deglutition, the intricate mechanics involved in the articulation of tooth surfaces (occlusal function) is a study in itself. Mastication calls on an integrated and precisely coordinated biologic system of bones, joints, ligaments, muscles, vessels, nerves, and glands that extends from the lips to the larynx and from the teeth to the esophagus. This system can be affected by disorders and complications without number."
>
> Welden E. Bell, DDS, FACD (1986)
> <u>Temporomandibular Disorders</u>

17. T.M.D. & OCCLUSION DISORDERS – HISTORY: SIGNS AND SYMPTOMS

T.M.D. and Occlusion Disorders
History: *Signs & Symptoms*
1. Joint Discomfort

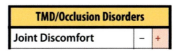

The Temporomandibular Joint (TM Joint) is a complex and very beautifully designed structure. It is important to understand the anatomy and function of the joint, in order to understand problems of the joint that cause discomfort. Let's build the essential form and function of the TM Joint:

- **The Bones**: The upper bone (temporal bone) forms a fixed socket (fossa) and a forward gliding ramp (eminence). The lower bone (mandible) has a ball (condyle) that sits in the upper socket. When opening the mouth, the condyle both rotates in the fossa (rotation), as well as glides forward and downward along the eminence ramp (translation).
- **The Disk**: The disk is a bow-tie shaped soft tissue pad that sits between the ball and socket. The disk is composed of dense fibro-cartilaginous tissue that is avascular and non-innervated in its load-bearing center portion. It acts as a shock absorber that protects the bones from wear and tear. The ball sits in the middle of the disk.

- **The Ligaments:** Ligaments are fibrous bands that connect bones together. In this joint, ligaments on the inward and outward sides join the upper and lower bones to each other (the medial & lateral capsular ligaments). There is a secondary ligament that joins the disk to the ball on the inside and outside (the medial and lateral diskal ligaments) so that the disk can rotate on top of the ball like a bucket handle or rotating bonnet. There is also a ligament attached to the back of the disk that tethers it to the neck of the lower bone behind the ball (the posterior ligament). This non-elastic ligament normally prevents the disk from shifting forward out of position and moving off the top of the ball. Elastic fibers bind the disk to the upper bone as well (the superior elastic stratum). The temporomandibular ligament is like a hammock, with the joint above it. It pushes the jaw forward on opening, in order to prevent cutting off the airway.
- **Superior Elastic Stratum or Retrodiskal Tissue:** Above and behind the disk and condyle is tissue that contains both nerves and blood vessels. This tissue engorges with blood when the jaw opens wide and the condyle glides down and forward. Like a sponge, it swells with fluid upon opening and compresses back down upon closing the mouth. This is an arterio-venous shunt, that fills and evacuates, preventing a vacuum in the joint on function.
- **Synovium:** There is both lubrication and nourishment provided to the disk and bone surfaces by the slippery synovial fluid that is produced so that it flows both over and under the disk. This fluid if the "WD-40" of the joint.
- **The Capsule:** The joint is a closed system with a paper bag-like envelope of soft connective tissue around it. This capsule prevents synovial fluids from leaking out.
- **Muscle:** There is muscle (the lateral pterygoid) attached to the condyle and usually the disk. This muscle pulls the condyle forward and toward the midline of the face when it contracts. It can also help position the disk on opening and closing.

The Shift

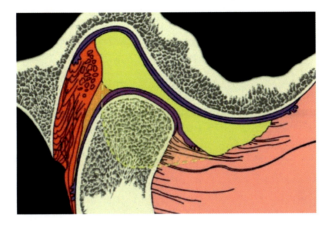

Figure[110]: The Temporomandibular Joint (TMJ) has a unique design.

What happens when a joint has discomfort?

Understanding the anatomy, physiology and function of the joint should help explain the reasons behind dysfunction and discomfort. It's important to understand that discomfort in the joint vicinity can come from either around the joint (outside of the closed capsular tissues) or inside the joint (inside the closed capsular tissues). Sometimes discomfort can come from both places at the same time. We divide TMJoint region discomfort into the following basic categories:

- **Extracapsular:** primarily muscle discomfort, especially from overusing the lateral pterygoid; bruxing (clenching or grinding); sore/inflamed temporalis, masseter, and medial pterygoid muscles; and referred pain from the anterior & posterior cervical (neck) muscles.
- **Intracapsular:** primarily disk misalignment, traumatic injury, inflammation, nerve pain, edema/effusion/fluid pressure, pressure on the retrodiskal nerves and blood vessels, bone & joint arthritides, and growths in the joint.
- **Combination – Extracapsular & Intracapsular:** muscle, inflammation, intracapsular damage or disease, overloading work of the muscles with damaging pressure inside the joint.

Specific tests will be described to help differentiate these sources of discomfort.

T.M.D. and Occlusion Disorders
History: *Signs & Symptoms*
2. Popping/Clicking/Limited Opening

The earliest sign of a problem in the temporomandibular joint (TMJ) is often the awareness of joint noises, when opening and closing the mouth.

TMD/Occlusion Disorders		
Joint Discomfort	−	+
Popping/Clicking	−	+
Limited Opening	−	+

What causes the jaw to pop or click?

Typically, when a TMJoint "pops" or "clicks", the soft tissue disk integrity is disturbed. If the attachment of the disk to the condyle becomes loose or detached, the disk can move off the top of the condyle, which is described as a **disk displacement.** Disks usually displace off the front end of the condyle, which is described as an **anterior disk displacement**. When opening, the condyle glides forward and slips back under the displaced disk, with a "click" or "pop". That is described as **recapturing the disk** or a **disk displacement with reduction**. This may happen again on closing, as the disk clicks off again, which is described as a **reciprocal click**. This can represent a **partial disk displacement** that may not get worse, or the beginning of a progressive problem which may lead to a **complete disk displacement** or **disk displacement without reduction** (also called a **closed lock**). If the disk becomes completely out of position, it's comparable to losing the disk pads in a car's brakes, resulting in future extensive internal wear and tear and inflammatory **osteoarthritis.**

Clicks can also occur in the presence of other pathology in the joint, such as bony benign tumors, called **osteochondromas.**

Limited Opening

When a **disk is displaced** in front of the condyle, either partially or completely, it can affect opening and closing movement. The jaw may open with a wiggle as the disk clicks back into alignment on opening, and wiggle again on closing, as it slips back out of position. If a displaced disk becomes misshapen, it can bunch up and create a "speed bump" in front of the condyle, which may limit opening. Sometimes there is scar tissue in the damaged joint, resulting in **fibrous and boney ankylosis**, which further limits free jaw movement. Very limited opening is referred to as a **closed lock**. Clicks can also occur without any pathology. When the eminence (ramp) of the socket is short, sometimes the condyle will glide forward and pop around the corner, resulting in a click. This is a type of joint dislocation, or **subluxation.** This click is described as an **eminence click**. The treatment for an eminence click in most cases is quite simple – just don't open that wide!

In some instances, such as when taking a big bite of a sandwich, the joint will dislocate (or "sublux") and result in an **open** lock, whereby the mouth is stuck open. This can be a frightening experience, but is usually minimally painful and without accompanying long-term damage. It may require manual manipulation of the jaw back into the socket to close the mouth.

T.M.D. and Occlusion Disorders
History: *Signs & Symptoms*
3. Sore Muscles

TMD/Occlusion Disorders		
Joint Discomfort	−	+
Popping/Clicking	−	+
Limited Opening	−	+
Sore Muscles	−	+

The muscles evaluated when considering possible T.M.D. and Occlusion Disorders consist of:
- **Posterior neck muscles**
- **Anterior neck muscles**
- **Elevator muscles of the face**
- **Positioner muscles of the jaw**

Muscles are most often sore due to overuse, so we want to understand when a muscle would be overused and, therefore, sore.
- **Posterior neck muscles** (trapezius, splenius capitis) can be sore for several reasons: a back or cervical (neck) problem creating a splinting/tightening of the muscles in a bracing activity; a forward head posture due to chest breathing and airway disturbances; whiplash-type injuries; and forward head posturing due to painful TMJs. Posterior neck muscle pain can radiate or refer pain up the back of the head, over the crown and down the front to the temples. This is a very common cause of temporal headaches after neck injuries.
- **Anterior neck muscles** (sternocleidomastoid, digastric, mylohyoid) are similar to posterior neck muscles and can be sore because of clenching, grinding and forward head posturing. They can refer pain across the TMJs, lower jaw, cheeks and temples.

- **Elevator muscles of the face** (superficial and deep masseter, temporalis, medial pterygoid) will often be sore when a patient is clenching and/or grinding. Obstructive Sleep Apnea (OSA) may potentially stimulate clenching activity during sleep to elevate the hyoid bone (Adam's apple), if it will improve airway space in the throat region.
- **Positioner muscles of the jaw** (lateral pterygoid) will be sore when the jaw is chronically positioning forward and/or laterally. The lateral pterygoid muscles are particularly hyperactive with bite misalignments, in individuals who hold their teeth together for prolonged periods of time, during the daytime or while sleeping at night. As mentioned, OSA and UARS may potentially create a forward jaw posturing in an attempt to open the airway.

Referred pain from muscles is very common. Janet Travell, MD, and David Simons, MD, did landmark work in the 1960s, mapping the referral patterns around the body. Their books, Myofascial Pain and Dysfunction: the Trigger Point Manual and the Travell and Simons' Trigger Point Flip Charts, are classic works. They demonstrate the very common referral patterns from the muscles of the cervical region of the spine to the three divisions of the trigeminal nerve – the upper and lower jaws (including teeth) and forehead regions. It is important to keep the possibility of referred pain in mind when evaluating TMD patients with a history of back and neck trauma or other issues. Muscles which are injured or overused may also demonstrate specific "hotspots" upon palpation, described by Travell and Simons as **trigger-points.** These represent specific muscle fibers that are inflamed, damaged and very sore to touch.

T.M.D. and Occlusion Disorders
History: *Signs & Symptoms*
4. Nerve Pain

TMD/Occlusion Disorders		
Joint Discomfort	-	+
Popping/Clicking	-	+
Limited Opening	-	+
Sore Muscles	-	+
Nerve Pain	-	+

Within the category of "Referred Pain", an overlapping condition is "Nerve Pain". When thinking about "pain", it's important to realize that sources of pain (whether from injuries/trauma to muscles, joints, or nerves) can sometimes produce a pain response which increases and spreads over time.

Neurologic pain, from excitement of the Sympathetic Nervous System, can become chronic and produce an elevated pain response, even if the original source of pain is reduced or eliminated. This is common with chronic pain patients.

Complex Regional Pain Syndrome (CRPS or "crips"):
The Mayo Clinic reports that "the cause of Complex Regional Pain Syndrome isn't completely understood. It's thought to be caused by an injury to or an abnormality of the peripheral and central nervous systems. CRPS typically occurs as a result of trauma or an injury."[111] They note that the "signs and symptoms of Complex Regional Pain Syndrome include:

- Continuous burning or throbbing pain, usually in the jaw, neck, shoulder, arm, leg, hand or foot
- Sensitivity to touch or cold
- Swelling of the painful area
- Changes in skin temperature – alternating between sweaty and cold
- Changes in skin color, ranging from white and mottled to red or blue
- Changes in skin texture, which may become tender, thin or shiny in the affected area
- Changes in hair and nail growth
- Joint stiffness, swelling and damage
- Muscle spasms, tremors, weakness and loss (atrophy)
- Decreased ability to move the affected body part" [112]

There are two known types of CRPS, with similar signs and symptoms but with different etiologies:

*Type 1 – Reflex Sympathetic Dystrophy (RSD): This type occurs after an illness or injury without direct damage to the nerves in the affected area. About 90 percent of people with CRPS are Type 1.

*Type 2 – Once referred to as "Causalgia", this type has similar symptoms to Type 1. Type 2 CRPS follows a distinct nerve injury.[113]

Chronic TMD patients, especially with significant joint involvement, frequently experience an elevated degree of pain, which is at times debilitating. The pain may radiate, for example, from the joint, face, and neck and out into the arm.

I'll never forget seeing a dear lady who was referred to me for an evaluation. She had come from Alabama with her husband because of her TMD/chronic pain concern. During our clinical evaluation, I had her open and close her mouth and palpated her head and neck muscles. As I was palpating her joints, she said, "There goes my ear again." Her husband smiled and said, "You won't believe this; it happens a lot." Within a few seconds, her right ear turned beet red and a flushed appearance extended down the right side of her neck. Mark Piper, MD, DMD, was consulted. He confirmed a diagnosis of CRPS. Stimulation of the region during our exam had provoked a SNS response of blood engorgement of her right ear and neck. We hear reports of these types of responses occurring in many situations, such as driving a car with the window down, exposure to cold weather, etc.

T.M.D. and Occlusion Disorders
History: *Signs & Symptoms*
5. Bruxism (Grind or Clench)

TMD/Occlusion Disorders		
Joint Discomfort	−	+
Popping/Clicking	−	+
Limited Opening	−	+
Sore Muscles	−	+
Nerve Pain	−	+
Bruxism (Grind or Clench)	−	+

This subject is one of great discussion and much current research. The International Classification of Sleep Disorders (ICSD) describes bruxism as *"a repetitive jaw-muscle activity characterized by clenching or grinding of the teeth and/or by bracing or thrusting of the mandible"*.[114]

Clenching and grinding are commonly related to the following: bite problems; airway issues; neurologic concerns such as Parkinson's bruxism; certain antipsychotic and anti-depressant medications such as selective serotonin reuptake inhibitors (SSRIs) like Prozac (fluoxetine), Zoloft (sertraline), and Paxil (paroxetine); illegal drugs such as cocaine, ecstasy, methamphetamine, and other amphetamines; psychosomatic anxiety; systemic stress in the Sympathetic Nervous System (SNS); alcohol consumption; cigarette smoking; caffeine; and fatigue.

A highly respected researcher, clinician and personal friend, Jeff Rouse, DDS, describes the "Bruxism Triad", in which a relationship has been established between bruxism, sleep disturbances and gastric reflux. Rouse reports, *"It has been demonstrated that a majority of dental patients present with tooth wear. However, sleep bruxers are a unique subset. Sleep bruxism is reflectively triggered by sleep micro-arousals. These disturbances in the sleep patterns are a natural occurrence but can also be caused by* *any **disruption of airway patency or a significant reduction of esophageal pH**. The bruxism triad is an attempt to explain the interlocking nature of bruxism, breathing, and erosion. These patients suffer a significant loss of tooth structure and restoration damage due to the increase in friction due to poor lubrication and roughened surfaces."*[115]

T.M.D. and Occlusion Disorders
History: *Signs & Symptoms*
6. Poor Bite/Malocclusion

TMD/Occlusion Disorders		
Joint Discomfort	−	+
Popping/Clicking	−	+
Limited Opening	−	+
Sore Muscles	−	+
Nerve Pain	−	+
Bruxism (Grind or Clench)	−	+
Poor Bite	−	+

To understand a poor bite, we must first understand a healthy bite relationship. There are two components to a "good bite":

1. **C.R. = M.I.P.**
   o When the muscles close the mouth, both TMJoints are seated and centered in their sockets. This is described in dental terminology as "Centric Relation" (C.R.).[116] Centric Relation is defined as the relationship between the mandible to the maxilla when the properly aligned condyle-disk assemblies are in the most superior position against the eminentiae (when the healthy ball is fully seated in the socket). When the upper and lower teeth mesh together completely, it is described in dental terminology as "Maximum Intercuspation Position" (M.I.P.). The first component of an ideal bite is that C.R. = M.I.P. When the joints are fully seated by the elevator muscles of the jaw, the bite should be fully seated too, with all teeth touching evenly at the same time.
   o When the teeth do not contact evenly when the joints are fully seated the result is a "hit and slide" in the bite. The teeth skid against each other, creating wear and tear over time. This can also create what is described as "occluso-muscle disharmony", in which the elevator muscles (those pulling the jaw up) and the positioner muscles (those pulling the jaw forward) are contracting at the same time. When this occurs in combination with chronic clenching (holding the teeth together), the muscles can become fatigued and sore.

2. **Anterior Guidance:**
    - How should the teeth touch when rubbing in or out – left, right and forward from centric relation? Many studies have reported that it's best to have only front teeth (anterior teeth) touch, with the back teeth (posterior teeth) completely separating when the jaw is moving in any of these directions.[117]
    - Electromyographic (EMG) studies of muscle activity have shown that the strong closing muscles tend to largely shut off when the back teeth are not touching.[118]
    - The important concept here is as follows: muscle activity is greatly decreased when only front teeth touch while rubbing the teeth together in any direction. Therefore, there is (1) much less wear and tear, if any, on the front teeth, and (2) no wear and tear on the back teeth, which don't touch at all. **Anterior Guidance** describes the goal of having only front teeth touch in all jaw movements, in order to protect the teeth and muscles and to reduce loading of the TMJoints.

Therefore, a poor bite can be created by:
- unseated or unhealthy TMJoints
- uneven contacts of all teeth in Centric Relation (with the joints fully seated)
- poor guidance on front teeth, when rubbing the teeth together
- heavy contact of back teeth, when rubbing the teeth together

A poor bite may demonstrate excessively worn teeth; loose or fractured teeth; drifting and shifting teeth; sore or sensitive teeth; impacted or partially-erupted wisdom teeth; crowded teeth; higher periodontal risk; sore muscles; clenching and grinding habits; headaches; and sore joints. These may be accompanied by TMJoint instability, nasal allergies, mouth breathing, tongue-tie, tongue thrusting, sleep disorders, swallowing disorders, gastric reflux, and problems of the cervical region of the spine.

A poor bite is a distortion of normal growth and development. There are several factors that influence a poor bite:

* **Joint health** is a major factor of bite stability or instability.

Mark Piper, MD, DMD, has been a true pioneer in temporomandibular diagnosis and surgical intervention. I have been privileged to work closely with Mark in St. Petersburg, Florida since 1983, witnessing hundreds of patients whose lives he has dramatically impacted. In 1992, he participated in a particularly significant study with Drs. Schellhas, Bessette and Wilkes.[119] Regarding subjects with retruded lower jaws (mandibular retrognathia) they reported,

> *One-hundred consecutive orthognathic surgery candidates with mandibular retrusion were selected for retrospective analysis. Patients had undergone imaging studies that included magnetic resonance imaging (MRI) of both temporomandibular joints to assess the presence or absence, stage, and activity of suspected internal derangement(s). Patients were divided into stable and unstable deformity groups based on the presence or absence of change in their facial contour and/or occlusal disturbances in the 24 months prior to evaluation. Each of the 58 unstable and 30 of 42 stable patients were found to have internal derangements of at least one temporomandibular joint. The degree of joint degeneration directly paralleled the severity of retrognathia in most cases. We concluded that* **temporomandibular joint internal derangement is common in cases of mandibular retrusion and leads to the facial morphology in a high percentage of patients.**[120]

88 out of 100 subjects in this study, who presented as retrognathic and with Class II malocclusions, were off the disk on one or both sides.[121]

Joint problems can arise for many reasons, including genetic anamolies; macro-trauma (from injuries, such as a fall or blow to the chin, or whiplash from a motor vehicle accident); micro-trauma (from years of overloading the joints through clenching or grinding the teeth); hormonal imbalances (creating inflammation and hard/soft tissue changes); rheumatoid and osteo-arthritis; and pathology (such as cysts and tumors). All of these can negatively impact the bite.

Stable temporomandibular joints are a primary foundation for bite stability. Unstable temporomandibular joints are a primary cause of poor bites.

Earl Pound, DDS (1901-1979), a pioneering prosthodontist and educator, often likened an ideal dental occlusion to an inverted tripod or three-legged stool: two legs are the fully seated temporo-mandibular joints, and the third leg is the fully seated bite. This creates a balance of forces and neuromuscular harmony. When the two joints are not fully seated or are damaged and unstable, the bite will also be unstable. The result is a poor bite.

It is impossible to have unstable TMJoint conditions and have a stable dental occlusion.

* <u>Genetic predisposition.</u> This generally-accepted premise may be a weaker link than other factors.

Lisa King, DDS, MS, Edward Harris, PhD, and Elizabeth Tolley, PhD, studied 104 pairs of siblings, prior to their having any orthodontic treatment. They report,

> *In this selected series of overt malocclusions, heritability estimates for craniometric variables were significantly lower than in a comparable series of adolescents with naturally occurring good occlusions, whereas heritability estimates for occlusal variations (e.g., rotations, crossbites, displacements) were significantly higher. This vindicates the clinical perception that siblings often present with similar malocclusions. We propose that the substantive measures of inter-sibling similarity for occlusal traits reflect similar responses to* **environmental factors** *common to both siblings. That is, given genetically influenced facial types and growth patterns, siblings are likely to respond to environmental factors (e.g.,* **reduced masticatory stress, chronic mouth breathing**) *in similar fashions.* **Malocclusions appear to be acquired, but the fundamental genetic control of craniofacial form often diverts siblings into comparable physiologic responses leading to development of similar malocclusions.**[122]

* <u>Environmental factors</u> can be involved, including nasal allergies, Upper Airway Resistance (UAR), and resulting mouth breathing. Much more research is needed to verify that airway and sleep disorders drive sleep bruxism. In reviewing the constantly-growing body of scientific information, Gary Klasser, DMD, Nathalie Rei, DMD, and Gilles Lavigne, DMD, PhD, summarize as follows:

> *The role of respiration in the genesis of sleep bruxism-RMMA (rhythmic masticatory muscle activity) is not fully understood, but recent evidence suggests that it may be relevant in some patients. RMMA tends to occur with large breaths, and oral appliances used to improve airway patency help to reduce sleep bruxism-RMMA frequency. However, before dental practitioners assume a direct role of respiration or a cause-and-*

effect relation between breathing disorders and sleep bruxism, more robust evidence is required.[123]

* Tongue-tie/Ankyloglossia

There appears to be a significant change in "neutral zone" muscle forces, between the tongue pressures forward and outward and the cheek and lip pressures inward, when the tongue is significantly tethered to the floor of the mandible. This change in neutral zone forces can potentially contribute to cranio-facial-respiratory changes, teeth crowding and a poor bite. This is supported by the findings of Drs. Srinivasan and Chitharanjan, researchers at Sri Ramachandra University, Porur, Chennai, India, who report the following regarding their tongue-tie (ankyloglossia) studies: "maxillary intermolar width and maxillary intercanine width are significantly reduced in subjects with ankyloglossia, suggesting maxillary constriction." Additionally they found that "overbite and mandibular plane angle changed with the severity of ankyloglossia."[124]

In summary, tongue-tie restricts the ability of the tongue to fill the roof of the mouth. Therefore, with reduced tongue pressure influencing the development of the upper bone arch and subsequent erupting teeth positions, the upper arch is narrower and the teeth are more constricted — resulting in more crowding and a poor bite.

T.M.D. and Occlusion Disorders
History: *Signs & Symptoms*
7. Worn Teeth

TMD/Occlusion Disorders		
Joint Discomfort	−	+
Popping/Clicking	−	+
Limited Opening	−	+
Sore Muscles	−	+
Nerve Pain	−	+
Bruxism (Grind or Clench)	−	+
Poor Bite	−	+
Worn Teeth	−	+

Worn teeth occur for several significant reasons, including the following:

- **Malocclusion**, with a failure to have evenly-distributed bite forces in the seated joint position (Centric Relation) and poor anterior guidance, will often result in pathologic wear on the teeth that touch excessively and unevenly.
- **Bruxism**, due to dental malocclusions, sleep micro-arousals, airway obstructions, lowered esophageal pH, neurologic disorders, medication and drug side effects.
- **Temporomandibular Joint instability,** such as a displaced disk or degenerative arthritis, will often create retrognathia and

a poor bite, in which the back teeth touch heavily and the front teeth may not touch at all (anterior open bite). The back teeth will subsequently wear excessively.

- **Gastric Reflux and eating disorders** can result in stomach acids damaging teeth, both on the biting surfaces and their side walls. The resulting wear produces cupped out incisal and occlusal tooth surfaces, which can erode through enamel and deep into dentin. Buccal and lingual tooth surfaces can also demonstrate severe changes on their smooth walls, penetrating through enamel and root cementum.

T.M.D. and Occlusion Disorders
History: *Signs & Symptoms*
8. Tongue Thrust

TMD/Occlusion Disorders		
Joint Discomfort	−	+
Popping/Clicking	−	+
Limited Opening	−	+
Sore Muscles	−	+
Nerve Pain	−	+
Bruxism (Grind or Clench)	−	+
Poor Bite	−	+
Worn Teeth	−	+
Tongue Thrust	−	+

A tongue thrust is the positioning of the tongue between the teeth on swallowing, usually forward between the front teeth. Lateral tongue thrusts can occur between back teeth as well. Tongue thrusts can adversely affect the position of the teeth and produce a poor bite. A person swallows from 1,200 to 2,400 times every 24 hours, with about four pounds of pressure each time. Tongue thrusting pressure tends to force the teeth out of alignment. A tongue thrust can produce an **open bite**, which is a space between the upper and lower teeth. The force of the tongue against the teeth is an important factor contributing to a malocclusion.

Tongue thrust is commonly associated with allergies, nasal congestion, mouth breathing, enlarged tonsils, and tongue-tie. It is also seen after prolonged therapy by Levodopa in the treatment of Parkinson's disease and as a side effect (acute muscular dystonia) after the use of Neuroleptics (Anti-Psychotics).

T.M.D. and Occlusion Disorders
History: *Signs & Symptoms*
9. Crooked/Crowded Teeth

TMD/Occlusion Disorders		
Joint Discomfort	−	+
Popping/Clicking	−	+
Limited Opening	−	+
Sore Muscles	−	+
Nerve Pain	−	+
Bruxism (Grind or Clench)	−	+
Poor Bite	−	+
Worn Teeth	−	+
Tongue Thrust	−	+
Crooked Teeth	−	+

Anthropologic studies of human skulls from museums around the world verify that for thousands of years it was normal to see well-developed dental arches, with uncrowded teeth, fully erupted wisdom teeth (3rd molars) and good bites.

Crowded teeth, impacted wisdom teeth and poor bites are a modern phenomenon since the Industrial Revolution when diets of soft processed food increased, allergies increased, and breastfeeding of infants decreased. This has resulted in a Western culture with generalized poor cranio-facial growth, inadequate development (of both hard and soft tissues) and widespread malocclusions.

Crowded teeth should alert the dentist to the possibility of maxillo-mandibular retrusion, poor anterior guidance, greater incidence of wear, abfractions (tooth root notching), gum recession, tooth mobility, airway problems (mouth breathing and/or breathing disordered sleep), allergies, tongue-tie, and periodontal compromise. Third molar impaction is also a sign of inadequate development of the dental arch.

Once a thorough written and verbal **History:** *Signs & Symptoms* is completed, proceed to **Evaluation:** *Clinical Signs* and then to **Screening & Testing.**

18. T.M.D. & OCCLUSION DISORDERS – EVALUATION, SCREENING & TESTING

Having obtained a thorough History of Signs and Symptoms regarding potential T.M.D. and Occlusion Disorders, at this point it is now appropriate to begin evaluating for Clinical Signs.

T.M.D. and Occlusion Disorders
Evaluation: *Clinical Signs*
1. ROM Atypical

ROM Atypical	–	+

Range of Movement (ROM) of the mandible is a helpful way to visually observe normal jaw excursions versus problems within the joints and muscles.

Normal ROM:
- **"Opening wide" (straight open): 40-50 millimeters**
    - Circular "rotation" of the condyle is possible up to approximately 20 mm of opening
    - Opening wider (beyond 20 mm) requires a gliding "translation" down and forward along the eminence of the fossa. This translation prevents the opening of the lower jaw from impinging on the airway in the throat region.

- **In left, right and forward excursions: 8-13 millimeters**
    - Normally, these movements should be free from tightness, discomfort, deviations, clicking/popping or locking.

Atypical ROM may have several sources:
- **Tight muscles** can limit comfortable wide opening. This is common when a history of clenching is present, in which the muscles may operate in a shortened, contracted state chronically and may feel uncomfortable initially with stretching movements.
- Muscles may appear to "splint" around hurting joints, immobilizing the uncomfortable or injured area.
- **Internal joint derangements** can alter ROM.
    - **Disk displacements with clicks** (reducible) may produce irregular opening and closing patterns. On opening, the jaw may "wiggle" to reposition the disk on top of the condylar head. It may wiggle again on closure, as the disk clicks off again.
    - **Disk displacements without click** (non-reducible) may produce a limitation of opening because of pain, fibrous and boney ankylosis (scar tissue), or disk interference to translation of the condyle (like a speed bump).

T.M.D. and Occlusion Disorders
Evaluation: *Clinical Signs*
2. Muscle Palpation

ROM Atypical	−	+
Muscle Palpation	−	+

Muscles of the shoulders, neck and face become tender to palpation due to inflammation, overuse or splinting to protect a damaged joint. Muscle pain or muscle soreness can range from acute discomfort, like a stiff neck or spasm, to the more severe Complex Regional Pain Syndrome.

Muscle pain is mainly due to tension, stress, overuse, and injuries.

***Common causes of local muscle pain include:**
- **Delayed-onset Muscle Soreness (DOMS)** – Pain and stiffness from strenuous exercise.
- **Muscle Cramp** – Sudden contraction of muscles (ex: jaw cramp).

- **Muscle Strain/Pull** – Hypertension of muscle fibers causing pain.
- **Repetitive Movement Strain** – Muscle which has been over fatigued, such as bruxism's chronic clenching and grinding over-activity.
- **Sprain** – Stretching or tearing of a ligament

***Common causes of Systemic muscle pain include:**
- **Myofascial Pain Syndrome** – A Complex Regional Pain Syndrome (CRPS) disorder, where trigger points in the muscles can cause pain in unrelated parts of the body. This is common in the head and neck region.
- **Fibromyalgia** – A generalized musculoskeletal pain, with a poorly understood etiology. The multiple sources of systemic inflammation should be considered and evaluated. Vitamin D deficiency is a common factor that may influence fibromyalgia-like symptoms. Breathing disordered sleep, including sleep apnea, has also been associated with fibromyalgia-like symptoms.
- **Lupus** – A long-term inflammatory disease
- **Rheumatoid Arthritis** – A chronic inflammatory disease that affects small joints in the hands, feet and TMJs.
- **Chronic Fatigue Syndrome** – Extreme fatigue disorder, similar to fibromyalgia, which is often made worse by physical activity.

*NOTE: All the common causes of systemic muscle pain have an *inflammatory* component. Please refer to the "Treatment" section of *The Great Fire* for management and resolution options.

A thorough clinical evaluation includes palpation of the major muscles of the head and neck region. These muscles may be palpated by regions:
- Posterior neck: **Trapezius** (shoulder); **Splenius Capitis** – Occipital Triangle (base of skull)
- Anterior neck: **Sternocleidomastoid** (diagonal to collarbone); **Digastric posterior belly** (beneath the angle of the mandible to the hyoid bone) & **anterior belly** (from the hyoid bone to the lower border of the mandible, near the midline)
- Elevator muscles of mastication: **Superficial Masseter** (the large clenching muscle, from the lower border of the

mandible to the cheekbone); **Deep Masseter** (from a depression beneath the back border of the Superficial Masseter, up to the cheekbone, just in front of the joint); **Temporalis** (fanning out from the cheekbone, above the eye and back to the ear); **Medial Pterygoid** (inside the mouth, behind the last molar teeth).
- Positioner muscles of mastication: **Lateral Pterygoid** (connecting the condyle & neck of the mandible to the pterygoid plate, at the junction of the hard and soft palate). This muscle is difficult to palpate, but it is often sore when the mandible shifts forward due to a poor bite and bruxism.

Patients are asked to rate any muscle tenderness to finger palpation on a scale of 0-3:
0 = no tenderness
1 = slight tenderness ("That feels good – I need a massage")
2 = moderate tenderness ("That's definitely tender to the touch")
3 = significant tenderness ("That's uncomfortable to the touch")

The importance of muscle palpation is that sore muscles are an indicator of the type of dysfunction that may be present. As an example, let's consider temporal headaches. These headaches may originate from several different muscle sources:
* **Clenching** – Elevator muscles will be sore, but not necessarily the Lateral Pterygoids or neck muscles.
* **Grinding** – Elevator and Lateral Pterygoid muscles are typically sore, and often the neck muscles.
* **Cervical neck injury** – Posterior & Anterior neck muscles are sore, with referred pain commonly radiating up the back & top of the head, to the temporal region. The Elevator & Positioner muscles may be sore.

In addition , it is important to remember that a *combination* of muscles may be sore, due to any of the following factors:
* Dental Malocclusion
* Temporomandibular Joint Disorders
* Cervical Neck Disorders
* Airway, Breathing & Sleep Disorders
* Neurologic Disorders
* Systemic Inflammatory Disorders

**T.M.D. and Occlusion Disorders
Evaluation:** *Clinical Signs*
3. Joint Palpation

ROM Atypical	−	+
Muscle Palpation	−	+
Joint Palpation	−	+

Focusing on the health of the Temporomandibular Joints is a primary responsibility for all dental professionals. A thorough history will review joint discomfort, popping, clicking and limited opening. Clinical evaluation of atypical ROM is followed by joint palpation.

Joint palpation involves three steps:
- **Closed mouth palpation** of the lateral pole of the joint.
    - Tenderness when palpating the outside of the condyle is typically indicative of inflammation, effusion (fluid build-up), and/or possible internal disruption of a healthy joint. Positive palpation tenderness may be loosely described as **"capsulitis"** – inflammation of the capsular tissue surrounding the joint.
- **Open mouth palpation** of the fossa (socket) area when the condyle is shifted/translated forward.
    - The joint space (retrodiscal tissue) fills with blood, like a sponge filled with water, when the mouth is opened. Positive palpation tenderness of this tissue may be loosely described as **"ligamentitis"** – inflammation of the ligaments and retrodiskal tissues inside the joint.
- **Through the ear cartilage on opening & closing: The Piper Test.**
    - Dr. Mark Piper developed a clinical evaluation test of the TM joint in which the little finger is placed in the ear. Pressing forward toward the joint, there should normally be an absence of tenderness. The patient then opens wide and closes. When a loose ligament connection is present between the disk and condyle, a click may be felt through the finger. This click is induced by the finger pressure in the presence of pre-existing discal ligament laxity. Joint palpation helps to assess both the presence of joint discomfort as well as the integrity of the condyle-disk assembly.

T.M.D. and Occlusion Disorders
Evaluation: *Clinical Signs*
4. TMJ Load Testing

ROM Atypical	–	+
Muscle Palpation	–	+
Joint Palpation	–	+
TMJ Load Testing	–	+

Another valuable joint assessment was developed by Dr. Peter Dawson, which he describes as **"Bilateral Manipulation"**.[125] Just as an orthopedic surgeon load tests a knee to check for any abnormal discomfort due to inflammation, tissue damage, or misalignment internally, so bilateral manipulation orthopedically load tests the TM joint. Using both hands to precisely cradle the mandible, the jaw is gently seated and the patient is asked, "Do you feel any sign of tension or tenderness in either joint?" *A positive response may indicate different possible causes:*

- The Lateral Pterygoid muscle is contracting, holding the condyle forward and resisting full seating of the joint(s). This may result in a patient reporting "tension" in front of the joint with load testing. This represents an **extra-capsular** problem. This is very common with unresolved bite problems and in bruxers.
- The joint has an **intra-capsular** problem. This may result in the patient reporting "tenderness" inside the joint with load testing. This is very common with unresolved inflammation (swelling), effusion (fluid), diskal displacements (loading vascular/innervated tissues), arthritides, and joint pathology.

Bimanual manipulation/load testing is an important clinical procedure for the evaluation of possible <u>joint conditions</u>. Bimanual manipulation is also a critical clinical procedure to correctly establish the physiologic <u>joint position</u> when the goal is occluso-muscle-CNS harmony. "Centric Relation" verification, utilizing bimanual manipulation, is a clinical skill that every dentist should understand and master. Some describe this skill as difficult to learn; however, over my years at the Dawson Academy, I have personally witnessed over 4,000 dentists learn this skill during specific lessons taught in a single day in our hands-on courses.

T.M.D. and Occlusion Disorders
Evaluation: *Clinical Signs*
5. C.R. to M.I.P. Slide

ROM Atypical	−	+
Muscle Palpation	−	+
Joint Palpation	−	+
TMJ Load Testing	−	+
CR to MIP Slide	−	+

Many TMD and occlusion concerns are related to functional disharmony of the masticatory system. Why?

When the mandible closes, the elevator muscles (masseters, temporalis and medial pterygoids) contract as a group, seating the joints completely into Centric Relation (C.R.). According to the extensive research of Lundeen and Gibbs, this occurs before the teeth contact.[126] C.R. is the repetitive, functional, neuro-muscular joint position on jaw closure. To maintain neuro-muscular harmony, it is necessary for the teeth to come together at the end of jaw closure, in coordination with centric relation (C.R.).

If the teeth do not come into Maximum Intercuspation Position (M.I.P.), with all teeth contacting, in harmony with full joint seating (C.R.), there can be a significant effect, creating neuro-muscular disharmony. The lateral pterygoids (the positioning muscles) will contract to bring the teeth fully together, while the elevator muscles are pulling the mandible in a different direction. This potential "tug of war", can create neuro-muscular disharmony, sore muscles, and inappropriate forces within the joints.

To clinically evaluate this important relationship, Bilateral Manipulation is utilized. Centric Relation (C.R.) is verified, when the joints are fully seated and load tested, with no signs of tension or tenderness in either joint, and a negative joint history.

Once C.R. is verified, the clinician continues bimanual manipulation seating of the joints while the mouth closes to first tooth contact. If all teeth touch simultaneously and completely, then C.R. = M.I.P. If there is a slide (shift) in the bite and jaw position (from first tooth contact to M.I.P.), this is recorded.

A C.R. to M.I.P. slide may be significantly coincident with several clinical signs and symptoms, including:
- Sore muscles (especially lateral pterygoids/elevator muscles)
- Clicking TMJoints – due to chronic contraction of the superior belly of the lateral pterygoid muscles and muscle overloading forces
- Worn, loose and/or sore teeth
- Periodontal complications, due to primary occlusal trauma
- Abfractions and/or gingival recession

Dawson's Classification can be used to analyze a dental occlusion in relation to the TMJs. The condition and position of the TMJs are determined before the occlusion can be analyzed.[127]

- **Dawson Type I:** Maximum intercuspation is in harmony with centric relation **[C.R. = M.I.P.]**
- **Dawson Type IA:** Maximum intercuspation occurs in harmony with adapted centric posture (A.C.P. = previously damaged joints that are now adapted) **[A.C.P. = M.I.P]**
- **Dawson Type II:** The condyles must displace from a verifiable centric relation for maximum intercuspation to occur. **[C.R. does not = M.I.P.]**
- **Dawson Type IIA:** The condyles must displace from an adapted centric posture for maximum intercuspation to occur. **[A.C.P. does not = M.I.P.]**
- **Dawson Type III:** Centric relation cannot be verified. (The joints are unable to be load tested without tension or tenderness, therefore the relationship to the bite cannot be determined until the joints are stabilized.) **[=possible joint instability]**
- **Dawson Type IV:** The occlusal relationship is in an active stage of progressive disorder because of pathologically unstable TMJs. (This is seen in cases of severe joint pathology, such as avascular necrosis, rheumatoid arthritis, condylar resorption.) **[=unstable joint pathology]**

Following routine review of **TMD/Occlusion History:** *Signs & Symptoms* and **Evaluation:** *Clinical Signs,* then routine and need-specific *Screening & Testing* is completed.

T.M.D. and Occlusion Disorders
Screening and Testing
1. Doppler Auscultation

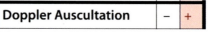

Thorough joint health assessment is critical in Integrative Dental Medicine. Doppler auscultation is a non-invasive ultrasound, which is essentially a stethoscope with a microphone incorporating the Doppler wave effect. The sounds indicate the presence of friction and the quality of lubrication within the joint.

Used throughout medicine to listen to vascular sounds, it was introduced to dentistry in the 1980s by Dr. Mark Piper. This closely coincided with **Piper's Classification of Intracapsular Disorders.**[128] To understand the value of Doppler auscultation, it is necessary to understand normal and abnormal joint function, as described in the Piper Classification.

In brief summary, **the Piper Classification has five stages**:

Stage I: A structurally intact TMJ
1. Properly aligned condyle-disk assembly.
2. Good synovial fluid lubrication inside the joint.

Stage II: Intermittent Click
1. Laxity of the lateral diskal ligament in combination with lateral pterygoid muscle hyperactivity, creating displacement tension on the disk. The disk displacement is reversible, if muscle coordination is re-established.
2. Good synovial fluid lubrication inside the joint.
3. No bone damage inside the joint.
4. Clicking occurs when muscle tension is present.

Stage IIIa: Lateral-Pole Click
1. Laxity of the lateral diskal ligament in combination with lateral pterygoid muscle hyperactivity, creating displacement tension on the disk. The disk displacement is sometimes reversible, if muscle coordination is re-established, depending on the severity of displacement and the degree of distortion of the disk anatomy.
2. Compromised synovial fluid lubrication to the lateral side of the joint internally.
3. Bone damage may be present on the lateral side of the condyle.
4. Clicking occurs on opening and closing chronically, as the lateral portion of the disk moves on and off the condyle.

Stage IIIb: Lateral-Pole Lock
1. Laxity of the lateral diskal ligament in combination with lateral pterygoid muscle hyperactivity, creating displacement tension on the disk. The disk displacement is partially reversible, if muscle coordination is re-established, depending on the severity of displacement and the degree of distortion of the disk anatomy.
2. Compromised synovial fluid lubrication to the lateral side of the joint internally.
3. Bone damage is present on the lateral side of the condyle.

4. Clicking previously occurred on opening and closing chronically, but now does not because the lateral disk tissue is locked in front of the condyle.

Stage IVa: Medial-Pole Click
   1. Laxity of the lateral, medial and posterior diskal ligament in combination with lateral pterygoid muscle hyperactivity, creating displacement tension on the disk. The disk displacement is partially reversible, if muscle coordination is re-established, depending on the severity of displacement and the degree of distortion of the disk anatomy.
   2. Compromised synovial fluid lubrication to the medial and lateral side of the joint internally.
   3. Bone damage is present on the medial and lateral side of the condyle.
   4. Clicking occurs on opening and closing chronically, but now comes from the medial aspect of the joint, while the lateral disk tissue remains locked in front of the condyle.
   5. Signs of changes in the dental occlusion, due to bone wear and loss of diskal padding, often producing an anterior open bite and posterior tooth wear.

Stage IVb: Medial-Pole Lock
   1. Laxity of the lateral, medial and posterior diskal ligament in combination with lateral pterygoid muscle hyperactivity, creating displacement tension on the disk. The disk displacement is often irreversible, depending on the severity of displacement and the degree of distortion of the disk anatomy.
   2. Compromised synovial fluid lubrication to the medial and lateral side of the joint internally.
   3. Bone damage is present on the medial and lateral side of the condyle.
   4. Previous clicking has ceased.
   5. Continual bite distortions.

Stage Va: Perforation with Acute Degenerative Joint Disease (DJD)
   1. A hole perforates through the retrodiskal tissue, creating early bone to bone contact.
   2. Minimal, if any, synovial fluid lubrication to the medial and lateral side of the joint internally.

3. Significant bone damage is present on the medial and lateral side of the condyle.
4. Osteoarthritic changes.
5. Bite distortions and retrognathic mandibular shifts.

Stage Vb: Perforation with Chronic Degenerative Joint Disease (DJD)

1. Bone to bone contact with severe flattening of both the condyle and fossa/eminence.
2. Lost synovial fluid lubrication to the medial and lateral side of the joint internally.
3. Significant bone damage is present on the medial and lateral sides of the condyle.
4. Advanced osteoarthritic changes.
5. Severe bite distortions and retrognathic mandibular shifts are typical.

Doppler Auscultation is useful in screening for different stages of the Piper Classification. How?
- **Amplification:** A Doppler will amplify clicking in the joint, so both the clinician and patient can audibly hear quieter clicks.
- **Doppler effect:** A change of frequency between contacting surfaces in motion, producing friction, is transmitted in an audible form. This results in mild, moderate or coarse crepitus (grating), which has a "sandpaper" sound.

With proper training, a Doppler provides valuable screening, especially for the presence of:
- **Clicking,** associated with **Piper Stages II, IIIa, and IVa**
- **Lateral Pole Crepitus,** associated with **Piper Stages III, IV, & V**
- **Medial Pole Crepitus,** associated with **Piper Stages IV, & V**

The Doppler is a valuable screening tool in identifying:
- healthy joints
- joints with hidden "red flags" for potential future problems
- joints with mild to moderate active problems, that should be addressed as a priority
- joints with severe problems, that may significantly impact treatment planning and complete health.

T.M.D. and Occlusion Disorders
Screening and Testing
2. Imaging (MRI/CBCT)

| Doppler Auscultation | - | + |
| Imaging (CBCT/MRI) | - | + |

The Dawson and Piper Classifications show us that proper treatment of TMD and dental malocclusions requires an accurate diagnosis of TMJoint conditions. Fortunately, with the sophistication of modern MRI and CBCT imaging, no joint conditions can hide from us.

Magnetic Resonance Imaging (MRI)
Painful and unstable joints are due to several causative factors that can be clearly revealed through MRIs, including:
* Disk position on both the lateral and medial sides of the condyle
* Joint spacing between the condyle and fossa/eminence
* Bone integrity of the cortical surfaces
* Osteoarthritis and/or Rheumatoid arthritis
* Pathology, such as osteomas (bony benign tumors)
* Fluid in the joint spaces, bone marrow, and muscle fibers
* Fibrous and bony ankylosis
* Skeletal effects related to abnormal craniofacial growth and development
* Airway and breathing compromise

MRIs represent an invaluable diagnostic tool. They are especially valuable when studying soft tissue related problems, such as disk displacements, joint effusion, and avascular necrosis.

*NOTE: Empirical clinical methods, that stop short of thorough diagnostic testing, risk missing the underlying cause producing the TMD signs and symptoms. It is always best practice policy to remember and implement:
WHEN IN DOUBT, GO FIND OUT.

Cone Beam Computed Tomography (CBCT)
Many TMD and occlusion changes are related to breakdown in the joints. Additionally, as we have seen, there is also currently a growing appreciation of the importance of diagnosing a healthy airway. Related questions include "Are the nasal passages patent and free of obstructions from the tip of the nose to the throat?" Potential problems could include:

* Deviated septum
* Enlarged adenoids in children
* Obstructing nasal turbinates
* Nasal polyps
* Enlarged and obstructing tonsils
* Narrow pharyngeal opening
* Masses in the nasal airway
* Sinus abnormalities
* Dental infections in the maxillary sinuses
* Growths in the mandible and maxilla — reports from both benign and malignant CBCTs represent a valuable diagnostic tool. They are especially valuable when studying hard tissue related changes in the TMJoints, maxilla, mandible & upper cervical spine; soft tissue related problems in the airway and sinuses; implant treatment planning; and endodontics (abscessed teeth and infected maxillary sinuses).

In utilizing MRIs and CBCTs to assess complex problems in the head and neck region, it is advisable to use imaging experts/services for diagnostic interpretation.

T.M.D. and Occlusion Disorders
Screening and Testing
3. Dawson Photo Series

Doppler Auscultation	−	+
Imaging (CBCT/MRI)	−	+
Dawson Photo Series		

Recording visual observations for further analysis, treatment planning, and review during consultations can be a valuable tool in complete care.

The Dawson Academy protocols include a series of 21 photographs that are utilized to study a number of important factors including maxillo-mandibular retrusion, facial asymmetry, occlusal irregularities, dental macro- & micro-esthetics, and dental arch form.[129]

Two additional photographs to consider for the appropriate cases include:

1. **Mallampati view**: Taken when the mouth is open wide, capturing the tongue form and the back of the throat. We know that patients with a scalloped tongue and Mallampati 3 or 4 are at high risk for airway, breathing and disturbed sleep concerns.

2. **Tongue-tie view**: Taken when the mouth is open wide and the tongue is raised as high as possible toward the maxillary incisive papilla. This can record tongue restriction that can be significant in malocclusions and dysfunctional breathing and swallowing.

T.M.D. and Occlusion Disorders Screening and Testing
4. Diagnostic Study Models

Doppler Auscultation	−	+
Imaging (CBCT/MRI)	−	+
Dawson Photo Series		
Diagnostic Study Models		

When studying dental malocclusions, evaluating esthetics, and treatment planning, diagnostic study models are an irreplaceable tool.[130] Whether using traditional plaster models or virtual models, the essential purpose of a diagnostic study model is to record:

- **The Hinge Axis**: obtained through an earbow or facebow recording of the correct arc of opening and closing.
- **Centric Relation:** traditionally obtained in the form of a bite record (with wax or bite registration material) of the tooth-to-tooth relationship of the maxilla and mandible, when the joints are fully seated.
- **Condylar Paths**: most often 20 degrees protrusive condylar path and 15 degrees lateral path.

It is beyond the purpose of this project to completely detail the complete principles of dental occlusion. Furthermore, these principles have already been masterfully communicated in Dr. Dawson's classic text, <u>Functional Occlusion from TMJ to Smile Design</u>. For further explanation of these principles, I would refer you to this excellent book. It is critical to understand that the analysis and correction of dental malocclusions is a very exact science. Any clinician involved in changing occlusions should be well versed in the principles of centric relation, anterior guidance, condylar guidance, the envelope of function, the neutral zone, vertical dimension of occlusion, incisal edge position, and the influence of tooth position on phonetics. All of these principles are reasons why properly mounted diagnostic study models are an important part of analyzing dental occlusions.

T.M.D. and Occlusion Disorders Screening and Testing
5. Dawson Wizard Analysis

Doppler Auscultation	−	+
Imaging (CBCT/MRI)	−	+
Dawson Photo Series		
Diagnostic Study Models		
Dawson Wizard Analysis		

The Dawson Wizard is a software program that helps guide the clinician through analysis and treatment planning decisions. Data gathered from the thorough patient examination, including the medical and dental history, clinical signs, Doppler auscultation, muscle palpation, TM joint load testing, diagnostic study models, 21 photographic series, and radiographic imaging are all included in the development of a restorative treatment plan. The purpose of the Wizard is to guide the dentist in developing a plan that is predictable both functionally and esthetically. It is also a tool that can be used during consultation with patients to help them visualize "before and after results of their proposed care.

We have seen many instances, over many years, where TMD and occlusal disorders have been "The Great Imposers", significantly affecting the quality of life for those suffering from their intrusion. When people suffer from sore facial and neck muscles, headaches, uncomfortable TMJoints, unstable bites, hyperactive neuromuscular responses, cervical neck issues, stressful breathing, tongue dysfunction, poor sleep, and chronic fatigue, their quality of life is severely compromised. It is a primary responsibility of those practicing the medical discipline of dentistry to recognize, screen, test, treat or refer for specialty care all those patients whose lives are being imposed upon by these disorders. This is the job description of "Physicians of the Masticatory System."

* * *

Following a thorough evaluation including:
- **History: Signs & Symptoms**
- **Evaluation: Clinical Signs**
- **Screening & Testing**

has yielded a **DIFFERENTIAL CONCLUSION**.

> This information determines that the patient presents either
> **NEGATIVE** or **POSITIVE** for
> TMD and/or Occlusion Disorders.
> If **POSITIVE**, proceed to the **TREATMENT** portion
> of the IDM Checklist.
> **The focus now turns to stabilizing the Temporomandibular Joints, Muscles, Occlusion, Neuromuscular harmony, Cervical Spine, Airway, and Complete Health.**

> "**Complete dentists add another circle:**
>
> As physicians of the masticatory system, complete dentists are responsible for how structures within the system affect the general health of each and every patient. In addition, it is an essential requirement of a complete examination to determine when and how structures within the system are affected by factors of health, disharmony and dysfunction that can disrupt masticatory system harmony.
>
> Clinical observation plus research has clarified the role of airway problems as both a cause and an effect of masticatory system disorders. So complete dentists must gain expertise in the possible interrelationships between a variety of airway related disorders and a variety of symptoms. It is not enough to just have a 'one size fits all' mentality that prescribes a cookie-cutter appliance as treatment. Airway problems require adherence to a standard of the Dawson Academy that has persisted for decades: 'First make a diagnosis.'
>
> The added airway circle is often a critical part of the diagnosis puzzle related not only to airway but also to occlusion, arch contour, bruxism and wear problems. It is also frequently related to problems of general health that go undiagnosed. The dentist's role as a gatekeeper for patients' health is an important dimension made practical because of frequent opportunities to observe patients in the typical dental practice.
>
> **CAUTION...New understanding of the varied effects of airway disorders does not diminish in any way the importance of occlusal disharmony as a factor in occlusal disease, including wear problems and certain types or orofacial pain such as occluso-muscle pain. Airway disorders should be considered as an additional focus of diagnosis, never as a substitute for occlusal analysis."**
>
> Peter Dawson, DDS, and John Cranham, DDS
> <u>The Complete Dentist Manual</u>

19. T.M.D. & OCCLUSION DISORDERS – TREATMENT

A **DIFFERENTIAL CONCLUSION,** from following the IDM Checklist History, Evaluation, Screening & Testing, has determined that the patient presents **POSITIVE** for TMD and/or Occlusal Disorders. We will next proceed to the **TREATMENT** portion of the IDM Checklist, where the focus now turns to stabilizing the TMJoints, muscles, occlusion, neuromuscular harmony, cervical region of the spine, airway, and complete health.

Remembering Our Mission:

*To educate each patient we serve about the multiple facets of the temporomandibular system and dental occlusion related to complete health.

*To empower them toward complete health, through counseling and treatment to establish a healthy masticatory system.

Let's explore these multiple facets of Masticatory System disorders and how we empower our patients toward complete health.

T.M.D. and Occlusion Disorders:
Treatment
1. "Form Follows Function"…

Louis Sullivan taught us to recognize, *"Form ever follows function, and this is the law. Where function does not change, form does not change."* We explored this profound principle of nature when considering airway and breathing. We saw that if the nasal airway functions normally, we breathe primarily through the nose. Nitric oxide, produced in the paranasal sinuses, destroys invading pathogens and dilates the airway. The air is sterilized, humidified, warmed and prepared to supply oxygen to the lungs and cardiovascular system. Meanwhile, the mouth is closed. The tongue postures both upward and forward against the palate and guides the developing boney and dental maxillary arch. This produces ideal formation of broad dental arches, with fully erupted third molars, plenty of room to house the tongue, and straight teeth. Form follows function to produce a stable, healthy masticatory system…in the ideal world.

We further discussed that if functional breathing changes to dysfunctional breathing, everything changes. Normal formation may change to deformation of the cranio-facial-respiratory structures, influencing dental malocclusions, crowded teeth, and locked out third molars. Therefore, we conclude:

**As Form follows Function,
so Deformation follows Dysfunction.**

This leads us into the analysis of TMD and Dental Occlusion Disorders. These disorders have an important early component of change that can significantly influence them: Temporomandibular Joint instability.

As previously discussed, the Schellas, Piper, Besette and Wilkes study reported that nearly 90% of patients presenting with retrognathic (retruded) mandibles are off the disk in one or both TM joints.[131] These joint derangements represent a deformation of hard and soft tissue integrity in the joints, as well as the developing dental occlusion. Joint derangements can produce dental malocclusions. These structural changes can influence compromised function of the neuromuscular system. Therefore, we conclude:

> As Function follows Form,
> so Dysfunction follows Deformation.

-or-

> As Function (dental occlusion and mastication)
> follows Form (joint development and health),
> so Dysfunction (malocclusion and TMD)
> follows Deformation (joint derangements).

We observe this in other parts of the body. For example, if one leg is shorter than the other, the compensating posture produces a change in gait with frequent problems of the knee, hip and back.

It is critical to appreciate the complexity of the masticatory system and not approach "TMD" as a one size fits all disorder.

Repeating for the sake of re-emphasizing:

DIAGNOSE – THEN TREAT

A thorough evaluation of the complete masticatory system, including the temporomandibular joints, cervical region of the spine, airway and breathing is critical to derive an accurate diagnosis and treatment plan. The diagnosis of dysfunctional airway and/or breathing and sleep should lead us to anticipate possible cranio-facial-respiratory and dental occlusal deformation, depending on the severity of the problem. We must also clearly understand that **deformation can precede dysfunction.** Deformation (internal derangement) of the temporomandibular joints can influence distortions of the cranio-facial-respiratory- occlusion-masticatory system complex; affect the airway; stimulate dysfunctional breathing; and lead to tongue dysfunction. We see this working in both directions:

> **As deformation follows dysfunction,**
> **so dysfunction follows deformation.**

When both dysfunction and deformation are diagnosed, what is the preferred treatment plan of action? Whenever possible, the preferred plan would be to correct both the dysfunction and the deformation.

Clinically speaking, planning can often be divided into two phases of treatment:

Management/Phase 1 & Resolution/Phase 2 Therapy

Management/Phase 1 Therapy for TMD and Occlusion Disorders is an initial strategy, utilizing modalities focused on:
- **reducing discomfort** – inflammation, muscle & joint soreness or pain
- **orthopedic stabilization** – harmonizing the joints, muscles, bite, and supporting the potential adaptive capacity of the individual system.

In some cases, Phase 1 Therapy may help clarify the diagnosis and final treatment plan.

Phase 1 Therapy may include occlusal splint therapy, physical therapy, chiropractic and/or orthopedic evaluation of the cervical neck and spine, trigger point injections in muscles, anti-inflammatory dietary changes (including nutritional supplements), anti-inflammatory medications, muscle relaxers, physical activity, airway/breathing and sleep hygiene, and oral myofunctional therapy.

Surgical consultation may be appropriate during this phase for Piper Stage IV and V joint conditions, depending on the MRI findings and the response to therapy.

TMD/Occlusion Disorders
Phase 1 / Phase 2 ↓
Phase 1
• Appropriate Orthotic
• Anti-inflammatory Meds/Diet
• Physical Therapy prn
• C1/C2 Therapy prn
• Injection Therapy prn
• Surgical Referral prn

Phase 1 Therapy is considered in some aspects to be a **"reversible phase"**, and it may be used to clarify the prognosis for more definitive, "irreversible" therapy.

For example, a patient presents with a sore and clicking right joint, diagnosed as a Piper Stage IIIa (reciprocal lateral pole click), reporting sore masseter and pterygoid muscles, and a slight bite discrepancy, with no apparent airway problem. Managing the condition, utilizing a C.R. acrylic bite splint to idealize the bite 24/7 and anti-inflammatory meds (Ibuprofen 400mg, 4 times/day), the patient experiences complete relief in the joint and muscles within a few days. The perfected bite on the splint remains stable for 6 weeks. This demonstrates both pain relief and orthopedic stability, during Phase 1 therapy. This outcome would positively influence a decision to consider irreversible bite therapy, such as a bite adjustment (equilibration) or orthodontics, in an effort to rebalance the apparent masticatory system imbalance.

Resolution/Phase 2 Therapy is a definitive strategy, utilizing modalities focused on **stabilizing the joints, bite and airway definitively and for the long term.**

Phase 2 therapy may include bite adjustment (equilibration), orthodontics (dental crowding, airway restrictions), restorative dentistry (crowns, bridges, implants), TMJoint surgery (such as a displaced, damaged disk repair), orthognathic surgery (jaw, bite, airway), and/or ENT surgery (upper airway, posterior airway, tongue-tie release).

The expanding model of Integrative Dental Medicine considers all the known co-factors of TMD and dental malocclusions in developing Phase 1 and Phase 2 treatment plans for each patient. There are numerous combinations of scenarios. Utilizing the **IDM Checklist** will help to ensure that no possible co-factors are missed and will help to identify the primary concerns to address.

TMD/Occlusion Disorders
Phase 1 / Phase 2 ↓
Phase 1 • Appropriate Orthotic • Anti-inflammatory Meds/Diet • Physical Therapy prn • C1/C2 Therapy prn • Injection Therapy prn • Surgical Referral prn
Phase 2 • Definitive Occlusal Therapy • Post Tx Orthotic prn

* * *

We will next discuss TMD and Occlusion Disorders *Management* and *Resolution*. The plan for managing these disorders depends on the preliminary diagnosis.

Using the **IDM: 7 Key Questions**, let's consider a few example clinical scenarios.

IDM: 7 Key Questions
The IDM Model seeks to answer 7 Key questions FOR EVERY PATIENT:

> 1. Does the **OCCLUSION** appear unstable?
> 2. Does the patient **BRUX**?
> 3. Does the patient have **SORE MUSCLES**?
> 4. Are there signs of **TMJ CHANGE**?
> 5. Could there be an **AIRWAY PROBLEM**?
> 6. Are there signs of local or systemic **INFLAMMATION**?
> 7. Is there an **UNESTHETIC SMILE** concern?

> "The question of whether genetic factors or environmental factors may be the primary agents causing dentofacial maldevelopment has been widely discussed in the past. The anthropological studies of Robert S. Corruccini...are a major contribution to finding the answer to this question. In certain populations the transition from predominantly good to predominantly bad occlusion occurred within one or two generations. This evidence throws the weight of suspicion toward environmental, non-genetic etiologic factors. This view is supported by correlative studies demonstrating that the process of industrialization is accompanied by an epidemiologic transition to high prevalence of such diseases as diabetes, cancer, stroke, and coronary heart afflictions. A genetic change of any kind can be ruled out as a factor in this change, as the change is simply too rapid."
>
> Rolf Frankel, MD, author of the *Preface* to
> How Anthropology Informs the Orthopedic
> Diagnosis of Malocclusion's Causes (1999)
> by Robert S. Corruccini, PhD

T.M.D. and Occlusion Disorders: Treatment
2. Examples of Management and Resolution of TMD and Occlusion Disorders

Scenario #1:

A 56 year old woman has no chief complaint, but the **OCCLUSION** appears unstable. The patient is unaware of grinding or clenching, has no sore muscles, no TMJ change, no airway problems, no apparent local or systemic inflammation, and no smile concerns. A thorough clinical examination is performed with the following conclusions:

IDM: 7 Key Questions:
1. Does the **OCCLUSION** appear unstable? …YES
2. Does the patient **BRUX**? …NO
3. Does the patient have **SORE MUSCLES**? …NO
4. Are there signs of **TMJ CHANGE**? …NO
5. Could there be an **AIRWAY PROBLEM**? …NO
6. Are there signs of local/systemic **INFLAMMATION**? …NO
7. Is there an **UNESTHETIC SMILE** concern? …NO

In this particular scenario, there are no symptoms, joint instability, or airway restrictions to address through Phase 1 Therapy. We will consider going directly to Resolution Therapy, which involves stabilization of the bite.

Dental occlusal stability has 3 basic requirements:
1. **Stable stops on all teeth, when the joints are fully seated in Centric Relation (C.R. = M.I.P.).** When the jaw closes and the joints are seated by the muscles, all the teeth should touch simultaneously with even force. Think of a door on its hinges, closing evenly within the frame, all the way around.
2. **Anterior teeth guidance, in harmony with the envelope of jaw function.** When the teeth rub together on opening or closing, only front teeth should contact, in harmony with normal jaw function in all directions.
3. **Disclusion (separation) of all posterior (back) teeth in protrusive (forward) and lateral (left & right) movements.** Just as only front teeth touch in jaw movements, so back teeth clearly separate in all jaw

movements (with rare exceptions). Muscle studies show that back teeth contacting, other than when the joints are fully seated, stimulates increased activity of the jaw muscles, which can create bite-related problems such as loose teeth, worn teeth, sore muscles, neuromuscular imbalance and overloaded TMJoints. One review showed that experimentally produced heavy tooth contacts may cause negative changes in jaw muscle contraction and change the muscle movement patterns of the jaw. The review summarizes that *"it is apparent that experimental occlusal interferences are associated with short-term clinical symptoms and signs, such as jaw muscle fatigue and pains, headaches, pains and clickings in the temporomandibular joints."*[132]

There are several signs of teeth that are unstable[133]:
* **Hypermobility** on one or more teeth
* **Excessive wear**
* **Migration** of tooth position, with teeth shifting horizontally, supra-erupting or intruding.

Analyzing an unstable occlusion begins with recognizing the signs of instability and understanding the basic requirements of a stable occlusion.

Fundamental dental occlusion principles to always consider are:
- **A stable occlusion begins with a healthy joint condition in a healthy joint position (CR).** If an unstable occlusion is observed, always ask:
    o What's the **condition of the joints** – healthy or unhealthy?
    o What's the **position of the joints** – seated or unseated?
- **A stable occlusion shares the biting forces over the maximum number of teeth, in Centric Relation (CR).** The more teeth that touch, when the joints are seated, the better the occlusion. An even distribution of force ensures that no one tooth is overloaded. Overloaded teeth are the sore ones, the loose ones, the ones with the most wear, and the ones that shift position the most. Furthermore, if one single tooth contacts first on closure, resulting in a "hit and slide" (a bite shift into a position where all the teeth touch), this turns on positioner muscles, the lateral pterygoids.

- Therefore, muscle imbalance can be created by a poor bite. **Muscle hyperactivity and fatigue, due to an uneven bite, is a major source of TMD complaints.**
- **A stable occlusion involves contact on only front teeth as soon as the jaw leaves centric relation.** Dr. Dawson teaches, "You can't wear what you don't touch." When back teeth do not touch other than on closing straight down, it's virtually impossible to wear them down or knock them loose, due to the bite.

Scenario #1 should be analyzed with these principles in mind.

Analysis includes studying the occlusion outside of the mouth by utilizing **diagnostic study models**. These models of the teeth and bite should be oriented on an instrument/articulator that can record the seated joint position (CR) and also the upper-to-lower bite relationship when the joints are seated. This will require the use of a semi-adjustable articulator, facebow or earbow, and centric relation interocclusal record.[134]

The 4 treatment options for correcting an unstable occlusion can be easily remembered as the **4 Rs**:

1. **RESHAPE:** Equalize the contact on each tooth in centric relation, all the way around the arch, on the maximum number of teeth possible. This can include either "reductive" or "additive" reshaping. Reductive reshaping is accomplished by gently and conservatively polishing the enamel of teeth that are in heavy contact, allowing other teeth to touch as well. Additive reshaping involves bonding composite resin material in specific sites to allow for better contact. It is very important that the front teeth both (1) touch in centric relation *and* (2) that they exclusively contact in left, right and forward jaw movements outward from centric relation, as well as back inward to centric relation. Reshaping teeth is the most conservative bite correction therapy. In dentistry, we refer to this procedure as **occlusal equilibration**.

   ***NOTE: Trial reshaping therapy (trial equilibration) should be first verified on the diagnostic study models as conservatively appropriate before any reshaping in the mouth. This procedure should never expose dentin or damage teeth.

2. **REPOSITION TEETH:** When it is impossible to achieve an ideal occlusion through reshaping teeth, the next most

conservative option is to reposition teeth through **orthodontics**. Rearranging tooth positions to establish C.R. = M.I.P. and ideal anterior guidance is the goal. It is imperative that all anterior teeth contact in C.R. at the end of orthodontic therapy, in order to achieve long term stability.

3. **RESTORE TEETH:** Unstable occlusions, bruxism, gastric reflux, eating disorders, or destructive habits result in significant destruction of the teeth. In these cases, it is necessary to rebuild the teeth and the bite together. Using the appropriate principles of both tooth protection and sound occlusal engineering ensures a stable long term result.

4. **REPOSITION BONE:** On the occasion that the upper and lower jawbones are severely mismatched, it may be impossible to establish an ideal bite through reshaping teeth, repositioning teeth, or restoring teeth. Repositioning bone involves a surgical procedure on the mandible, maxilla, or both, to reestablish anatomic and functional bite harmony. This is described as **orthognathic surgery**. This surgery can also move the jaw positions forward (anteriorly), significantly increasing the airway volume in the back of the throat. In light of current thinking, **"Cranio-facial-ortho-respiratory (C-FOR) surgery"** better describes this procedure.

In some cases, a combination of two or more of the **4 Rs** may be required to produce an ideal occlusion.

***NOTE: The treatment options are listed from the simplest to the most complex: 1. Reshape Teeth → 2. Reposition Teeth → 3. Restore Teeth → 4. Reposition Bone

Resolving occlusal problems will require an interdisciplinary team. The general dentist serves as the team captain, coordinating the overall plan. Key team members include the dental hygienist, periodontist, orthodontist, endodontist, oral surgeon, and oral-myofunctional therapist. Several medical specialists will be enlisted including: allergists, ENTs, gastroenterologists, endocrinologists, chiropractors, physical therapists, and sleep physicians. Communication and coordination between team members is a critical component of complete care. Developing a great team is a top priority in all phases of Integrative Dental Medicine.

Scenario #2:

A 37 year old man has a chief complaint of **SORE MUSCLES, GRINDING** and **CLENCHING, WORN TEETH** and an **UNEVEN BITE.** The patient has no TMJ changes, no airway problems, no systemic inflammation, and no smile concerns. A thorough clinical examination is performed with the following conclusions:

IDM: 7 Key Questions
1. Does the **OCCLUSION** appear unstable? ...**YES**
2. Does the patient **BRUX**? ...**YES**
3. Does the patient have **SORE MUSCLES**? ...**YES**
4. Are there signs of **TMJ CHANGE**? ...**NO**
5. Could there be an **AIRWAY PROBLEM**? ...**NO**
6. Are there signs of local/systemic **INFLAMMATION**?...**NO**
7. Is there an **UNESTHETIC SMILE** concern? ...**NO**

Since we've ruled out airway and TMJ changes, including an overnight Home Sleep Test (HST), the problem will be addressed as an **occluso-muscle** problem. Since symptoms are present which include sore muscles and parafunctional clenching and grinding, we will consider Phase 1 Therapy initially.

What are our objectives in this scenario?
1. Relieve sore muscles
2. Reduce bruxing
3. Stabilize the occlusion

We need effective therapeutic aids that will directly address these concerns. What tools are available to assist in accomplishing these objectives?

Occlusal Splints (in the form of bite guards, orthotics, and/or appliances) are acrylic overlays on the teeth that can change the occlusion and influence muscle activity. There are several different occlusal splint designs.

We will discuss **3 specific occlusal splint designs** and explain their purpose:
    1. Anterior Contact Splint (ACS)
        a. This design contacts exclusively on the front teeth when biting together. A horizontally flat acrylic anterior "discluding element" allows smooth side-to-side and forward movement of the mandible.

The design principle is based on a few simple concepts:
  i. Separating the back teeth of bruxers typically provides relief for sore muscles.
  ii. Muscle EMG studies demonstrate that when front teeth touch exclusively, elevator muscle activity (notably the masseter and temporalis) is significantly reduced.[135]
b. Our unpublished findings, when recording EMG muscle activity with anterior contact splints, demonstrated elevator muscle activity on clenching was typically reduced by 70-80%.
c. Lateral pterygoid muscles are often hyperactive and sore in the presence of malocclusions. Anterior contact splints, designed with a flat horizontal surface, allow the joints to seat in centric relation as the lateral pterygoid muscles release contraction.
d. On a historic note, anterior deprogrammers have been used in clinical dentistry for many decades. Cotton rolls, leaf gauges, NTIs, Lucia jigs, and B Splints all separate the back teeth. Patients experiencing severe muscle tension will typically report significant relief, often within a few minutes, when these aids are placed between their teeth. This has been described as **"clearing the dance floor"** of any noxious tooth contacts that may stimulate hyper-activate muscle responses.

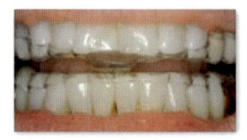

Figure: B splint/ACS

  i. Jim Boyd, DDS, a highly respected colleague and friend in San Diego, California, designed the NTI device, which received FDA approval for the treatment of headaches and TMD in 1998. In his research with Andrew Blumenfeld, MD, (Neurologist and Migraine Headache Specialist), they identified that both certain types of migraines and tension-type headaches were often effectively treated with their anterior contact splint design. They theorized that noxious afferent (incoming) messages to the CNS, from sore temporalis muscles in clenchers, can stimulate a sympathetic nervous system (SNS) response, producing blood flow changes in the head, activating migraine and migraine-like symptoms. The NTI (Nocioceptive Trigeminal Inhibition) device, similar to botox injections used by Dr. Blumenfeld, reduces temporalis muscle activity, decreasing the noxious incoming messages to the CNS, thus minimizing SNS responses of blood flow change, and therefore suppressing both migraine and tension type headaches in many cases. Thousands of patients have experienced dramatic relief from debilitating headaches, using this simple splint and other designs similar to it.

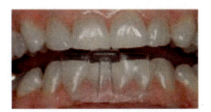

Figure: NTI/ACS splint

ii. The NTI splint has received criticism from some clinicians, who are concerned that its design (which only covers the incisors of one arch) may produce bite changes if worn long term. Patients have presented with intruded anterior teeth and supra-erupted posterior teeth. It is doubtful that intrusion and supra-eruption of teeth

occurs when an NTI is worn only 7-8 hours per day, as prescribed. It is likely that such changes occur due to extended usage. It is possible that a patient experiencing headaches might leave an NTI in during the daytime or even several days. Therefore, in my private practice, we use the NTI primarily for acute care and have designed a full coverage, dual arch appliance, with an anterior discluding element, called a B (Bruxism) Splint, for extended usage.
   e. **These splints are preferred when the joints are healthy (Piper Stage I,II), muscles are sore, and the bite may be a factor.**
2. **Superior Repositioning Splint (SRS)**
   a. Also known as a **Centric Relation Splint**, it covers all the teeth of either the upper or lower arch, contacts on all teeth, and has a ramp from canine to canine, providing immediate anterior guidance in all excursions. This splint's purpose is to create **"an idealized occlusion in a reversible manner"**.

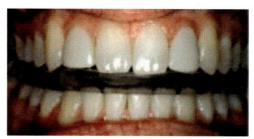

Figure: Lower SRS splint

   b. The design principle is based on the following concepts:
      i. Fully seated joints in centric relation
      ii. Perfected occlusion in centric relation
      iii. Anterior guidance in all excursive movements
      iv. Immediate disclusion of the posterior teeth in all excursive movements

- v. This splint will distribute biting forces around the dental arch and minimize forces through the TM joints.
- vi. This provides a way to test out the role of malocclusion in symptoms that may be described by patients.
- vii. This is most useful if definitive occlusal therapy is being considered to resolve a symptomatic problem (the 4 Rs).
- viii. This is a tool to reduce joint loading in damaged joints. This can be helpful to differentiate damaged joints that may "adapt" when the joint-muscle-bite system is harmonized, versus those painful joints that are "non-adaptive" and may require surgical intervention.

c. **These splints are preferred when the joints are unhealthy (Piper Stage III-V), muscles are sore, and the bite may be a factor.**

3. **Anterior Repositioning Splint (ARS)**
   a. This splint is designed to position the mandible forward. There are two primary reasons to anteriorly reposition the mandible forward:
      i. For patients who fall into **Piper Stages IV and V**, respositioning the condyle down and forward may relieve pain and pressure on the vascular, **innervated retrodiskal** joint tissues, which are impinged upon when the joint is seated and the disk is out of position (forwardly displaced off the condyle). This repositioning, down and forward, may also allow the displaced disk to recapture on top of the condyle, in some cases.
      ii. Repositioning the mandible and tongue base forward during sleep can aid attempts to open the collapsed airway in the back of the throat.

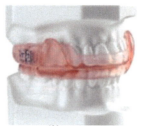

Figure[136]: ARS splint

    b. An ARS is the same splint design as a **Sleep/Airway/Breathing Appliance.**
    c. These splints are preferred when the joints are very unhealthy and uncomfortable (Piper Stage IV-V), or when airway issues are present during sleep.

In review:

Splint Design	Piper Classification
Anterior Contact Splint (ACS)	Stage I-II
Superior Repositioning Splint (SRS)	Stage III-V
Anterior Repositioning Splint (ARS)	Stage IV-V

    In Scenario #2, the patient has a chief complaint of **SORE MUSCLES, GRINDING and CLENCHING and the OCCLUSION appears to be unstable.** The patient has no TMJ change, no airway problems and no systemic inflammation. Utilizing the tools available to us, let's develop a Phase 1 and Phase 2 plan.

    Phase 1 Therapy is about getting the patient's symptoms under control. The symptoms are sore muscles, with grinding and clenching, in the absence of a joint problem.

    The splint of choice would be an anterior contact splint (ACS), such as an NTI or B Splint. The splint would be worn 24/7, taken out for meals and brushing. The duration of usage would be 48 hours to 7 days, depending on symptom relief. Anti-inflammatory medications would be recommended over the course of treatment: Ibuprofen 400 mg, four times per day. (Additionally, other anti-inflammatory diet and lifestyle changes would ideally be recommended, as appropriate; please see the "Treatment" chapter in the *Great Fire* for further details.)

Phase 2 Therapy: Evaluate the dental occlusion with mounted diagnostic study models.
Consider the 4 Rs: Reshape, Reposition teeth, Restore, Reposition bone. Select the most conservative option that will idealize the occlusion. Utilize a dual arch B Splint during sleep, only if nighttime symptoms or para-function continue after the completion of Phase 2 treatment.

Scenario #3:
A 23 year old woman has a chief complaint of **SORE MUSCLES, BRUXING,** the **OCCLUSION** feels increasingly uneven, right **TMJ** clicking, constant soreness and occasional closed lock (difficulty opening). There are no airway problems, systemic inflammation, or smile concerns. A thorough clinical examination is performed with the following conclusions:

IDM: 7 Key Questions
1. Does the **OCCLUSION** appear unstable?...**YES**
2. Does the patient **BRUX?**...**YES**
3. Does the patient have **SORE MUSCLES?**...**YES**
4. Are there signs of **TMJ CHANGE?** ...**YES**
5. Could there be an **AIRWAY PROBLEM?** ...**NO**
6. Are there signs of local or systemic **INFLAMMATION?**...**NO**
7. Is there an **UNESTHETIC SMILE** concern?...**NO**

Two critical foundations for **masticatory system stability** are (1) **TMJoint health** and (2) **Airway/Breathing health**. Scenario #3 will require a thorough diagnostic analysis of the uncomfortable, clicking and occasionally locking right TMJoint. The analysis and findings in Scenario #3 include
- Palpation = Right joint: Capsulitits and Ligamentitis
- Range of Motion = Limited opening, favoring the right side
- Load Testing = Sore in the right joint to moderate loading
- Doppler Auscultation = Right joint: reciprocal click, lateral pole mild crepitus; Left joint: quiet – no clicking or crepitus

*<u>Preliminary Diagnosis</u> = Right joint: Piper Stage IVa (medial pole disk displacement with click); Left joint: Piper Stage 1

*Further Testing: MRI and Imaging Report
  • Right joint: complete anteriorly displaced disk on both medial and lateral views, with recapture on opening, and joint effusion (fluid) in the anterior and superior joint space
  • Left joint: normal disk alignment in closed and open joint views, no joint effusion or pathology
  • The right joint disk shape is biconcave (normal) with an ideal disk position/alignment on wide opening.

*Diagnosis: Piper Stage IVa on Right; Piper Stage 1 on Left

*Treatment Plan: Due to the presence of a complete disk displacement, with soreness and occasional locking, and complete recapture with normal disk anatomy, surgical disk repair is recommended as a definitive therapy. If pain were intractable, joint surgery may be considered immediately. Furthermore, the sooner the surgery is performed, the better the prognosis. Over time, the disk will continue to deform, and inflammatory hard and soft tissue damage will progress, making surgery more complex.

Phase 1 Therapy: After confirming the right joint can be loaded without significant discomfort:
  * A **Superior Repositioning Splint (SRS)** is utilized, in order to evenly distribute a high percentage of the loading forces on the splint, idealize the occlusion in harmony with the elevator muscles, and separate the posterior teeth in excursive movements of the mandible. The SRS will be worn 24/7, as long as the right joint is comfortable and improving. It should be immediately removed if joint pain develops. It will be removed only for meals and tooth brushing.
  * **Anti-inflammatory Medication:** Medrol Dosepak (Methylprednisolone) – per instructions on label for 5 days, followed by Ibuprofen 400 mg, 4 times/day, to reduce joint effusion and muscle soreness. (Additionally, other anti-inflammatory diet and lifestyle changes would ideally be recommended, as appropriate; please see the "Treatment" chapter in the *Great Fire* for further details.)
  * Weekly appointments will allow for evaluation of comfort and the occlusion on the splint. Occasionally, with reduction of joint effusion, muscle relaxation and disk repositioning, the disorder may reverse to a Piper Stage III, in which the disk is partially recaptured and manageable without surgical

intervention. If the occlusion on the splint stabilizes, over a minimum of 3 months, Phase 2 occlusal therapy can be considered. If the disk displacement remains a Piper IVa, surgery should be considered.

*Phase 2 Therapy is initiated only after the joints are considered stable, either through extended occlusal splint therapy or joint surgery. Evaluate the dental occlusion with mounted diagnostic study models. Consider the 4 Rs: Reshape, Reposition teeth, Restore, Reposition bone. Select the most conservative option that will idealize the occlusion. Utilize the splint only if nighttime symptoms or parafunction continue after the completion of Phase 2 treatment.

* * *

A Central Theme of Integrative Dental Medicine is TMD & Occlusion Disorders. These *Great Imposers* are being addressed more and more effectively as we learn how all the cofactors of systemic inflammation, airway & breathing disorders, TMJoint internal derangements, and dental malocclusions produce weary, hurting, discouraged, sore, tired, headachy, misunderstood and generally beaten up friends, neighbors and family members.

Managing TMD & Occlusion Disorders, and understanding how they relate to other systemic concerns, is a critical role of Integrative Dental Medicine.

Part V:
Integrative Dental Medicine's
7 Key Questions

20. INTEGRATIVE DENTAL MEDICINE'S 7 KEY QUESTIONS

> *"The physician of the masticatory system*
> *must understand how all the interrelated parts*
> *of the total masticatory system work in harmony...*
> *and if one part of the system*
> *gets out of harmony all*
> *the other parts are affected."*
>
> *Peter E. Dawson, DDS*

As we have seen, *The Shift* of focus toward Integrative Dental Medicine requires careful attention to several key factors of oral and systemic health. Focusing on IDM's "7 Key Questions" ensures a truly comprehensive approach, and following the IDM Checklist enables dentists to address each of the topics involved in these questions. This chapter provides a summary guide of IDM's 7 Key Questions, designed specifically for dentists seeking to implement these principles.

Integrative Dental Medicine's 7 Key Questions:
1. Does the **DENTAL OCCLUSION** appear unstable?
2. Does the patient **BRUX**?
3. Does the patient have **SORE MUSCLES**?
4. Are there signs of **TMJOINT CHANGES**?
5. Could there be an **AIRWAY PROBLEM**?
6. Are there signs of local or systemic **INFLAMMATION**?
7. Is there an **UNESTHETIC SMILE** concern?

Let's review each key question, in order to understand why it is significant and how it is evaluated.

1. Does the **DENTAL OCCLUSION** appear unstable?

"The Masticatory System" refers to the dynamic structures that work in a synchronized manner for chewing, swallowing and breathing: the maxilla and mandible, the teeth with their supporting structures, the temporomandibular joints, the muscles of mastication (including the major jaw muscles) the tongue, the lips, the cheeks, and the neuromuscular system. How the upper and lower teeth come together, or occlude, during function, is a key factor in the stability of the whole masticatory system.

A **malocclusion** is present when the teeth are out of alignment due to:
- poor arch form – this can be related to genetically and/or epigenetically crowded teeth, malpositioned teeth, mouth breathing with dysfunctional tongue posturing, swallowing dysfunction, tongue thrust, and cranio-facial-respiratory deformation.
- poor arch to arch relationship – this can be related to a discrepancy between the seated joints and fully seated bite, a size mismatch between the dental arches, malposition of the upper and lower teeth relative to each other, inadequate anterior guidance and posterior disclusion.

Dr. Sigurd P. Ramfjord (1909-1997), a world-renowned dental occlusion authority, taught that "the goal of all occlusal therapy (bite stabilization therapy) is to create a peaceful neuromusculature." An unstable occlusion may produce an imbalance in the masticatory system, creating muscle hyperactivity.

*What are possible signs of an unstable dental occlusion?
- **Sore muscles:** this can include soreness of the masseters, temporalis, medial pterygoids, lateral pterygoids, anterior & posterior neck muscles and can be related to headaches
- **Sore teeth:** due to excessive vertical and horizontal forces
- **Loose, worn and/or broken teeth:** due to traumatic occlusal forces
- **Drifting teeth:** due to the lack of stabilizing bite contacts and muscle influences
- **Sore TMJoints:** due to excessive loading
- **TMJoint clicking:** due to tension from the lateral pterygoid muscle, when maximum intercuspation of the teeth is anterior to centric relation

*Clinical assessment of dental occlusions includes the following:
- A history review for sore teeth, perceived malocclusion, broken and worn teeth, muscle and joint symptoms.
- Visual observation of wear facets (caused by opposing teeth rubbing against other and producing flattened, worn surfaces), chipping, mobility, drifting, and dental abfractions (root notching).
- Verification of Centric Relation (C.R.) joint position and comfort through bilateral manipulation, identifying the first tooth contact on closure in C.R., and observing any shift in the occlusion from C.R. to maximum intercuspation position (M.I.P.) of the teeth.
- Observation of which teeth contact in left, right and protrusive excursions, to determine if acceptable anterior guidance and posterior disclusion is present.

It is a primary responsibility of the Physician of the Masticatory System to evaluate and resolve dental occlusal problems, which can significantly impact total masticatory system stability.

2. Does the patient **BRUX (GRIND OR CLENCH)?**

The term "bruxism" is defined as a "repetitive jaw muscle activity characterized by clenching or grinding of the teeth and/or by bracing or thrusting of the mandible."[137]

Muscle hyperactivity is a sign of an overactive neuromuscular system. This can be manifested during the daytime as well as during sleep. It may result in muscle hypertrophy (enlargement) in the absence of reported symptoms, or it may create muscle soreness, pain and headaches. It may occur in episodic time periods, or may persist chronically and daily. It may be related to dental malocclusions, or may remain after occlusions are perfected. A published research review by Dr. Giles Lavigne, a preeminent researcher in pain, bruxism, and sleep at the University of Montreal, and his cohort, include the following summary:[138]

- Awake bruxism, with an awareness of jaw clenching, is reported to be 20% among the adult population.
- During sleep, awareness of tooth grinding, as noted by sleep partner or family members, is reported by 8% of the population.
- Sleep bruxism is a behavior that was recently classified as a 'sleep-related movement disorder'.
- Recent publications suggest that sleep bruxism is secondary to sleep-related micro-arousals, defined by a rise in autonomic cardiac and respiratory activity, that tends to be repeated 8-14 times per hour of sleep.
- The putative roles of hereditary factors and of upper airway resistance in the genesis of rhythmic masticatory muscle activity and of sleep bruxism are under investigation.
- Rhythmic masticatory muscle activity in sleep bruxism peaks in the minutes before rapid eye movement sleep, which suggests that some mechanism related to sleep stage transitions exerts an influence on the motor neurons that facilitate the onset of sleep bruxism.

***Clinical assessment** for bruxing includes the following:
- A history review for an awareness of bruxing (clenching and/or grinding), sore muscles, and/or headaches
- Palpation for sore and hypertrophied (enlarged) muscles
- Visual observation for matching wear facets on teeth, chipping, mobility and dental abfractions (root notching)

Bruxing (clenching and/or grinding) represents an example of the interconnected nature of Integrative Dental Medicine as we observe associations ranging from malocclusions, normal sleep transitions, sleep disorders, neurologic disorders, and medication side effects.

3. Does the patient have **SORE MUSCLES**?

Muscles can become sore for a variety of reasons, including the following:
- **Fatigue** from over-usage in the presence of bruxing, clenching, and chronic adaptive reposturing – such as a bite "hit and slide" or chronic forward head posture
- **Stress** from sympathetic dysregulation (fight or flight response) with chronic release of stress hormones, such as cortisol, in the bloodstream
- **Inflammation** from infection, injury, autoimmune conditions, poor nutrition, and drug side effects
- **Chemical deficiency** such as hypocalcemia (low blood calcium level) with or without low vitamin D levels.
- **Muscle damage** such as chronic myofascial pain (CMP), in which damage occurs to muscle fibers and surrounding fascia. The origin is unknown, but is thought to relate to overuse, fatigue, inflammation, and strain. CMP is referred to as "regional fibromyalgia" and is characterized by the presence of muscle trigger points and is commonly associated with referred pain patterns.

***Clinical assessment** for sore muscles includes the following:
- A history review for an awareness of sore muscles and/or headaches.
- Muscle palpation tenderness on a scale of 1-3
    - 1 = "That feels good – I need a massage!"
    - 2 = "That's definitely sore to the touch"
    - 3 = "That's very sore; I wish you weren't touching it"
- Sore muscles are not normal. They most typically reveal an imbalance in function of the Masticatory System, or reflect a systemic disorder related to inflammation and/or breathing disordered sleep.

4. Are there signs of **TMJOINT CHANGES**?

TMJoint health is foundational to both a stable dental occlusion and to Masticatory System health. TMJoint changes can occur for several reasons, including:

- **Trauma:** both macro and micro
    - **Macro-trauma:** the sources of macro-trauma can include a blow to the jaw, a fall on the chin, or a whiplash type injury. If the patient can't recall such an injury, look for a telltale scar on the chin.
    - **Micro-trauma:** the sources of micro-trauma can include constant overloading of the joint, sustained clenching, and cyclic bruxing: these are detrimental to the TMJ disk – producing an overload that can lead to severe damage of the tissue.[139]
- **Hormonal changes**
    - Different studies have provided compelling information on the relevant effects of estrogen deficiency on joints. Although much of the attention has focused on the effects of estrogen on articular cartilage, estrogen deficiency also affects other joint tissues during the course of osteoarthritis, such as the periarticular bone, synovial lining, muscles, ligaments and the capsule.[140]

***Clinical assessment** of TMJoint changes includes the following:
- A history review for jaw trauma, bruxism, signs such as popping, clicking and locking, symptoms of soreness and/or pain, and progressively developing malocclusion.
- Visual assessment of mandibular range of movement patterns.
    - Normal:
        - Maximum opening range: 40-50mm, smooth, straight and comfortable
        - Maximum lateral movement, left and right: 8-13 mm, smooth and comfortable
        - Maximum protrusive movement: 8-13 mm, smooth and comfortable
    - TMJoint internal changes produce limited, irregular, and sometimes uncomfortable movement patterns
- Palpation of the lateral joint capsule, posterior joint ligament, and verification of Centric Relation (C.R.) joint position and comfort through bilateral manipulation.

- Doppler auscultation for joint sounds, including clicks, crepitus (related to boney changes), and joint rhonchi, (which are rattling-type sounds related to scar tissue).
- Imaging (MRI, CBCT) of the joints is obtained following positive signs and/or symptoms which require further clarification to finalize a diagnosis and treatment strategy.

Unstable TMJoints can significantly affect growth and development of the cranio-facial-respiratory complex and negatively affect the airway. It is not possible to stabilize a dental malocclusion if the TMJoints are not stable. TMJoint changes can affect Masticatory System health and dramatically alter complete health.

Every dental patient, of every age, should be screened for temporomandibular joint disorders. TM joint health is a fundamental factor of both oral and complete health.

5. Could there be an AIRWAY PROBLEM?

Airway obstructions from the tip of the nose to the bottom of the pharynx can significantly affect breathing. When airway obstructions exist in the nasal airway, a conversion to mouth breathing may occur. Mouth breathing affects normal tongue function and can negatively altar craniofacial development, dental occlusion and respiration.

***Clinical assessment** of the airway includes the following:
- General screening through the use of written evaluations such as the Epworth Sleepiness Scale (ESS) and the STOP-BANG questionnaires.
- A history review of the IDM Checklist including mouth breathing, snoring, sleep apnea, daytime sleepiness, poor sleep quality, nasal congestion, forward head posture, tongue tie, chronic cough and deviated septum.
- Visual assessment, utilizing the IDM Checklist, includes neck circumference, Mallampati score, tongue scalloping, tongue mobility restriction, nasal stenosis, and skeletal profile.
- Screening and testing through overnight high resolution pulse oximetry (HRPO), home sleep testing (HST), heart rate variability (HRV), or sleep center polysomnography (PSG).

Every dental patient, of every age, should be screened for airway and breathing disorders. Airway, breathing and respiration represent fundamental factors of both oral and complete health.

6. Are there signs of local or systemic **INFLAMMATION**?

The inflammatory response is the body's defense mechanism to protect from threatening infection and injury. The purpose is to localize and eliminate the injurious agent and to remove damaged tissue components so that the body can begin to heal. When working within ideal limits, this is important both for increased health of the oral hard and soft tissues and for increased health throughout the body. In contrast, chronic inflammation, both orally (locally) and systemically, weakens the body's immune response and is considered the most important factor contributing to atherosclerosis and accelerated aging. We must remember the reality that oral health and systemic health are not separate entities but are intimately related.

***Clinical assessment** of inflammation includes the following:
- A review of the Inflammation and Infection "History – Signs & Symptoms" section of the IDM Checklist, which can include caries, toothaches, bleeding gums, oral sores, tobacco use, toxins exposure, high blood pressure, a pro-inflammatory diet, chronic pain, chronic stress, diabetes, gastric reflux, and physical inactivity.
- Clinical assessment, utilizing the IDM Checklist, includes visual inspection, periodontal probing, lymph node palpation, and tonsilar evaluation.
- Screening and testing may include a full mouth series of radiographs, HbA1c blood glucose fingerstick test, salivary testing for oral pathogens, oral cancer screening, and the Koufman Reflux Index screening. (In addition, some patients may need to be referred to their medical physicians for further screening and/or testing regarding systemic inflammation.)

Inflammation is a subject of great importance that should be discussed with patients daily regarding a variety of concerns including periodontal disease, blood sugar levels, nutrition, breathing disordered sleep, stress, nicotine usage, gastric reflux, and physical inactivity.

> "INSULIN RESISTANCE:
> THE REAL CAUSE OF DIABESITY
>
> When your diet is full of empty calories and an abundance of quickly absorbed sugars, liquid calories (sodas, juices, sports drinks, or vitamin waters), and refined carbohydrates (bread, pasta, rice, and potatoes), your cells slowly become resistant or numb to the effects of insulin, and need more and more of it to keep your blood sugar levels balanced. This problem is known as **insulin resistance**. A high insulin level is the first sign of a problem. Unfortunately, most doctors never test this. The higher your insulin levels are, the worse your insulin resistance. As the problem worsens, your body starts to lose muscle, gain fat, become inflamed, and you rapidly age and deteriorate. In fact, insulin resistance is the single most important phenomenon that leads to rapid and premature aging and all its resultant diseases, including heart disease, stroke, dementia, and cancer."
>
> Mark Hyman, MD
> <u>The Blood Sugar Solution</u>

7. Is there an <u>**UNESTHETIC SMILE** concern?</u>

Dentistry is an amazing and unique profession, combining the science of medicine, the construction principles of engineering, and the beauty of art. An unesthetic smile can communicate advanced aging and poor hygiene. A beautiful smile communicates youthfulness and health. An unesthetic smile can produce embarrassment and self-consciousness. A beautiful smile produces a sense of comfort and increased self-confidence. Therefore, smile esthetics is a very important consideration for most people.

*Clinical assessment of smile esthetics includes the following:
- **Understanding the patient's concern** about their present smile and future esthetic goals. It is helpful to ask simple esthetics-related questions on new patient forms, such as: **"Are you happy with the appearance of your smile?"**

- Ask for clarification when the answer is "No", such as *How can your smile be improved? Shade? Straighter? Shape? Size?*
- **Photographic Series:** For every new patient a series of 21 photographs are taken to analyze macro (full smile) and micro (tooth by tooth) esthetics, tooth conditions and occlusion, as taught at the Dawson Academy. These photos are reviewed with the patient to evaluate and discuss any concerns that are observed.
- **Dawson Wizard Software Analysis:** The 21-photo series is imported into the software program to visually evaluate each patient's esthetic profile and determine a plan to idealize both the esthetics and the occlusion. This is reviewed with the patient to "co-diagnose" together the concerns that will be addressed along with possible solutions.

Integrative Dental Medicine addresses functional esthetics that create both "engineering" stability and "artistic" beauty. Integrative Dental Medicine proactively addresses the "medical health" of the bite, the muscles, the joints, and the airway, while simultaneously focusing on creating a confident, beautiful smile.

Utilizing the 7 Key Questions for each patient will initiate an Integrative Dental Medicine model of care that can change smiles and lives! Therefore we must always remember to ask:

1. Does the **DENTAL OCCLUSION** appear unstable?
2. Does the patient **BRUX (GRIND or CLENCH)**?
3. Does the patient have **SORE MUSCLES**?
4. Are there signs of **TMJOINT CHANGES**?
5. Could there be an **AIRWAY PROBLEM**?
6. Are there signs of local or systemic **INFLAMMATION**?
7. Is there an **UNESTHETIC SMILE** concern?

Part VI:
The Shift –
In Closing

21. *THE SHIFT* – A LOOK BACK, A LOOK AHEAD BY GARY KADI

Gary Kadi is the CEO of Next Level Practice, based in Manhattan, New York. He created Next Level Practice to implement the Complete Health Dentistry business model, where teams willingly embrace and implement change, patients consider their best treatment opportunities and invest in their health, and doctors enjoy practicing the way they envisioned when they graduated from dental school. Gary and his team have worked with hundreds of dental practices all over the United States. He has produced the documentary Say Ahh: The Cavity in Healthcare Reform and authored 3 books.

Gary is a wonderful advocate, coach and personal friend. We asked Gary to contribute his thoughts to *The Shift* by taking a look back and a look ahead. Enjoy Gary's experienced perspective!

* * *

Looking back, Hippocrates (460 BC) held the belief that the body must be treated as a whole and not just a series of parts. He held the belief that illness had a physical and a rational explanation.

At some point, teaching institutions and practitioners changed from "root cause", Integrative Medicine to symptomatic, reactive sick-care, and the neck became the body's Mason-Dixon Line.

My journey in the world of Integrative Medicine began as

a traditional dental practice management consultant. I remember it so well; it was a cold, snowy day, and I was working with a general dental practice in New York. That day, while training beside hygienists, I began sharing my passion and dedication as an "accidental expert" in oral-systemic health. The following day, my dad had quintuple bypass surgery. One of the hygienists asked, "How was his perio?" My response was, "My dad had a heart attack…what does perio have to do with heart attacks?"

> *"Though the world does not change with a change of paradigm, the scientist afterward works in a different world." (Kuhn)*

I could not un-fry this egg. I now saw through different eyes. As a business and team development expert, I went on a clinical research crusade to understand what I thought was the holy grail for the traditional, recurring problems in a dental practice. That "ah-ha" moment led me to the most profound, courageous and smart healthcare pioneers.

Over the past 11 years, I've realized the need to build the practice of the future, bringing together all the latest preventive modalities, with the goal of helping 30 million people get healthier by 2020. Doing the research for several books and filming <u>Say Ahh: The Cavity in Healthcare Reform</u>, I have had the privilege of meeting incredible men and women, like Dr. Wilkerson, from across the globe who are on a mission to transform dentistry, medicine and our broken healthcare system.

With the help of Dr. Wilkerson and his colleagues, we have collaborated to create Healthcare 2.0. Along this journey, we have failed and succeeded; we have taken arrows in the back. We have experienced the equivalent of Edison's 9999 ways not to create a lightbulb. Each year we get closer to creating a model that allows the patient and the practitioner to win.

Looking ahead, there are three areas that we continue to refine for the ideal "triple win" (patient, practitioner and company) integrated business model:
- New mindset – to create a delivery system that breaks down past based thinking.
- New clinical practice models – fully integrated; not built on top of a dental or medical chassis, but rather from a blank canvas focused on Complete Health® visits.
- New, easier payment models – that reward positive healthcare

outcomes and each practitioner accordingly.

There are <u>problems</u> that can be fixed with a short-term fix or a long-term solution. Playing in this field and on this path is addressing a <u>predicament</u>. Like all scientists, these pioneers keep bumping up against challenges and keep searching for solutions, and after countless tries the scientist has a breakthrough and a new world opens up. **I see this new world of complete health through dentistry opening up more and more, each and every day!**

I love waking up each day with the possibility that in our lifetime we will experience a breakthrough in how mainstream healthcare is delivered and, most importantly, reduce healthcare costs and extend productive healthy lives.

Looking ahead, I see a very bright future for every dentist and dental team willing to engage in *the shift* to complete health care. Reading, studying, and implementing *The Shift* will surely inspire that pursuit.

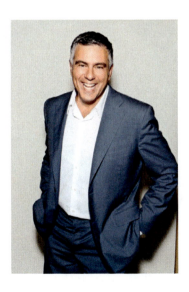

> "Doctors will be the first ones to tell you that they can't keep you from getting heart disease, or put sunblock on your nose before a noontime run, or snatch that third Twinkie out of your paw before you torpedo it down your throat.
>
> ***But you can.***
>
> You can control your health destiny. While you can't always control what happens to you (no matter how fit you are), there are some things that you can control: your attitude, your determination and…your willingness to take your health into your own hands and know as much about your body as possible."
>
> Michael F. Roizen, MD, and Mahmet C. Oz, MD,
> <u>YOU: The Owner's Manual</u>

22. PERSONAL REFLECTIONS BY DEWITT WILKERSON, DMD

I'm a firm believer that each person's life is significant and important.

Our in-depth study of the systems of the human body support that belief. We've seen the magnificent design of the respiratory system. Nitric oxide gas, produced in the paranasal sinuses, is a superstar molecule that destroys invading pathogens in the nose, dilates the respiratory tract, and relaxes the smooth muscles around arteries to improve blood flow and prevent atherosclerosis. The temporomandibular joint is an amazing design of engineering genius. The immune system represents a super-sophisticated protection against thousands of insults each day. The human brain is able to process and store more information than the largest computer ever designed. The complexity of the nucleus of one single cell and the DNA contained within is mind boggling. Studying the brilliant design of the five senses of sight, hearing, smell, taste, and touch leaves us in wonderment.

I'm continuously awed by the wonderful design of our bodies, and how they beautifully function. The more I study, the more I embrace the words of the Biblical Psalmist:

> "For you created my inmost being;
> you knit me together in my mother's womb.
> I praise you because I am fearfully (reverently)
> and wonderfully made;
> your works are wonderful, I know that full well.
> My frame was not hidden from you
> when I was made in the secret place,
> when I was woven together in the depths of the earth.
> Your eyes saw my unformed body;
> all the days ordained for me were written in your book
> before one of them came to be.
> How precious to me are your thoughts, God!
> How vast is the sum of them!
> Were I to count them, they would
> outnumber the grains of sand..."
> (Psalm 139:13-18)

Each of us is reverently and wonderfully made by our Creator, with lives of great significance and importance. How encouraging! Anne Graham Lotz reflects on Psalm 139 in her book God's Story as follows:

"We can only imagine the concentrated thoughts that occupied the divine Mind and the gentle, skillful touch of the divine Hand that first shaped man from the dust. Where did the Creator begin? Did He start with a skeletal frame? Did He then cover it with an outside layer of skin, which at no place is thicker than three-sixteenths of an inch, is packed with nerve endings to enable man to feel the outside world, and is virtually waterproof? Into the skin stretched over the frame did He next place the heart that pumps seventy-two times a minute, forty million times a year? When did He hang the lungs in their sealed compartments so that the rivers of blood necessary for life can deposit the carbon dioxide and pick up oxygen to be carried to every single one of the more than twenty-six trillion cells in the body? When did He place the brain inside the bony skull and program it to send messages that travel faster than three hundred miles an hour along the nervous system to the entire body? Truly, we are fearfully and wonderfully and lovingly and personally created by an awe-inspiring, loving Creator!"[141]

Dr. Pete Dawson, in his must-read biography, A Better Way, thoughtfully articulates, "So here is what I now believe with total confidence: God Himself wrote the instructions in my DNA code at the moment of conception. He designed me for a purpose, and He ordained my days to fulfill His purpose."[142]

As a lifelong student of both science and Scripture, I've learned that each of us is complexly and wonderfully created with a **Body**, a **Soul**, and a **Spirit**. *The Shift* has heavily emphasized the health of the **Body**, as we have studied inflammation, infection, nutrition, physical activity, toxins, airway, breathing, sleep, TMJ disorders and dental occlusion.

The Shift has also referenced the **Soul**, which is our psyche, mind, emotions and will. We've seen that stress is a major factor affecting complete health. Dr. Robert Sapolsky, Professor of Neurology at Stanford University, in his book entitled <u>Why Zebras Don't Get Ulcers,</u> explains how prolonged stress in humans causes or intensifies a range of physical and mental afflictions, including depression, ulcers, colitis, heart disease, and more. We have discussed the importance of recognizing and addressing stress, both physically and mentally, as an important consideration of complete health.

As we close our discussion of *The Shift*, we also want to recognize the central role of the **Spirit** for complete health. The Spirit is the very core of our being. It's the real person and personality deep inside, that extends beyond matter and mind. The Spirit connects us with God's Holy Spirit and eternity. Let me share 3 Scriptural verses that explain so much better than I can:

> "The Spirit of God has made me, and the breath
> of the Almighty gives me life."
> (Job 33:4)

> "May the God of hope fill you with all joy and peace in believing, so that by the power of the Holy Spirit you may abound in hope."
> (Romans 15:13)

> "The fruit of the Spirit is love, joy, peace, patience, kindness, goodness, faithfulness, gentleness, and self-control."
> (Galatians 5:22-23)

Jesus encouraged his followers with these words, referring to the Holy Spirit, "I am leaving you with a gift – peace of mind and heart! And the peace I give isn't fragile like the peace the world gives. So don't be troubled or afraid." (John 14:27) What's the value of that promised gift? Priceless!

Along with freedom from infection and inflammation and the health that comes from exercise and good nutrition, open airways and great sleep, healthy TMJs and stable dental occlusions, I'm convinced that we were designed for loving relationships, peace of mind and heart, hope, joy, purpose and encouragement, both for today and for eternity.

Like 3 circles that intersect, "Complete Health" speaks of a healthy body, a healthy mind, and a healthy spirit. My hope and prayer is that *The Shift* will encourage many on their significant and important pilgrimage toward complete health.

23. PERSONAL REFLECTIONS BY SHANLEY LESTINI, DDS

The foundation of my passion for the message of *The Shift* is a very personal one. There are many people in my life whom I know and love who suffer from chronic illness and debilitating pain. Much of their suffering comes from circumstances beyond their control, but thanks to the advances in medicine and dentistry that are the backbone of *The Shift*, it is my hope and prayer that the information in these pages can help alleviate, reverse or prevent their present or future struggles. Many of them are pushing past their limitations to continue serving others and sharing their gifts despite their physical challenges. However, many of these physical conditions rob them of time, energy and resources that I know they would like to be pouring into their work and relationships.

It is my personal belief that we were created for relationship – both with those around us and ultimately with our Creator. Like any masterful artist, I believe He created us to function in certain ideal ways – spiritually, emotionally, and physically. Within medicine and dentistry, we have learned (and are continuing to learn) more about the ideal physical functioning of our bodies than we could have imagined possible in years past – thanks to the tireless work of countless researchers and practitioners. This research and information provides us with new opportunities to live lives with less pain, fewer limitations, and more energy. We now know that we can have more abundant lives because of the choices we can make.

It is, however, my personal hope and prayer that the abundant life of everyone reading this text does not have to be restricted to the merely physical. Regardless of circumstances, I have personally found that it is my relationship with my Creator that is my true source of abundant life. When Jesus spoke these words, *"I have come that they may have life and have it abundantly"* (John 10:10), calling any who would seek His love and forgiveness to draw near to Him, I know He intended countless blessings for those who would call upon Him – both now and, most importantly, eternally. In Him, I have found that true abundant life is grounded in His saving grace and in fixing my eyes on His promises, no matter what situations arise. Personally, I cannot thank Him enough for His love and for the forgiveness, peace and purpose He gives me. It is my hope that everyone who reads these words will come to experience the true meaning of "abundant life," in all its forms – not only physically, but beyond that as well.

There is so much pain and heartache in life that is unavoidable. However, thanks to these recent advances in medicine and dentistry, we now know that we have more control over our health than we ever previously imagined. When people are set free from pain and illness that can be reversed or prevented, then they are better able to live out the meaningful work and relationships for which they were created. I believe the message of *The Shift* can be a part of helping us live more abundant lives, and because of that, I am deeply humbled and grateful to have been able to participate in this work.

* * *

> "Dear friend, I hope all is well with you and that you are as healthy in body as you are strong in spirit."
> (3 John 1:2)

> "Jesus stood and said in a loud voice,
> 'Whoever believes in me, as Scripture has said, rivers of living water will flow from within them.'"
> (John 7:37-38)

Part VII:
Appendix and
Further Resources

Further Resources

The Shift is intentionally written to be very reader-friendly. For health professionals pursuing Integrative Dental Medicine who would like to go deeper into the science and implementations of these topics, the following resources are provided for you in this Appendix.

Kim Kutsch, DMD, is an internationally-recognized authority on the subject of dental caries diagnosis and therapy. He has graciously provided an outstanding thesis on caries etiology, assessment, diagnostics, and therapeutic strategies entitled, "The Disease of Caries – Intervention and Treatment" (Chapter 24).

Tom Nabors, DDS, is a true pioneer on the subject of the oral-systemic connection, the role of oral pathogenic bacteria and their destructive effects clinically. He has graciously provided a very thorough contribution to this project entitled, "A Medical Model for Diagnosing and Treating Periodontal and Peri-Implant Diseases" (Chapter 25).

Further resources include the 2017 American Dental Association Policy Statement entitled, "The Role of Dentistry in the Treatment of Sleep-Related Breathing Disorders" (Chapter 26). Rachaele Carver Morin, DMD, is an outstanding clinician who has implemented a very effective anti-microbial therapy, which she has graciously outlined in her contribution entitled, "Ozone Therapy" (Chapter 27).

24. THE DISEASE OF CARIES – INTERVENTION AND TREATMENT, BY KIM KUTSCH, DMD

Outline
Introduction
Dental Caries: a Biofilm Disease Model
Caries Risk Assessment
CAMBRA
Salivary diagnostics
Intervention/Treatment Strategies
    Reparative Strategies
    Restoration
    Remineralization
    Therapeutic Strategies
    Antimicrobial
    Fluoride
    pH
    Xylitol
    Remineralization HA
    Silver Diamine Fluoride
    Probiotics
    Behavioral Strategies
    Homecare: Brushing and flossing
    Diet
    Wellness Coaching

Special Needs
Medications
Patient Examples
Conclusion
References
Figures

Introduction

Dental caries is understood to be a pandemic, transmissible, bacterial infection of the teeth that produces prolonged periods of low pH and demineralization of the hard tissue with net mineral loss, leading to pulpal death. Originally thought to be caused by just two different bacterial species, *Mutans streptococci* and *Lactobacillus*, we now consider dental caries to be a complex multifactorial disease influenced by diverse bacterial, dietary, environmental, socioeconomic and physiological risk factors. In simple terms, dental caries is a **disease process**. We tend to think of "dental caries" as a cavity in a tooth, where in reality it is the disease that caused the cavity. The cavity itself is just a sign or symptom of the disease. Unfortunately, the dental profession has become more disease-oriented than health-oriented — more surgically-oriented than medically-oriented. The profession has addressed and re-addressed how best to identify or "diagnose" a cavity, how best to fill or restore a cavity, which material to use, what preparation design to employ, what bonding system to recommend and then what toothpaste or mouth rinse to use. Our recommendations typically come down to fluoride and "don't eat sweets". We focus on the cavity as if it were the disease, all the while ignoring the actual disease process responsible for the cavity. As a result, our patients continue to experience cavities throughout their lifetime, until they run out of teeth or die.

Dental Caries: a Biofilm Disease Model

The old disease model of dental caries involved just two bacteria, *Mutans streptococci* and *Lactobacillus*, as the agents responsible for tooth decay. Recent scientific evidence from biofilm research now indicates there are more than fifty different bacteria that play a role in dental caries, and the list continues to grow. Therefore the old disease model no longer adequately accounts for the complexity of this disease. Among some of the newly identified cavity-causing bacteria, *Bifidobacteria* is of particular concern because this same species has also been suggested as a probiotic to prevent this disease. Other scientific evidence indicates that, much like periodontal disease, dental caries also has potential systemic effects. Studies have demonstrated that caries-causing bacteria are the most commonly found bacteria in heart arteries and heart valve plaque. Additional studies have implicated cavity-causing bacteria in contributing to impaired mental function, ulcerative colitis and infections following surgery. Dental caries also appears to have a genetic component, and numerous studies have now identified different genes that make a patient more susceptible to this disease. Then there is a long list of known risk factors (such as a lack of saliva) that further complicate the picture. But regardless of how complex the dental caries disease model becomes, it still comes down to prolonged periods of acidic conditions in the mouth, resulting in mineral loss of the teeth, followed by the invasion of the bacteria into the tooth and the resulting creation of the cavity. Now the challenge becomes how to identify specifically what is causing an individual patient's cavities, so that we can target our therapeutic approach. Rather than just identifying how many cavities a patient has, our goal can (and should be) figuring out *why* they have cavities and addressing that underlying cause instead.

Caries Risk Assessment (CRA)

As the scientific evidence base has grown, the dental profession has progressed from the "drill and fill" model of fixing cavities to a model that includes some anti-cavity strategies (like fluoride). Continued growth in the evidence base will lead us into a future of precision medicine, where the cause of the cavities is identified or diagnosed, can be measured, and then can be targeted for therapy. A six year clinical study conducted in 2011 on 12,954 patients at the UCSF School of Dentistry identified different risk factors involved in the creation of cavities and then also validated the use of a caries risk assessment form as a diagnostic tool to help identify patients' specific risk factors, as well as their resulting risk of getting additional cavities if untreated.[1] This concept of using a risk assessment form has been given the name "CAMBRA" (Caries Management By Risk Assessment). In this study, they identified the odds that each risk factor contributed to the disease risk and also identified indicators of the disease. The disease indicators identified

---

[1] Validation of the CDA CAMBRA caries risk assessment--a six-year retrospective study. Doméjean S, White JM, Featherstone JD. J Calif Dent Assoc. 2011 Oct;39(10):709-15.

include visible cavities, radiographic lesions penetrating to the dentin, active white spot lesions, and a history of a restored cavity in the previous three years. Risk factors identified in the study include noticeable plaque build-up on the teeth, frequent snacking, hypo-salivation, exposed roots, deep pits and fissures and recreational drug usage. In simple terms, we *can* identify common risk patterns for this disease. These common patterns include the following factors:
1. bacteria (the patient either has too much bacterial plaque load on their teeth, or they have too high a level of acid output of those bacteria);
2. diet (the patient either has too much sugar in their diet or they are snacking too frequently);
3. saliva (the patient either doesn't have enough salivary flow, or their saliva is not able to adequately buffer the acid that the bacteria are producing).

CAMBRA

With this simple foundation in mind, CAMBRA can be a simple process as well. It consists of three separate steps:
1. assessment
2. diagnosis
3. prescription/intervention

The caries risk assessment (CRA) form can either be filled out by the patient (allowing them to self-identify their specific risk factors, which can then be evaluated/reviewed by the dental professional), or the form can be filled out via an "interview" style by the dental professional. There are a number of these different clinical forms available from the American Dental Association, the California Dental Association Foundation, the American Academy of Pediatric Dentistry and Carifree, (Fig. 1). The assessment process consists of identifying the risk factors and disease indicators for the patient. Combining this information with all other data obtained from the oral exam, radiographs, bacterial testing, and the patient's history will then allow an accurate diagnosis of the patient's caries risk to be established. In this model, identifying cavities and restoring them is the treatment for the *symptom* we call "cavities"; identifying, understanding and addressing the specific risk factors for each patient is the treatment for managing the *disease* of dental caries.

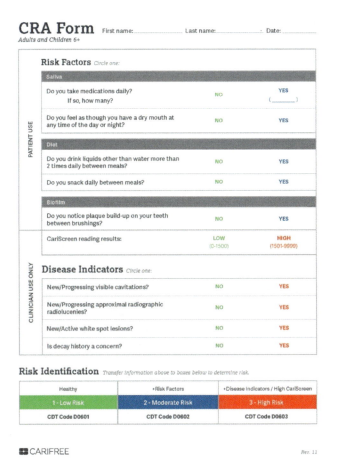

Figure 1. A caries risk assessment form that identifies the patient's attitude toward dental caries, and also has them self-report their risk factors, making the process more efficient from a time-management standpoint in the hygiene operatory.

Salivary Analysis and Biometrics

As has been mentioned, saliva is a major protective factor against dental caries. Human saliva contains 2260 proteins and various minerals, and it has an alkaline pH – all of which enable it to protect the teeth. Current tests for saliva include measuring the following:

 -salivary flow, both unstimulated and stimulated
 -salivary pH, both resting and stimulated
 -buffering capacity of the saliva

- bacterial pathogen presence, including *Mutans streptococci* and *Lactobacillus*
- plaque cariogenic potential
- biofilm activity level measured by ATP bioluminescence

The challenge facing dentistry today is finding a valid chair-side test for dental caries that is time-efficient, cost-effective and predictive of caries presence and progression. Such a salivary or biofilm test is desirable clinically to first establish a baseline for the patient; measure outcomes during and after therapies aimed at managing the patient's individual risk factors; and, finally, to monitor progress.

Salivary flow is easy to measure via simple collection techniques, as is salivary pH. However, neither of these chair-side tests are very predictive for measuring dental caries, so while it provides nice educational information, it doesn't help predict the patient's risk for cavities. Research data has long established a strong predictive relationship between levels of salivary *Mutans streptococci* and *Lactobacillus* and a higher risk of caries. To evaluate their levels, a sample of the patient's saliva can be collected and then cultured in an oven for 48 hours. However, it is a management challenge to schedule patients and recall them for the results of the test; additionally, of all the commercial culture tests available, none of them accurately identifies the levels of cavity-causing bacteria. Newer technology measures DNA for *Mutans streptococci* and *mitis*, and *Lactobacillus casei* from a saliva sample and more accurately assesses levels of those bacteria in the patient's mouth. This test needs to be mailed to a laboratory for analysis.

ATP Bioluminescence is a technology that has been around for a long time. It involves a testing swab and a meter. ATP is the fuel molecule for all living cells, and measuring for ATP on the teeth gives an immediate report of the bacterial levels present. Additionally, cavity-causing bacteria survive and thrive in an acidic pH; their adaptive mechanisms to accomplish this acidic pH end up resulting in a high use of energy, or ATP. Numerous studies have validated ATP Bioluminescence as a chair-side test to measure bacterial levels on the teeth (and cavity-causing bacteria specifically). ATP bioluminescence is a simple chair-side test that involves swabbing a specific site on the teeth and then a 15 second measurement with a meter. It is efficient, effective and provides reasonable predictability. The ATP bioluminescence test is a great patient educational tool and can also be used to motivate a patient to pursue treatment immediately.

One of the challenges to incorporating CAMBRA into clinical practice stems from the lack of time available to perform this task, as it is usually assigned to an already-burdened hygiene appointment. A recent CRA form developed for clinical practice addresses this time capacity issue, beginning with three motivational interview questions denoted on the form, followed by self-reporting of risk factors by the patient, (Fig. 1). This form can be filled out in the reception area prior to the hygiene visit. Then the dental professional can identify disease indicators present and discuss the risk factors with the patient.

The caries diagnosis is made by examining all of the data obtained from the patient: the CRA form, the oral examination, radiographs, history with the patient, and any tests used (such as ATP Bioluminescence). The ADA Council of Scientific Affairs published definitions for the different risk categories for children and adults in a special supplement to JADA in 2006. Once the caries diagnosis is determined, the next step is to design therapeutic strategies for the individual patient, specifically targeting their individual risk factors.

Intervention/Treatment Strategies

Intervention or prescriptive strategies for managing dental caries can be organized into three categories: (1) reparative strategies, (2) therapeutic materials, and (3) behavioral changes.

1. Reparative Strategies
Reparative strategies (such as "drill and fill" and fluoride) are well developed by the dental profession and include remineralization and restoration.

- **Reparative Strategies via Restorations**: The dentist may decide to stage the restorative treatment of lesions on the high caries risk patient, first restoring all lesions with an intermediate material like glass ionomer (GIC) during the period in which they are working with the patient while they attempt to modify the biofilm and behaviors. In the Wellness Coaching model, the decisions on when and how to proceed with restorative treatments are best determined by a well-informed patient. In this case, the dental professional just needs to communicate very clearly with the patient that this restorative phase is merely the beginning, and that their risk factors must be addressed to help them achieve a successful, stable and healthy outcome. In this situation, risk management becomes a strategy of protecting the teeth and the newly-placed restorations.

- **<u>Reparative Strategies via Remineralization</u>**: Dental caries lesions that are not cavitated on the enamel surface do not require fillings and can be remineralized (Fig 2). Most scientific evidence on therapeutic remineralization involves the use of fluoride. Additional evidence indicates that xylitol also influences remineralization and potentiates the effects of even small amounts of fluoride. Furthermore, there are a number of forms of calcium phosphate that have been used in remineralization strategies. The process by which these work is based upon the fact that saliva is supersaturated with hydroxyapatite and fluorapatite mineral, which are what the body uses to protect and remineralize the teeth. If the patient has a dry mouth or suffers from hypo-salivation/xerostomia, it would make sense to address this problem by adding fluoride and xylitol to the patient's daily routine. This routine could range from being very minimal to very involved. A more minimal routine could simply be making sure the patient is brushing twice a day with a standard fluoride toothpaste (1100ppm fluoride); a more involved routine could include recommending they incorporate the use of a 5000ppm fluoride gel once or twice a day (or as a replacement to dentifrice). Another strategy might be to add xylitol with the fluoride strategy as a gel or rinse. Additionally the professional might consider a product that contains a form of calcium phosphate. For the extreme high caries risk patients that also have dry mouth, another recommended strategy would include using a neutral/alkaline 5000ppm gel in a tray for up to 8 hours during the day or night. Some products include all of these components in one gel, rinse or delivery.

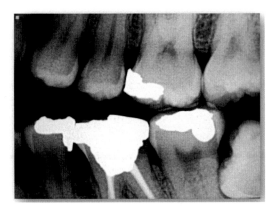

Figure 2. Radiograph demonstrating cavities E2/D1 that must be restored and D1/D2 white spot lesions that can be remineralized.

2. Therapeutic Strategies

Therapeutic strategies include the following categories: antimicrobials, fluoride, pH-management, remineralization, metabolic aids, Silver Diamine Fluoride, and (potentially) probiotics.

- **Antimicrobial Strategies**: Traditionally, Chlorhexidine (CHX) has been the gold standard antimicrobial strategy for dental caries and is used to reduce bacterial levels on the teeth. It is very effective on *Mutans streptococci*, but it has little effect on other bacteria (such as *Lactobacillus*). Recent reviews of studies and recommendations by the ADA in 2011 have virtually eliminated the use of CHX as an antimicrobial agent for dental caries. Aside from CHX-thymol varnish every 3 months for root surface caries, all other CHX — in any form, for any lesion site, for any age — is not recommended. That realistically leaves sodium hypochlorite as an antimicrobial rinse. It has been proposed that using 0.1—0.5% sodium hypochlorite rinses as antiseptics for patient self-care have significantly broader spectra of antimicrobial action and are less likely to induce development of resistant bacteria and adverse host reactions. Additionally, a recent study of 0.25% sodium hypochlorite demonstrated a dramatic reduction in plaque build-up from all surfaces of the teeth. For the high caries risk patient with a bacterial risk factor, the recommendation would be to place the patient on an antimicrobial rinse once or twice daily and plan the therapy for 2 years duration, monitoring the effectiveness every 3 months.

- **Fluoride**: While fluoridated water has been demonstrated to reduce the overall decay rate in populations, the best form of professionally-applied fluoride is fluoride varnish. Patient-applied fluoride is best in the form of a 0.05% fluoride rinse or 5000ppm fluoride gel. For high caries risk patients, the recommendation for fluoride varnish application is every three months, and more frequent varnish application does not demonstrate an improved benefit. For the high caries risk patient with dry mouth, it would make sense to recommend daily use of a fluoride product and also to include some form of calcium phosphate. This therapy would be a life-long, ongoing recommendation (as long as the patient's dry mouth symptoms remained).

- **pH management**: In a healthy individual, there is an ongoing balance between episodes of acidic pH (demineralization) and alkaline pH (remineralization), with no resulting loss of mineral from the teeth. After an acid challenge, buffering agents in the saliva and bacteria in the mouth return the pH to a healthy level. This normal pH cycling in the mouth provides a dynamic stability, where mineral is lost during periods of low pH and returns to the teeth during periods of higher pH. Conversely, dental caries results when this system is out of balance and there are more periods of low pH (and mineral loss) than periods of high pH (and remineralization). In this sense, dental caries is a simple "pH-specific" disease. As the byproducts of the cavity-causing bacteria are acidic, managing pH can play an important role in intervention strategies.
    o For the dry mouth patient, it is very important to consider the loss of the protective value of the normally-alkaline saliva. To address this risk factor, it is important for the patient to stay well-hydrated, and it is important that the patient understand the effects eating and drinking can have on the pH within the mouth, as well as the potential demineralization of the teeth. Based on the pH balance, eating too frequently can be disastrous for

this patient. Furthermore, it is important for the patient to understand that if they drink bottled water frequently throughout the day, they must make sure it has a neutral or alkaline pH (as about half of the commercially-bottled waters have an acidic pH of about 4.0). Additional pH-management strategies would include recommending oral care products that are alkaline, since, for patients with inadequate saliva, neutralization strategies supplement the protective role of the saliva.

- **Remineralization with hydroxyapatite (HA):** Fluoride alone as a remineralization strategy has not been shown to be sufficient to prevent dental caries. Various forms of calcium phosphate have also been included with fluoride in some oral care products. Tricalcium phosphate, amorphous calcium phosphate and CPP/ACP (casein phospho-peptide coated amorphous calcium phosphate) are currently available in products, as well as nano-particle hydroxyapatite. Especially for the high caries risk patient with dry mouth, adding a calcium phosphate product in addition to fluoride strategies is a good recommendation.

- **Xylitol:** One other potential, metabolic strategy for managing the cavity-causing bacteria is xylitol. Xylitol has been shown to potentiate even small amounts of fluoride, so it might make sense to combine xylitol with fluoride strategies. However, there is conflicting evidence for xylitol. Therefore, the incorporation of xylitol could be considered a useful strategy when applied in a combination with other strategies targeted to the patient's specific risk factors, but it might be ineffective as a solo strategy. There currently are products available that combine xylitol, fluoride, pH-management, remineralization and antimicrobial strategies. These can be helpful, as it makes sense to recommend therapies that don't involve too many steps and procedures. The more complicated the recommendations are, the more challenging it is for the patient to create sustainable behavioral change and successful outcomes.

- **Silver Diamine Fluoride (SDF):** Silver Diamine fluoride has recently been approved by the FDA as a desensitizing agent, although the majority of practitioners use it off-label as an anticaries agent. It comes in a solution and is applied directly to active lesions. The silver ion is a strong antimicrobial agent and after a couple of applications of the solution, the SDF performs very well in minimizing the continued progress of the lesion. There are two suggestions on its mode of action. The fluoride ion readily helps create fluorapatite in the lesion, and there is evidence that the silver precipitates in the tubules as microwires. Both would explain the relative immediate increase in surface hardness of the lesion. The only downside to this agent is that it turns the lesions dark black. That being said, it provides a great opportunity to halt lesion progression, but at the cost of short-term esthetic issues. With this in mind, SDF can play an important role in treating lesions in small children and all the way through older adults.

- **Probiotics**: Probiotics deserve mention as one of the options for therapeutic interventions. Probiotics, by definition from the World Health Organization (WHO) and the United Nations Food/Agriculture Organization (FAO),[2] must meet the following criteria: they must be living microorganisms or bacteria; they must be safe for human consumption; and when ingested they must have beneficial effects beyond basic nutrition. Early use of probiotics has demonstrated great efficiency in treating gastro-intestinal disorders, such as Crohn's disease or ulcerative colitis. However, attempts to use probiotic bacteria therapeutically to control dental caries have had mixed results. To date, no studies indicate that the probiotic bacteria become permanent members of the oral biofilm or that they impact dental caries incidence in the

---

[2] Magdalena Araya, Catherine Stanton, Lorenzo Morelli, Gregor Reid, Maya Pineiro, et al., 2006, "Probiotics in food: health and nutritional properties and guidelines for evaluation," Combined Report of a Joint FAO/WHO Expert Consultation on Evaluation of Health and Nutritional Properties of Probiotics in Food Including Powder Milk with Live Lactic Acid Bacteria, Cordoba, Argentina, 1–4 October 2001, and Report of a Joint FAO/WHO Working Group on Drafting Guidelines for the Evaluation of Probiotics in Food, London, Ontario, Canada, 30 April–1 May 2002 [FAO Food and Nutrition paper 85], pp. 1–50, Rome, Italy: World Health Organization (WHO), Food and Agricultural Organization (FAO) [of the United Nations], ISBN 9251055130, see [1], accessed 11 June 2015.

long term. While probiotics are an interesting option and offer a potential additional strategy for the future, currently more research is indicated. For the high caries risk patient, it is fine to recommend probiotics, but it wouldn't make sense to rely on this as a stand-alone strategy.

3. Behavioral Strategies

Behavioral strategies include methods (a) to alter behavior and also (b) to account for risks that cannot be modified. Some behaviors are theoretically modifiable while others are not, and this reality must be taken into account.

a. **Modifiable Behaviors**

Diet and home care both play major roles in the incidence of dental caries. Too much plaque build-up on teeth accompanied by infrequent disruption by brushing and flossing leads to site-specific demineralization of the teeth. Home care instructions, daily brushing, and flossing continue to be important recommendations for a healthy mouth. Most dental professionals are well-versed in making recommendations for tooth brushing techniques with either manual or electric brushes and also for daily flossing protocols. Nevertheless, effective home care habits remain a challenge (and, therefore, risk factor) for many patients. The challenge here is that telling somebody what they should be doing and how they should be doing it doesn't ultimately change their behavior.

Dietary issues involved in the development of dental caries tend to stem from too much sugar intake or from snacking too frequently. Americans consume a tremendous amount of sugar (about 23 teaspoons per day on average) and are number one in high fructose corn syrup consumption (at 51 pounds per person per year). For most high risk patients, they are either eating too much sugar (which is basically true for most Americans) or they are eating/snacking too frequently. When xerostomia caused by medications or aging is added into this equation, it becomes a perfect storm for dental caries. Both of these behaviors (sugar consumption and snacking frequency) should be modifiable, but human behavioral change is not easy – nor is it linear. Additionally, sugar is very addictive. It is important to make good dietary recommendations to the high caries risk patient and to help them understand how their behaviors contribute to their decay issues.

Motivational Interviewing and Wellness Coaching principles can help patients manage their own behavioral changes, but realistically these changes take time and require consistent reinforcement. The best approach is for the dental professional to view the patient as a whole, complete, and capable person who suffers from a disease. The dental profession has been very good at educating patients on proper home care and diets, but we have also been equally good at making patients feel judged, guilty or ashamed about their condition. To speak in plain terms, what we've been doing hasn't worked. This approach has not led to successful behavioral change for many patients, even though, sadly, dental caries is largely a preventable disease. A Wellness Coaching approach provides non-judgmental assessment and reporting of findings to the patient, and then engages their participation while focusing on their wants, needs and benefits. Wellness Coaching uses open ended and non-judgmental questions to draw the patient into the process. Too often dental professionals create elaborate treatment plans and stage the treatment based on their own ideas, rather than including the patient. Give the patient control, let them lay out the solution, and then fiercely support them and advocate for them.

b. **Non-modifiable Behaviors**

Non-modifiable issues typically involve medication-induced hyposalivation, aging, reduced cognitive or physical function, and special needs. Dry mouth is a major risk factor for dental caries and most often is related to prescription medications. The more medications are involved, the greater the risk and severity of dry mouth. It would be important for the hyposalivation patient to be given appropriate recommendations on hydration, eating, and the role of pH and their dental caries risk. Typically these patients present with multiple root surface lesions, and appropriate recommendations would include 5000ppm fluoride gel daily along with xylitol mints.

Other non-modifiable behavioral strategies include those needed when helping patients with special needs. There is mixed data surrounding this population. Some studies indicate that special needs patients have increased salivary flow while other studies conclude that they have reduced salivary flow. They certainly are at a higher risk for caries based on their levels of dexterity and home care capabilities, and they may be limited by the level of skill, care, knowledge and judgment of their care providers or facilities.

Patient Examples

Designing the appropriate and effective treatment strategy for an individual patient is straightforward. The patient's individual risk factors drive the treatment strategies. The patient in Figure 3 is high risk for dental caries, as is the patient in Figure 4. However, the risk factors associated with these two patients are significantly different and require a targeted approach for their treatment to be successful. If the patient has a bacterial issue (Fig. 3), it should be addressed with antimicrobial materials, pH modification and home care instructions. For the patient with a dietary issue, the strategy should focus on modifying their sugar consumption or snacking habits. The hyposalivation patient (Fig. 4) will likely benefit from maintaining hydration levels and pH neutralization materials which support a healthy oral environment. The patient with a genetic risk for dental caries (Fig. 5) may be harder to diagnose but will benefit from minimizing acid exposures during the day and from supporting wellness.

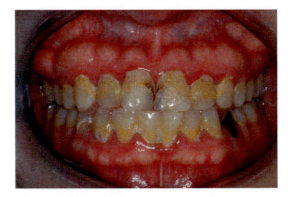

Figure 3. High caries risk patient with plaque build-up and dietary issues. The patient chose to work on the dietary issue first during the Wellness Coaching conversation.

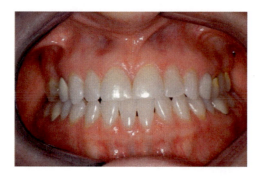

Figure 4. High caries risk patient with hyposalivation related to medications.

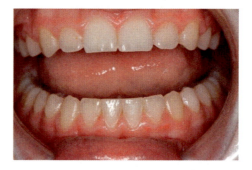

Figure 5. High caries risk patient with LYZL2 salivary bacteriolytic enzyme deficiency and geographic pattern of decay limited to mandibular incisors.

Conclusion

The key to creating successful and predictable treatment outcomes in managing dental caries is to correctly identify the risk factors driving the disease for the patient. While dental caries is a multifactorial disease, typical patterns of the disease do emerge, and identifying these patterns simplifies the creation of the strategies for intervention. CAMBRA represents best practices and provides the next step toward precision medicine, promising more effective and predictable treatment outcomes for dental caries in clinical practice.

Kim Kutsch, DDS

* * *

Kim is an Albany/Corvallis area native and received his dental degree from the University of Oregon. He is an internationally recognized expert in cavity prevention and minimally invasive dentistry. He has dedicated his entire career to the development of new technologies and treatment methods in dentistry. A lifelong inventor, he holds numerous patents relative to the dental profession. He helped develop the Carifree® system, which diagnoses and eliminates tooth decay. He is a mentor at the Kois Center in Seattle, Washington. Dr. Kutsch is a published author and speaker at dental meetings throughout the world.

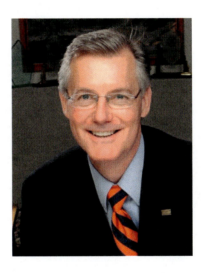

25. A MEDICAL MODEL FOR DIAGNOSING AND TREATING PERIODONTAL AND PERI-IMPLANT DISEASES, BY THOMAS W. NABORS, DDS, FACD

Introduction:

A few years ago, I had the privilege of addressing the attendees of the International Academy of Periodontology in a scientific presentation. Periodontists from around the world had gathered to hear the latest in science and to review the latest in technology.

My talk was designed to introduce our new clinical laboratory and a number of new saliva tests that we had developed. Our saliva tests were (and are) designed to improve clinical examination by providing important information that the traditional examination cannot provide. After the presentation, I had time for a few questions. Most of the questions were interesting and quite good. However, the most surprising question came from a frequent speaker on the topic of periodontal disease treatment. His question was, **"Why do I need testing? After all, I can see periodontal disease."** The following is a brief summary of my answer as to why salvia testing is more important than relying on what we can see.

1. What we "see" is not the disease; we see the <u>symptoms</u> of the disease.

*Today, we recognize that "symptoms" and "causative agents" of disease vary from person to person – and that specific microorganisms, along with genetics/epigenetics, influence symptoms. A lab test can detect both causative agents as well as genetic variations (Colombo, et al; J Perio Vol 83 Number 10; Oct.,2012; 1279-1287).

2. A diagnosis based purely on symptoms assumes that "symptoms" represent the "targets of treatment". Furthermore, when using only clinical signs, we are diagnosing and treating late-stage disease in most cases.

*The literature clearly states that pathogenic organisms are the "target of treatment" (not symptoms) and that we should be diagnosing and treating these infections sooner.

3. Lastly, and most importantly, this question did not address the potential impact of periodontal pathogens to vascular health and disease. Since "symptoms" of periodontal disease are not recognized as being connected to systemic inflammation, but specific periodontal pathogens are, it behooves us to consider lab testing to discover the pathogen burden relative to systemic inflammation.

*A primary goal of periodontal therapy is to prevent the potential risk of periodontal pathogens increasing systemic inflammation. Since different pathogens influence inflammation differently, testing helps to predict the influence they have on systemic inflammation. (We must remember, we are not all the same).

Why we must change our beliefs regarding the importance of periodontal infections...

In 2008, a meta-analysis was examined regarding the impact of periodontal infections on coronary heart disease (CHD). The conclusion of this analysis by the United States Preventative Services Task Force (USPSTF) is that periodontal disease is a **risk factor or marker for coronary heart disease (CHD) that is independent of other CHD risk factors, including socioeconomic status** (Humphrey et al.: Periodontal Disease and Coronary Heart Disease Risk; JGIM). This conclusion should be extremely important to patients as well as to all health professionals – those that treat these infections and those that treat heart disease, diabetes, and other systemic diseases.

Many additional studies since then have shown that periodontal disease is not just an oral health problem. It is, in fact, a much broader health care issue that may affect the entire vascular system, including the vessels in the heart and the brain. The debate over this issue has become even more relevant with indications that specific periodontal infections may actually cause heart disease (including increased risk for heart attack and stroke).

Another important fact in this discussion is that the traditional model for diagnosis and treatment of periodontal disease (e.g. based on clinical signs) does not make the connection to heart disease. The most powerful influence of periodontal infection to CHD is from those infections with high concentration of pathogenic bacteria. And, since these infections vary from person to person based on oral pathogen profiles, it behooves the dental and medical professions to not only recognize the potential for systemic risk, but to recognize how to differentiate infections based first and foremost on the most important aspect of the infection: the pathogen profile of the patient that may cause vascular injury.

Are we there yet?

Unfortunately, for most clinicians in both the oral health and general health realms, we are not. The traditional model for diagnosis and treatment of these infections does not yet achieve both desired goals: oral health and the reduction of the systemic risk.

However, there are many in both fields of health that are indeed there. And, armed with this important information and new diagnostic tests, these clinicians can differentiate and recognize those at risk for CHD and treat the infection with both important goals in mind.

Another significant point here is that traditional models of diagnosis and treatment often fail to resolve the infection. When that happens, we often hear the statement that…"periodontal diseases cannot be cured, only managed."

This statement is not accurate, as many of these infections can, in fact, be cured. And, more importantly, we can verify if our treatment has resolved the infection as well as the potential systemic effects of the infection. Thus, this chapter gives some insight to how the diagnosis and treatment end-points should be improved based on 21st century knowledge of these serious infections.

How and Why Testing for Periodontal Pathogens Changes the Game:

> **"The ultimate risk factor for any infectious disease is the causative agent(s) of that disease"**
> (Haffajee, et al. 2006)

With the above statement in mind, **risk factors and causative agents** are both important relative to understanding infections and diseases. So, what's the difference between the two?

By definition, a **risk factor** is something that increases a person's chances of developing a disease. For example, cigarette smoking is a **risk factor** for lung cancer, and obesity is a **risk factor** for heart disease.

The term **causative agent** usually refers to the biological pathogen that **causes a disease**, such as a **virus, parasite, fungus, or bacterium**. Technically, the term can also refer to a toxin or toxic chemical that **causes illness.**

In summary, a risk factor does not cause an infectious disease; a causative agent does.

So, the initial quote simply states a clear fact; risk factors are important in understanding infectious diseases, but **causative agents of disease become the ultimate risk factor.**

An important note: By identifying causative agents prior to the manifestation of the disease, we have the potential to actually prevent the disease. And, when clinical signs of any inflammation (gingivitis, early periodontitis, peri-implantitis, etc.) *are* visible, it is important to test for the specific oral pathogens that will indicate risk for more aggressive disease as well as the potential for vascular disease. Additionally, an antimicrobial treatment plan to reduce or remove the "causative agents" of disease should be planned.

Periodontal & Peri-implant infections:
Risk factors & Causative Agents

Why testing is so important:

In some diseases, there is more than one causative agent. Periodontal and peri-implant diseases are excellent examples in which there are multiple causative agents. Based on decades of microbiological research, we understand that these serious infections are biofilm infections that are made up of many different species and billions of microbial agents that develop and mature over time. Additionally, the pathogenic potential of some biofilms is more aggressive than others.

However, there are potentially hundreds of different species that may be found in an individual oral biofilm infection when examining different individuals (Biekler, et. al., 2005). While some biofilms are made up of different species that may produce inflammation and slight tissue damage, other biofilms are made up of highly toxic species that produce massive local inflammation and systemic inflammation, as well as severe tissue damage.

It is well understood within periodontal medicine that there are important risk factors to be taken into account, including smoking, diabetes, obesity, immunosuppressive diseases, and others. Traditionally, though, we have not understood the "causative agents" on a person-to-person basis. However, it has become imperative that those attempting to prevent and treat periodontal and peri-implant disease understand the "causative agents" at play.

It is also important to understand that the "systemic effects" are based upon understanding "true etiology" of periodontitis and peri-implantitis. Current findings from multiple reviews from the medical and dental literature confirm the importance of understanding these connections. (For further details, see the *Journal of American Heart Association, Circulation, Stroke, Journal of Clinical Periodontology, Periodontology 2000,* and *Cell Biology,* to name a few.)

Periodontitis, Peri-implantitis, and The Systemic Effects: A Short Review

These conditions have been called "infections," "diseases," "illnesses," and "infectious diseases" …and all of them fit the definitions of periodontitis and peri-implantitis. As is the case here, science is always ahead of clinical practice, so it behooves the clinician to keep up with current science. It is more from the medical literature (rather than the dental) that we would expect to find the connections between oral health and its impact on systemic health. Thus, we will use medical literature, as well as some dental literature, to support this chapter.

A main difference when defining periodontal disease in the medical literature today is the emphasis on etiology and the pathogens that create the greatest risk to systemic disease. The traditional model of basing diagnosis and treatment on clinical signs such as bleeding on probing, pocket depths, plaque scores, etc. does have good support for systemic influence, especially when there is frank disease.

However, the biological presentation of these diseases based on causation (the number and specificity of pathogens) has become a source of medical research. Furthermore, depending on the etiological agents, many of our patients have periodontal infections that place them at risk for systemic diseases such as diabetes and arterial diseases including heart disease, heart attacks, and stroke. Thus it is important to know that we finally have the ability to use modern science in our day-to-day patient care within this model of etiology and systemic effects in order to define these diseases based on "true causation".

We should also remember that these are chronic infections and that they differ from the traditional model of "infectious diseases." However, the fact that they may present as low-grade infections does not diminish their important role in systemic disease. The chronic condition of inflammation has the potential to be extremely serious; periodontitis is one of the causes of chronic inflammation. Additionally, the diseases of this discussion are transmissible from person to person through saliva contact: from parents to children, from spouse to spouse, from children to children, and so on.

The understanding of chronic infections such as periodontitis and peri-implantitis has changed the model of infectious diseases. We know that anyone we "share our saliva with" will receive a few of our microbes as well. While risk factors such as smoking, diabetes, genetics, poor home-care, etc. are very important and bend the "risk curve" toward disease, they are not "causative agents." So, what do we need to know more specifically about these causative agents?

Pathogens Vs. Non-pathogens: Defining the "Ultimate Risk Factor"

Not all bacteria are created equal. And, within healthy people, there is a balance between good bacteria and bad bacteria (symbiosis). When the good ones outnumber the bad ones, we typically have health. However, when the balance shifts from good to bad, we tend to shift from health to disease (dysbiosis).

While most oral microbes are helpful with little potential to cause disease, there are others that are "true pathogens" and can actually cause bone loss, eventual tooth loss, vascular injury and systemic inflammation.

The original word "pathogen" comes from the words "pathos" and "genesis" and literally means "the beginning of disease." Thus, some bacteria are non-pathogenic (do not cause disease) while others are pathogenic (cause disease). When a person has an imbalance (dysbiosis), the bad bacteria (pathogens) shift the balance of the entire microbial community within the mouth. These pathogens will cause periodontitis and peri-implantitis when in sufficient quantity regardless of the genetic make-up of the individual. The concept of the "susceptible individual" is certainly relevant. However, it is not primary in this causation experience in most people.

For us to get a handle on this, we should realize that it is not just the accumulation of dental plaque or bleeding on probing that will determine bone loss and the systemic link, but more importantly, it is the species of bacteria, as well as the genetic influence, which will determine bone loss and the systemic link. Many species can cause the gingival tissues to become inflamed and bleed, but they lack the ability to cause bone loss. It is the "true pathogen(s)" and their ability to create such a massive immune response which will cause the body to eventually dissolve bone and "extract" teeth if necessary, in order to wall off these true infections and prevent them from further invasion.

Biofilm vs. Pathogens:

"Oral biofilm" is easily visible within the mouth. However, the concept that biofilm is the same from patient to patient is incorrect. It may look the same, but based on DNA profiles of the bacterial species within the biofilm, it may be very different. The simple point here is that the soft plaque (biofilm) that we observe within the mouths of our patients varies in species and in quantity of "pathogen profiles" from patient to patient. In fact, the most serious biofilm is not visible to us because it tends to live within the tissues. Thus, today, we know that "plaque" is very unique and personal.

The good news is that these "biofilm differences" can be measured quite easily using a saliva or subgingival sample. By using saliva or subgingival samples, we can send patient samples to a clinical laboratory that uses DNA technology to determine a more relevant and accurate diagnosis of what lies within the biofilm. With this knowledge, one can determine risk of bone loss and even risk for systemic inflammation. Interestingly – and very importantly – you don't have to wait for bone loss to occur to discover this information. Even early signs of disease may be an indicator that you should find out if "true etiology" is present in each patient.

This ability to view every patient with this unique information changes our concept of risk associated with bone loss around teeth and implants, and more importantly, it changes our concept of risk associated with arterial diseases.

> **"There are no average people."**
> Muin Khoury, MD,
> Centers for Disease Control (CDC), June 2014

This recent statement is important for all health care providers. Dr. Khoury continues: "For personalized medicine to continue its advance toward treating patients ..., clinicians and scientists are going to have to get over thinking of people in terms of averages. There are no average people".

This statement is true for all human disorders including cancer, heart disease, and diabetes. It also includes periodontitis and implantitis. Genetics (the study of DNA of humans) and metagenomics (the study of microbial communities and their influence on human health) have changed the way we define diseases because each person has differences in both their disease patterns and how they respond to treatment.

In other words, **"one size does not fit all" in any form of medicine today. This includes the diagnosis and management of periodontal infections in all of its forms.** As clinicians, we have all observed that people respond differently to periodontal therapy. Some will do well; others will only "get better"; and others will show little difference after therapy. The understanding of etiology and systemic effects will answer most of these questions regarding why patients vary so much.

The most important paradigm shifts regarding periodontal infections are that (1) what you see clinically is not the disease; (2) periodontal disease occurs sub-clinically long before we can "see it"; (3) targets of therapy have changed; (4) early periodontal diseases can be cured; and (5) the "end-point" of treatment varies based on testing, not on clinical signs. All of these shifts in thinking require an understanding of etiology and causation.

Bacterial "Fingerprints":

The bacterial component of health and disease cannot be over emphasized. By definition, periodontal diseases are inflammatory diseases that **are caused by bacteria** (Carranza, et. al. Clinical Periodontology, 2002). Other newer definitions include susceptibility as well as genetic variations. However, the most basic definition of causation is that periodontal infections are bacterial in nature and vary from patient to patient.

While we understand that bone loss occurs due to the immune response, it is those bacteria known as pathogens that cause the immune response that results in bone loss. Therefore, it makes sense to know what causes the immune response in each patient and how severe it can become. However, since the types of bacteria that cause these diseases vary from person to person, those with disease cannot be classified as "average." These infections and the damage they cause are the result of **specific bacterial induced inflammatory responses involving both the innate and adaptive arms of the immune system** (Dentino, et. al. 2013). Gingival infections that do not resolve, periodontitis in all of its forms, and infections around implants all fall within this same definition.

Today, most clinicians are **treating the symptoms** of disease. Doesn't it make more sense to treat the cause? We have assumed that it is technique only or a method of therapy that is coming into play. Actually, while these are important, even the best methods of therapy do not always work. Thus, it makes sense to know and treat the **cause** in every patient in order to help the body heal. Thus, as clinicians, we should know more about causation than any other component of the disease because, arguably, we have more control over bacteria than we do over any other component of these diseases.

Another important fact to remember is that different oral pathogens live in different locations. Some live within the biofilm that attaches to the teeth and others actually live within the gingival tissues, tongue, tonsils, endothelial cells, and other mucosal surfaces. So, if we only treat "the teeth', we may miss reducing or eradicating the most dangerous species that live within other niches.

Refractory disease:

Our term "refractory disease" needs to be redefined. Refractory disease should not be "progressive disease based on bone loss," but rather it should be based on the return of any symptom of disease. If bleeding returns, you, the clinician, should know why. Healthy gums do not bleed, and our goal is to make sure they are healthy! Refractory disease (as seen in bleeding on probing) is often the result of our treatment's inability to accomplish the goal of removing the causative agents of the disease (infection) or because the patient is being continually re-infected by another person.

This concept explains why simply removing soft plaque, hard deposits, and giving more hygiene instructions is insufficient in many cases to accomplish the return to total health signified by the absence of clinical signs of inflammation, bleeding, bone loss, and and symptoms).

Multiple diseases:

Periodontitis is not a single disease and our classification system based on pocket depths does not explain the microbial and genetic differences between its variations. So, when we go back to the previously made statement that there are no "average" people, we find further support in science teaching us today that the pathogens causing these diseases are specific to the individual. Thus, each person is dealing with their own definition of disease. We should realize that general terms of "infection" or "biofilm" do not apply to the individual nature of the diseases that we see and treat. We must define differently those diseases that do not respond to treatment; therefore, a more specific diagnosis based on etiology is needed.

Think of this concept in more common terms, such as that of your own "fingerprint". Just as each of us has our own unique fingerprint patterns, we also have our own unique DNA patterns. These genetic differences are being utilized more and more in modern medicine.

Similarly, we each have our own "bacterial fingerprint patterns" in our bodies and in our mouths. When people have healthy mouths, their "oral bacterial fingerprint" is composed of those microorganisms that are consistent with supporting health.

Thus, our goal for ourselves and for our patients is to have "bacterial fingerprints" comprised of health-associated organisms. Consider this: today, it is possible to know, at any age, what your own "oral bacterial fingerprint" is. Armed with that information, it is possible to prevent periodontal disease, predict future disease, and treat these diseases based on the individual needs of each patient. This is amazing new science.

We must remember that, when our patients present with clinical signs of periodontal disease, they each have a unique "bacterial fingerprint." In these patients, there is an imbalance (dysbiosis) in the bacterial species and the number of organisms. Each "bacterial fingerprint" is unique to each disease state, and each person has their own pattern of response when the oral microorganisms are out of balance. Their risk factors are not causal; they simply increase or decrease that patient's risk.

CSI

Some may remember the TV series *Crime Scene Investigators (CSI)*. Much of that series was designed to show how DNA can be used to solve crimes. In a real sense, the clinician who understands this disease will become an "investigator," determining the unique qualities of each patient (including the medical and dental histories) and then designing a treatment and maintenance plan for each individual. This will include a diagnosis based on etiology and additional risk factors for each patient. Then, when an individual member of a family is diagnosed using DNA, the other family members may need evaluation for treatment as well. Thus, periodontal disease often becomes a family therapy plan, not a "single member of the family" plan.

The good news is that, today, we have the same tools as *CSI* – that is, our ability to use DNA. This means that we can discover and measure these unique "human DNA" and "bacterial fingerprints." We can record those differences from patient to patient. In healthy mouths, we will see a consistent pattern of oral microorganisms that are working together and actually promoting a healthy mouth. In an unhealthy person, we will see a pattern of oral microorganisms that include a variety of oral pathogens.

It is also important to underscore that clinical signs are insufficient to determine this unique "bacterial fingerprint pattern." In fact, clinical signs alone cannot predict disease status or long-term treatment strategy. We cannot "guess" and just use the same treatment strategy for every patient. While the basic principles of biofilm disruption still continue (e.g. SRP), based on current scientific knowledge, it is imperative that an antimicrobial model be included after the DNA report is obtained. By determining the "bacterial fingerprint" via a saliva sample, we can diagnose more accurately, predict disease progression, and even predict bone loss around both teeth and implants before it happens. We can also design an antimicrobial therapy and home-care model appropriate for each patient regardless of where they are in the disease state.

When a patient's "bacterial fingerprint" is composed primarily of "oral pathogens," we have a problem. This "fingerprint" will cause disease, and the disease will continue until someone does the "right thing" to help that patient make the shift toward a healthy "fingerprint." This shift may include antimicrobial therapy; you will know which therapy is appropriate after you learn the "bacterial fingerprint" of that patient.

When to move patients into periodontal therapy vs. another prophy?

We must consider the medical risks involved for each patient when answering this question. Using traditional information based purely on clinical signs is always a guessing game, and, additionally, it does not sufficiently take into account the potential for systemic risks. When basing treatment only on clinical signs, there are many shades of gray. For example, the patient in room #1 presents with a few 4mm pockets but with little bleeding. The patient in room #2 presents with a few 4mm pockets with lots of bleeding. Do they have the same disease or not? Do you treat them the same or not? Should their home care be the same? Is either patient (or are they both) at risk for heart attack or stroke? How do you bring the medical history into this decision? Without understanding causation, we would still be playing a guessing game and not be up to date with current science.

In contrast, using a DNA report provides an independent "investigator" that looks at the disease from the "inside," not the outside. Thus, when you discover the power of DNA, you will know every time which patients need periodontal therapy, regardless of pocket depths. When any patient presents a DNA report that reveals the presence of high-risk oral pathogens, that patient will receive appropriate comprehensive therapy, while those that present with low-risk pathogens are at low risk and will receive appropriate therapy as well. The DNA report also provides valuable information regarding the specific pathogens and their role in arterial damage and systemic risk. The lab report becomes the critical link for making perio treatment decisions as well as decisions regarding the patient's general health.

Really Good News...

The good news is that when a saliva sample report reveals that pathogens are present, you clearly know that you should not perform another standard six-month prophy. More specific treatment can make it possible to reverse the disease process and to later determine whether or not you have accomplished your goals. By the elimination of the pathogens through a "personalized plan" with the goal to restore a "bacterial fingerprint" that is consistent with a healthy mouth, you can be confident that your treatment is effective and that the oral condition of your patient is not contributing to their potential systemic disease.

Metagenomics:

> **"Metagenomics is turning medical knowledge on its head."**
> (T. Marshall, PhD; 8th Annual Conference on Inflammation and Autoimmune diseases; Grenada, Spain, 2012)

So, why spend so much time talking about oral pathogens? The impact of chronic infections, the specific members of biofilms, and their ability to cause disease are clearly shedding new light on health and disease. The sheer numbers of microorganisms that live on us and in us have the ability to overpower even our own genetics. Simply put, properly understanding oral pathogens is critically important in understanding human health and disease.

The study of the microorganisms in humans and how they control health and disease has become an extremely important topic. The National Institute of Health (NIH) allocated $180 million dollars to this project. Their findings include the fact that we have 10 times more bacteria living "in and on" us than we have human cells. Most are helpful and help sustain life. However, when "shifts" occur from "non-pathogens" to "pathogens," bacteria will be the causative agents for disease (dysbiosis). We now know that when you have large numbers of bacterial species working together, their combined genetic influence is more impactful on our health and disease than our own genetic influence! No wonder they are important.

The five chronic infectious diseases known to cause systemic inflammation include:

1. Periodontitis
2. Otitis media
3. Bacterial vaginosis
4. Gastro-esophageal disease
5. Inflammatory bowel disease/obesity

The presence of significant quantities of oral pathogens represents an "oral dysbiosis." The new field of metagenomics (the study of large numbers of microorganisms and their influence on human health and disease) is revealing the unique and critically important role that this "oral dysbiosis" has on our day-to-day lives.

The study of bacteria on a person-specific basis has changed the way we view health and disease. Today, a dentist's ability to "study the oral bacteria" in each patient's mouth is incredibly important for both that patient's oral health and for their general health. **Steps to help apply these principles clinically include the following:**

- Plan to attend a course that teaches this model
- Learn how to send saliva samples or subgingival samples to clinical laboratories that specialize in oral pathogen detection using DNA technology
- Learn how to use the result report and the important information that it contains
- Remember that it is important for all team members to know and understand these principles

The "Ultimate" Risk Factor

Each bacterial species is unique. Each also has different capabilities to cause disease based on virulent characteristics, biofilm shifts, volume shifts, and host modifying factors. Together with volume shifts, different species may have the ability to form synergistic or dysbiotic communities of biofilm. The immune system of the host has the ability to recognize pathogens and virulent differences. When the biofilm matures toward disease-associated bacteria, the response is determined by the perceived threat with the release of an inflammatory cascade of cytokines, chemokines and matrix metalloproteinases (MMP's). Certain species play distinct roles in the shift from a health-related biofilm community to a disease-causing biofilm community.

Research initiatives have confirmed and validated the following bacterial species that are important players in these shifts toward disease. As such, these species have been designated as **"targets" of therapy**. Based on the current level of evidence, the **"ultimate risk factors"** for periodontal-associated diseases (endangering teeth and implants) include the following: *Aggregatibacter actinomycetemcomitans, Porphyromonas gingivalis, Tannerella forsythia, Treponema denticola, Eikenella corrodens, Fusobacterium nucleatum, Campylobacter rectus, Micromonas micra, Eubacterium spp., and Prevotella intermedia.* The first four, called the "Red complex," are considered to be "keystone" pathogens due to their unique and significant ability to shift the entire genetic balance away from health and toward disease. Keystone pathogens have the genetic influence to surpass the genetic influence of the host. **Clinical application steps to keep in mind regarding these principles are as follows:**

- **Test patients that are not responding to treatment with a saliva or subgingival sample.**
- **Personalize therapy based on etiology, history, and risk factors.**
- **"High-risk bacteria":** *Aggregatibacter actinomycetemcomitans, Porphyromonas gingivalis, Tannerella forsythia, Treponema denticola, Fusobacterium nucleatum, Streptococcus viridans, Streptococcus mutans.*
- **Remember the following for "high-risk Bacteria":**
  - **For Periodontal risk**: These bacteria, when in sufficient quantity, cause bone loss around teeth and implants. They should be eliminated or at least reduced to very low levels. The lab test will determine their presence and their quantity. It will also address potential antimicrobial strategies. Ideally, a follow-up test is recommended to

determine if the periodontal therapy was successful in eliminating the high-risk bacteria, especially since they have a direct connection to systemic inflammation.
- o **For systemic inflammation**: These bacteria are directly involved in vascular injury. Patients that have them, in sufficient quantity, may be at greater risk for heart disease, heart attack and stroke.
- o **These high-risk pathogens represent the most consistent relationship between periodontal disease and vascular disease including coronary heart disease, heart attack and stroke.** (For further information, see the last six articles in the bibliography).
- o When these bacteria are present, ideally, the patient's dentist and physician(s) should work together toward identifying systemic inflammation through blood and urine tests.

- "Moderate-risk" Bacteria: *Eikenella corrodens, Campylobacter rectus, Micromonas micra, Eubacterium spp., and Prevotella intermedia.*
- Remember the following for "moderate-risk" bacteria:
  - o **For Periodontol Risk**: These bacteria represent a risk for bone loss but not at the same level of risk as the Red Complex. However, some patients can have very serious disease when these are present.
  - o **For Systemic Inflammation**: While we can't be completely sure, it appears that these bacteria do not present the same systemic risk as do the high-risk species.
  - o **Mixed infections**: All periodontal infections will have a mixture of High Risk and Moderate Risk pathogens.

Genetics: "Be careful how you choose your parents."

Actually, this humorous statement doesn't really apply to periodontitis. Humans are not born with periodontal disease, nor do they ultimately lose their teeth "because Mother and Father did." Periodontal disease is not a genetic disease in the real sense of Mendelian genetics (e.g. diseases passed down from parent to child). While genetic factors influence these diseases, they are very complex, and they still are not completely understood at this time. We do know that the subject of genetics plays an important role in chronic diseases such as periodontitis. Another way to say this is that our "gene expression" (how we respond to infections) varies depending on how our DNA is arranged. It also varies depending on the type of "oral pathogens" and the overall health of the patient. These genetic variations do influence how we react to microbial invasion.

We do have strong evidence that a genetic variation (single nucleotide polymorphisms or SNP) associated with the interleukin 1 gene pool is a player as a specific genetic trait that contributes to a more severe inflammatory response and thus more tissue and bone damage in periodontitis. A recent meta-analysis concluded that this genetic variation is significantly associated with chronic periodontitis. It is estimated that 30-35% of the American population has this genetic variation. The immune response is therefore more aggressive or less aggressive, with varying levels of the resulting clinical signs (such as bleeding and loss of alveolar bone). Risk factors, such as smoking, diabetes, obesity, poor oral hygiene, and certain medications are well recognized as influencers that can modify the response but are not causative. Clinical application steps to implement these principles include the following:

- This genotype (along with bacterial variations) is measureable from a saliva sample. Patients who are genotype positive (IL-1 positive) have an increased risk for more aggressive forms of periodontal diseases. This is especially important in smokers that are genotype positive.
- Remember, the genetic expression is caused by the invasion of pathogens. If the patient and the clinician can contain this invasion, there is little reason for the genotype positive individual to have a greater risk than one who does not have this genetic variation.
- Test for pathogens more often
- Inform implant patients of their increased risk for implant infections if they are genotype 1 positive.
- Other genetic tests that include additional genetic markers may present a clearer picture for future use. (Interleukin 6, for an example)

"To Set on Fire":

> **Definition of "Inflammation":**
> Latin, īnflammō,
> "to ignite, set alight", "to set on fire"

Inflammation is the central theme of the oral / systemic connection. However, by itself, simply using the term "systemic inflammation" does little to change our understanding of the disease process. With a better understanding of the specific causes of these diseases, the clinician will have a clearer understanding of both local and systemic inflammation.

As we have seen, this is where a saliva sample is so helpful. Not only does a saliva sample provide information regarding the "bacterial fingerprint," but it provides a clearer understanding of the relationships between these chronic inflammatory diseases and the cumulative effect of inflammation relative to periodontal inflammation, systemic inflammation (endothelial dysfunction) and other systemic inflammatory diseases.

Recent data demonstrates a strong positive association between "oral pathogen burden", periodontitis, and vascular inflammation (injury). The "oral pathogen burden" is based on the combined colonization levels of five periodontal microbes: *Aggregatibacter actinomycetemcomitans, Porphyromonas gingivalis, Treponema denticola, Tannerella forsythia, and Fusobacterium nucleatum* with vascular injury. These bacteria are known to be causative agents of periodontitis.

Using medical tests such as ultra-sound carotid intermedia thickness (c-IMT) and serum markers of inflammation including CRP, MPO, and Lp-PLA2, our physician colleagues can measure the level of systemic inflammation that may be present, as well as the level of atherosclerosis. The results of these tests and those from saliva testing should be considered as important information for the dentist, physician, periodontist, hygienist, and nurse practitioner.

For example, in some periodontal infections, even early on in the inflammatory process, with little to no bone loss and with pockets of 3mm or less, specific oral pathogens can cause severe oral inflammation and, more importantly, vascular injury that may increase the risk for atherosclerosis (Desvarieux, et al. 2013).

Interestingly, these highly pathogenic bacteria can be found even in shallow periodontal spaces that we commonly consider to be "safe". In other words, these bacteria have the ability to create systemic inflammation even before the tissue has exhibited the commonly accepted clinical signs of frank periodontal disease. Thus, the importance of "subclinical periodontal infections" highlights the significance of a clinician's role in recognizing this relationship between periodontal infection and increased cardiovascular disease risk. Relatively shallow periodontal sites not only have the potential to develop gingivitis and subsequent periodontitis, but the may also be undergoing subclinical pathological processes that have systemic effects. Those shallow periodontal sites that contain these pathogenic microbes in sufficient concentration might actually be considered to be "nascent systemic disease" (Demmer, et al., 2010, Desvarieux, et al., 2013). A real eye-opening statement from the medical literature states that **"even periodontal probe measurements of ≤3mm (when these microbes are detected in sufficient quantity) are not considered safe from a systemic health view-point."** (Demmer, et al., 2013). That statement alone changes everything about the importance of early detection of periodontal infections.

These recent scientific findings, as reported in the journals of the *American Heart Association* and *Circulation* have forever impacted the important role that the oral health clinician plays in health care and how important oral health is to over-all health. It is important to remember that these illnesses trigger aggressive forms of chronic inflammation with subsequent systemic vascular injury serious enough to trigger heart attacks and strokes (Pessi, et al. 2013). It is clear that periodontal disease is significantly more important than we ever knew. **Practical application of these principles includes remembering the following:**

- Inflammation is "link" that connects oral and systemic disease.
- The clinical signs, while important, are not as important as understanding what drives periodontal inflammation and disease: pathogenic microbes.
- **Periodontal disease:** All periodontal diseases are driven by specific bacterial pathogen patterns. Periodontal inflammation must be understood by understanding first the "Bacterial Finger-Print" as the driver of bone loss, bleeding, etc.
- **Systemic inflammation:** High risk bacteria are the primary drivers of systemic inflammation derived from

periodontal infections and the connection between oral disease and systemic disease.
- There are courses that teach this important relationship between oral and systemic health and attending one can be extremely beneficial.

Threshold:

A DNA analysis from a saliva sample, as discussed, will reveal the presence or absence of very specific periodontal pathogens and quantify each one. Once the clinician learns the value of this information, the report will provide a clear understanding of the patient's risk for alveolar bone loss over the next six months if these pathogens are allowed to remain. This unique information from the clinical lab report provides the practitioner with critical information that will determine which patient is infected with true pathogens at any given point in time – even before clinical attachment loss occurs (Bartold, et. al. 1998).

This provides excellent opportunities for prevention and early intervention founded on a diagnosis based on causative agents. While not all gingivitis proceeds to periodontitis, it is true that some gingivitis patients are "primed" toward periodontitis. Since not all gingivitis patients have these pathogens in high numbers, it is the presence of specific pathogen profiles "at threshold" that deserves immediate attention. The therapy plan then becomes clear: to eliminate the pathogens or reduce them to "host acceptable levels".

"Threshold" from an oral health perspective:

We all have small quantities of pathogens in many areas of our bodies that have the potential to cause disease; yet, we remain healthy. In other words, we can have very small numbers of potentially pathogenic organisms and not be sick. An example would include the MRSA bacterium. This "bad boy" can cause disease rapidly, with devastating tissue loss and even death, in a matter of hours and days. Our own epithelial cells have an antibiotic property, allowing them to keep pathogens at low numbers and to keep us healthy, when we are in good health and have minimal additional risk factors. However, if a shift in bacterial species occurs and the pathogens are allowed to grow in quantity; bacteria can cause acute as well as chronic infections.

Our bodies defend themselves against infections in many ways, including keeping the "sheer numbers" of pathogens very low. However, the concept of "over-whelming" the immune system is very real. Additionally, the "threshold" point is significantly important. A very important concept to remember is that the "threshold" can vary from person to person, especially when the patient is challenged with additional risk factors (such as smoking, diabetes, engagement with an infected partner, etc.). Even though the threshold varies from one patient to another and that no two people are exactly alike, the literature does give us some potential guidelines for oral pathogens in regards to threshold (Socransky, et. al., 1994, 2006). The lab report will give a basic guideline regarding this threshold concept, but, remember, each patient is different even with similar levels of bacteria. One person may become very ill while another may be only moderately ill with similar levels of bacteria.

It is worthwhile to further discuss the principles involving quantity of pathogens and quantity. While very important, the mere presence of pathogenic species is not the ultimate risk factor, but instead the ability of species to accumulate to volumes that turn the immune response into high-gear (thus creating chronic or over exuberant inflammation) is what is most important. And, remember, each patient is different. Those that have the Interleukin variation (IL-1b) will have more inflammation even at relatively low bacterial burden. Interestingly, the signs of inflammation may not be visible for some time (hence the term "subclinical infection"). Earlier studies that stated pathogens may be present in non-diseased patients failed to recognize the importance of concentration (thresholds), duration, and other differences relative to subclinical disease. Today, we understand that it is most desirable for the level of specific oral pathogens be very low or undetectable, as evidenced on the laboratory report after completion of the salivary sample.

Systemic Disease and Threshold:

Increased threshold levels of specific oral pathogens are known to increase risk for atherosclerosis, arterial injury, endothelial dysfunction as well as alveolar bone loss. Additionally, it is interesting to note that recent discoveries show that some periodontopathogenic species require this "threshold" concept in triggering vascular endothelial cell inflammatory response and "cross talk" with mononuclear cells via Interleukin-6 and Toll-Like receptor 4 activation. While not the topic for this discussion, the importance of this lies not just within the boundaries of periodontal disease inflammatory expression, but also in vascular endothelial inflammatory expression. We cannot "feel" this happening, of course. However, when specific pathogens such as the Red Complex are present, the literature states that the risk is very high for systemic inflammation.

Subclinical infections:

Literature confirms that periodontal infections occur long before the presence of clinical or anatomical changes (Bartold, et. al., 1998). The following statement from their 1998 study is helpful: "The factors associated with the development of periodontal infections include (1) Infection, (2) Genetic response, (3) Metabolic response, and (4) Anatomical changes." Our traditional model has looked only at stage (4) in this disease process. Instead, when specific microbes at "threshold" values (as seen on the report) are present, they typically present a clear and present danger to both systemic and oral health at even subclinical and early disease states. The threshold values can also serve as potential "risks" for bone loss based on "relative risks" even prior to the presentation of periodontitis (Teles, et. al, 2006).

This approach of early detection of specific microbes that are causally related to periodontitis at threshold values has the ability to prevent and even cure early periodontal infections. We can prevent attachment loss and can ensure that the oral cavity is not a continual source of systemic inflammatory burden. While the objective is not to "sterilize" the mouth or even to eliminate all biofilm populations, our objective should be to re-balance the oral organisms into a healthy relationship between their members. This requires saliva samples to determine what organisms are present and what your disease therapy targets are for each patient.

What is "active disease"?

For those patients with attachment loss, it is important to determine: "is the disease active disease or not." Clinical signs cannot reveal this. However, the clinician can determine the specifics of oral pathogens and threshold values based on saliva sampling with subsequent laboratory findings. Once the causative agents are defined (providing a diagnosis), then the clinician can design a plan with systemic risk in mind. Additionally, the clinician can design a therapeutic approach that can "prove" an acceptable end-point of therapy (hence the importance of before and after reports). This is important both for oral health but also for the determination of active disease prior to general surgery that would involve joint replacement, heart surgery, etc.

Collaboration with other health care professionals:

More than any other oral disease, periodontal infections (and the sheer numbers of patients with these infections) should encourage a collaborative relationship between oral medicine and general medicine practitioners. While not commonly known by most dentists and physicians, this model of shared responsibility of treating periodontal disease and understanding these relationships between preventing heart attacks and strokes is the model for present and future health care. While still in its infancy, this model is being taught today to dentists, physicians and nurse practitioners to create a local working model for this collaboration (Bale, Doneen, Nabors 2012).

Important points to remember for clinical application of these principles include:
- Use saliva or subgingival samples to determine presence or absence of oral pathogens. The traditional model of using only clinical signs of disease (bleeding on probing, pocket depth, plaque, etc.) and a treatment model that is based purely on "procedures" (e.g. SRP, lasers, trays, prophies, etc.) often fails to remove the cause of the illness and leaves many patients at risk for continual systemic inflammatory burden and refractory disease.
- End-point of therapy requires knowing if the treatment has eliminated or significantly reduced pathogen burden to a host acceptable level (absence of clinical signs). A follow-up test is important to determine if therapy accomplished the intended goals. This is typically done 4-6 weeks post therapy.
- The goals of periodontal therapy today include both clinical and microbiological stability as well as the elimination of vascular inflammation that may have been caused by specific pathogens (Columbo et. al., 2012).

The Clinical Laboratory and Periodontal Medicine

Oral health must include excellent periodontal health. Additionally, periodontal disease detection and treatment is at the heart of periodontal medicine. The statistics, relative to the incidence of these diseases and relative to the importance to general health, show that clinicians should view the important role of the "saliva sample" just as the physician views the important role of blood testing.

Consider how this plays out in medicine. As patients ourselves, we would be astonished if our physician never took a blood sample and never looked to a lab report for information. Simply put, clinical laboratory testing of blood and urine has become a requirement and an indisputable partner for every practitioner of medicine. Sixty to seventy percent of all clinical decisions in general medicine are based upon the biological information within these body fluids. From detection of subclinical disease, to diagnosis, and then to prognosis: the clinical lab is the only model that can provide this information.

Saliva is a body fluid that has immediate clinical application for periodontal and peri-implant infections. It is the body fluid of choice that defines the biological differences in patients at risk and in patients with disease.

The two important contributions within salivary diagnostics are (1) information within saliva relative to "systemic inflammation", and (2) information within saliva relevant to "oral disease". The need is important with regards to both health categories, as both have the potential to affect the patient in a bidirectional manner. Today, there are tests that are immediately relevant to oral and systemic health using the DNA from both the human and the bacterial content. Saliva has become an indisputable partner in oral medicine and general medicine due to the development of DNA laboratories that specialize in these areas. Dentists, periodontists, hygienists, pediatric dentists, cosmetic dentists, physicians, etc. and all other health related practitioners are recognizing the critical information that we have at our disposal by sending a saliva sample to the clinical lab. Saliva tests for systemic diseases are being developed but not ready for clinical use. However, the clinician who starts today in learning about this important model will be far ahead of the curve.

Today's role of "Whole saliva" in health-care:

Saliva contains many forms of information for improving the diagnosis for oral diseases including; gingival crevicular fluid, mucosal fluid, and fluid from all of the major and minor salivary glands. It is a storehouse of significant biological information regarding both the individual microbiological nature of periodontal diseases as well as the individual influence of the host response. Today, the most common information is from the DNA found within an oral rinse sample. This DNA information includes genetic sequences of oral bacterial species and human cells. DNA of each helps to define the unique differences in patient diseases as well as how they respond to therapy.

Current knowledge of oral "biofilm infections" has advanced our understanding of how specific infections cause specific host immune responses. The work of microbiologists over the past decade has brought a new understanding of the specific nature of these communities of microorganisms. Funding from the National Institutes of Health (NIH) for the human microbiome project ($180 million) has brought new attention to the impact that all microorganisms have on our health and disease. In oral health, a shift in microorganisms is diagnostically important for understanding causation of periodontal and peri-implant diseases. These infections, based on specific microbiota as opposed to purely clinical signs, are independently associated with risk in arterial diseases. New definitions of disease are now based on "dysbiosis", or a shift of health related bacteria to disease related microbiota and biofilm communities.

At the Cellular Level:

With any specific pathogenic species, an antibody and a cell-mediated response will come into play. Both are important for defense against the pathogen. The immune responses are tailored to the pathogen and to where the pathogen resides. Cells in primary defense (the innate immune system) include phagocytic cells (monocyte/macrophages and PMNs), NK cells, basophils, mast cells, eosinophiles and platelets.

The virulent characteristics of specific microorganisms (specifically the "Red" complex (*Aa, Pg, Tf, Td*) and *Fn* have virulent factors that create aggressive immune responses. Some of these characteristics include leukotoxins, epithelial toxins, lipopolysaccharides (LPS), fimbriae, host evasion capacity, collagenase, and other components. All are recognizable by designated cells due to highly specific patterns of recognition and patterns of response. It is interesting to note that each microbe has a unique molecular pattern (Pathogen Associated Molecular Pattern or PAMP). This molecular pattern is recognizable by defensive immune cells. The molecular patterns of each microbial species are recognized by specific receptors on the surface of the immune cells: called Pattern Recognition Receptors (PRR's). **The type and strength of the cellular response (relative to inflammation) are determined by these receptors.**

The host immune response is a "measured response" based on the perceived threat. Recognition receptors are also called Toll-Like Receptors or TLR's. Thus some receptors recognize non-pathogens, some recognize true pathogens, some recognize viruses, and some recognize specific patterns that represent highly virulent strains such as lipopolysaccharides (LPS). The response is based upon the interaction between the molecular pattern (PAMP), the pattern receptor (PRR), genetic profiles, and the condition of the patient. The "pattern to receptor" mechanisms are species specific. These "patterns" and "receptors" resemble "lock-and-key" mechanisms where the unique "key" fits precisely into the unique "receptor". Remarkably, the immune response will not be the same for each patient, as we are all different.

The virulent capacity of the microbial community, the type of response, and length of time of response determines the strength of response and thus the type of injury. Significant amounts of inflammatory proteins are released into the surrounding tissue, including the interleukin family, TNFα, PGE2, MMP's, and chemokines. Also, it is important to note that billions of bacteria may be involved in these infections. Viruses are also recognized, again at different receptor sites. The host responds by releasing powerful cytokines intended to kill the invaders. However, when these powerful "killers of pathogens" continue working for long periods of time (e.g. chronic infections), they cause a detrimental impact on the host.

Other important cells, not typically defined as defensive cells, have similar capacity to initiate the inflammation cycle. A recent discovery involving Toll-Like Receptor 4 (TLR 4) presents another window into how the human immune system reacts to activation by specific microbes and their virulent potential. Recent discovery reveals that even endothelial cells, gingival epithelial cells and the cells included within the gingival attachment apparatus are also highly active in the protective process.

Interestingly, the activation of TLR 4 has significant importance to our understanding of the role of inflammation within the endothelial lining of all blood vessels. When this receptor is activated, multiple inflammatory cytokines are released that contribute to the development of atherosclerosis and arterial plaque instability. Among other causes of activation, TLR 4 is also activated by lipopolysaccharide (LPG) —an important defensive component of *P. gingivalis* and *A. actinomycetemcomitans*. When LPG stimulates microvascular and macrovascular endothelial cells, large amounts of inflammatory mediators are released including cytokines, chemokines, growth factors and adhesions molecules (to name a few). This factor confirms that oral pathogens that contain LPS are uniquely important to our understanding of the role of specific oral bacteria in connection to the atherosclerotic process. These findings support recent discoveries underscoring the importance of understanding that **specific oral pathogens are more relevant to the oral/systemic connection than are merely recording clinical signs of periodontal disease.**

Summary: What Clinicians Need to Know

Chronic forms of gingivitis, periodontitis, and peri-implant infections are serious infections. They often present with the same manifestations when measuring clinical signs of inflammation including bleeding, color, and pocket depths, etc. However, these diseases are very personal and different, even when clinical signs are the same. Today, the literature encourages a more definitive recognition of causation in conjunction with clinical factors. Clinical presentation is very misleading as it relates to the serious nature of the infection; regardless of the pocket depth.

A "one-size-fits-all" mentality is inappropriate with the evidenced-based science of today.

Ideally, individual differences of even the beginning stages of disease should be detected early. Based on specific bacterial profiles, and genetic differences, the patient response to the bacterial challenge will trend toward three different predictable patterns: (1) a response toward chronic gingivitis, (2) a response toward chronic periodontitis, (3) a response toward advanced disease. The type and concentration of multiple oral pathogen species are very important pieces of information to help determine the risk. Genetic variations and additional risk factors will influence the immune response as well.

It behooves the clinician to recognize the uniqueness of the individual disease, and of the patient, in order to best design an appropriate and personal prevention and treatment strategy. Both the health of the mouth and the overall health of the patient will be at a greater risk than when these decisions are based purely on traditional clinical signs of disease and without specific bacterial information.

Final thoughts:

It is my firm belief that an important role for Periodontal Medicine in general health-care includes a greater understanding of the infections we aim to treat. An exciting future for dentistry includes our ability and desire to adopt to the clinical laboratory model (as general medicine has already done). We must change our phenotypical model of diagnosis and treatment that is based purely on clinical signs to one that uses a biological model. Salvia gives us a unique diagnosis, prognosis and treatment strategy that is based on evidence – not symptoms. These lab reports provide critical information for the clinician, for the patient, and for our communication with other colleagues from general medicine. Dentists, dental hygienists, and periodontists should be "on the front lines" of health care.

Understanding the "biological nature" of these serious infections/diseases based on causative agents and genetic differences, and their relationships to systemic disease, are important first steps. They require that we use the clinical laboratory. Therefore, a new reliance on saliva sampling, with a highly accurate clinical lab report, is an important *shift* in our thinking and an important step toward improving the overall health of each of our patients.

Thomas Nabors Sr. DDS, FACD

* * *

Tom received his degree from the University of Tennessee College of Dentistry. He served in the U.S. Navy and on the medical staff of Baptist Memorial Hospital in the Oral Surgery and Dental Division for approximately 25 years.

In 2004, he co-founded and served as CEO for Advanced Dental Diagnostics, LLC.

In 2008, he founded OralDNA® Labs: a salivary diagnostics clinical laboratory.

Tom is a true pioneer in the field of the oral-systemic connection. He has studied the role of oral pathogenic bacteria and their destructive effects clinically, for over 45 years.

Tom is a legend among researchers and clinicians alike, receiving the first life achievement award from the American Academy of Oral and Systemic Health (AAOSH), in 2012, for his invaluable work. You will learn more about periodontal disease, it's etiology, testing, and treatment from Tom, than anyone else we know!

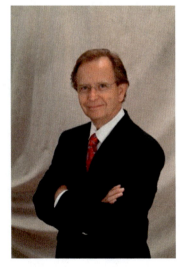

Bibliography:

- Andrew Dentino, Seokwoo Lee, Jason Mailhot, Arthur F. Hefti; Principles of periodontology; *Periodontology 2000, Vol. 61, 2013, 16-53*
- Frank Schwarz, Jürgen Becker; PERI-IMPLANT INFECTION: *Etiology, Diagnosis and Treatment*; Quintessence Publishing Col. Ltd.; ©2010
- Offenbacher, Barros, Beck; Re-thinking Periodontal Inflammation; J Periodont. August 2008 (Supplement) 1577-91;
- Mantyla, Buhlin, Paju, Persson, Nieminen, Sinisalo, Pussinen; Subgingival A. actinomycetemcomitans associates with the risk of coronary artery disease; *Journal of Periodontology*, March 2013, doi:10.1111/jcpe.12098
- Sinem Esra Sahingur, Xia-Juan Xia, Robert E. Schifferie; Oral Bacterial DNA Differ in Their Ability to Induce Inflammatory Responses in Human Monocytic Cell Lines: *J Periodontol* Aug. 2012; 1069-1077
- Anne D. Haffajee, Ridardo P. Teles, Sigmund S. Socransky; The effect of periodontal therapy on the composition of the subgingival microbiota; *Periodontology 2000, Vol. 42, 2006, 219-258*
- Roberto Teles, Anne D. Haffajee, Sigmund S. Socransky; Microbiological goals of periodontal therapy; *Periodontology 2000, Vol. 42, 2006, 180-218*
- Paul I. Eke, Roy C. Page, Liang Wei, Gina Thornton-Evans, Robert J. Genco; Update of the Case Definitions for Population-Based Surveillance of Periodontitis; *J Periodontol 2012; 83: 1449-1454*
- S. J. Byrne, S. G. Dashper, I. B. Darby, G. G. Adams, B. Hoffmann, E. C. Reynolds; Progression of chronic periodontitis can be predicted by the levels of Porphyromonas gingivalis and Treponema denticola in subgingival plaque: Molecular Oral Microbiology, 12 OCT 2009, 469-477
- Beck, et al., Periodontal Disease and Coronary Heart Disease; A Reappraisal of the Exposure; *Circulation. 2005;112:19-24*
- Spahr, et al; Role of Periodontal Bacteria and Importance of Total Pathogen Burden in the Coronary Event and Periodontal disease (CORODONT) Study; ARCH INTERN MED; Vol. 166, 2006;66(5):554-559.
- Healthcare Innovation, Center for Health Studies; Chronic Disease Management; American College of Physicians, 2012
- McPherson, RA, et al; Analysis of Body Fluids in Clinical Chemistry: Approved Guideline; C49-A, ISBN 1-56238-638-7; Vol 27, Number 14; Clinical and Laboratory Standards Institute
- Thomas F. Flemmig, Thomas Beikler; Control of oral biofilms; *Periodontology 2000, Vol. 55, 2011, 9-15*

- Zimmerman, Park, Wong; Annals of New York Academy of Sciences; Vol. 1098; Oral-Based Diagnostics, 2007
- Mariano Sanz, Arie Jan van Winkelhoff, Group 1 Seventh European Workshop; Periodontal infections: understanding the complexity-Consensus of the Seventh European Workshop on Periodontology; *J Clin Periodontol* 2011; 38 (Suppl.11): 3-6
- JØrgen Slots, Henrik Slots; Bacterial and viral pathogens in saliva: disease relationship and infectious risk; *Periodontology 2000, Vol. 55, 2011, 48-69*
- Desvarieux. ,M., MD, PhD, Demmer, RT., MPH, Rundek, T., MD, PhD, Boden-Albala, B., DrPH, Jacobs, DR., PhD, Sacco, RL., MD, MS, Papapanou, DDS, PhD; Periodontal Microbiota and Carotid Intima-Media Thickness: The Oral Infections and Vascular Disease Epidemiology Study (INVEST); Circulation, 2005, February 8; 111(5): 576-589
- M. Desvarieux, RT Demmer, DR Jacobs ; Periodontal bacteria and hypertension: the oral infections and vascular disease epidemiology study (INVEST); Journal of Hypertension 2010, 28: 1413-1421
- G. Hajishengallis, R.J. Lamont; Beyond the red complex and into more complexity: the polymicrobial synergy and dysbiosis (PSD) model of periodontal disease etiology; Molecular Oral Microbiology; July 2012; 406-409
- Unpublished data from the authors research; patient samples of 40,684 individuals; ages ranging from 7 – 84 yrs; exhibiting varying degrees of inflammation and bleeding; localized and generalized; pocket depth ave. 5.9mm; medical histories
- Thomas F. Flemmig, Thomas Beikler; Control of oral biofilms; *Periodontology 2000: Vol 55, Issue 1; pages 36-47*, Dec 2011
- JØrgen Slots, Henrik Slots; Bacterial and viral pathogens in saliva: disease relationship and infectious risk; *Periodontology 2000, Vol. 55, 2011, 48-69*
- Zhongyang Lu, Yanchun Li, Junfei Jin, Xiaoming Zhang, Maria F. Lope-Virella, Yan Huang; Toll-Like Receptor 4 Activation in Microvascular Endothelial Cells Triggers a Robust Inflammatory Response and Cross Talk With Mononuclear Cells via Interleukin-6; Arteriosclerosis, Thrombosis, and Vascular Biology; Ma7 17, 2012:32;1696-1706
- Nadeem Y. Karimbux, Veeral M. Saraiya, Satheesh Elangovan, Veerasathpurush Allareddy, Taru Kinnunen, Kenneth S. Kornman and Gordon W. Duff; Interleukin-1 Gene Polymorphisms and Chronic Periodontitis in Adult Whites: A Systematic Review and Meta-Analysis. Journal of Periodontology Nov 2012, Vol. 83, No. 11, Pages 1407-1419
- Moise Desvarieux MD, PhD, Ryan T. Demmer PhD, MPH, David R. Jacobs, Jr, PhD; Panos N. Papapanou DDS, PhD,

- Ralph L. Sacco MD, MS, Tatjana Rundek MD, PhD; Changes in Clinical and Microbiological Periodontal Profiles Related to Progression of Carotid Intima-Media Thickness: The Oral Infections and Vascular Disease Epidemiology Study; J Am Heart Assoc. 2013; 2:e000254; October 28, 2013; d0i: 10.1161/JAHA.113.000254
- Tanja Pessi, Vesa Karhunen, Pasi P. Karjalainen, Antti Ylitalo, Juhani K. Airaksinen, Matti Niemi, Mikko Pietila, Kari Laounatmaa, Teppo Haapaniemi, Terho Lehtimaki, Reijo Laaksonen, Pekka J. Karhunen, Jessi Mikkelsson; Bacterial Signatures in Thrombus Aspirates of Patients With Myocardial Infarction; *Circulation* 2013; 127: 1219-1228
- Ryan T Demmer, Panos N Papapanou, David R Jacobs, Jr, Moise Desvarieux; Evaluating clinical periodontal measures as surrogates for bacterial exposure: The Oral Infections and Vascular Disease Epidemiology Study (INVEST); *BMC Med Res Methodol.* 2010; 10: 2. doi: 10.1186/1471-2288-10-2
- Mena Soory; Chromic Periodontitis as a Risk Marker for Systemic Diseases with Reference to Cardiometabolic Disorders: Common Pathways in their Progression; *Immunology and Immunogenetics Insights: 2010:2 7-21*
- Demmer RT, Papapanou RN, Jacobs DR Jr., Desvarieux M.; Bleeding on probing differentially relates to bacterial profiles: the Oral Infections and Vascular Disease Epidemiology Study (INVEST); *J Clin Periodontol 2008; 35: 479-486*
- Moise Desvarieux, MD, PhD, Ryan T. Demmer, MPH, Tatjana Rundek, MD, PhD, Bernadette Boden-Albala, DrPH, David R. Jacobs Jr, PhD, Ralph L. Sacco, MD, MS, Panos N. Papapanou, DDS, PhD; Periodontal Microbiota and Carotid Intima-Media Thickness: The Oral Infections and Vascular Disease Epidemiology Study (INVEST); *Circulation* 2005 February 8; 111(5): 117; 576. Doi: 10.1161/01. CIR.0000154583.37101.15

Bacterial Laboratories that support saliva or subgingival samples:
Hain Diagnostics.com
OralDNA Labs.com

26. POLICY STATEMENT: "THE ROLE OF DENTISTRY IN THE TREATMENT OF SLEEP RELATED BREATHING DISORDERS" – ADOPTED BY THE ADA'S 2017 HOUSE OF DELEGATES

"Sleep related breathing disorders (SRBD) are disorders characterized by disruptions in normal breathing patterns. SRBDs are potentially serious medical conditions caused by anatomical airway collapse and altered respiratory control mechanisms. Common SRBDs include snoring, upper airway resistance syndrome (UARS) and obstructive sleep apnea (OSA). OSA has been associated with metabolic, cardiovascular, respiratory, dental and other diseases. In children, undiagnosed and/or untreated OSA can be associated with cardiovascular problems, impaired growth as well as learning and behavioral problems.

Dentists can and do play an essential role in the multidisciplinary care of patients with certain sleep related breathing disorders and are well positioned to identify patients at greater risk of SRBD. SRBD can be caused by a number of multifactorial medical issues and are therefore best treated through a collaborative model. Working in conjunction with our colleagues in medicine, dentists have various methods of mitigating these disorders. In children, the dentist's recognition of suboptimal early craniofacial growth and development or other risk factors may lead to medical referral or orthodontic/orthopedic intervention to treat and/or prevent SRBD. Various surgical modalities exist to treat SRBD. Oral appliances, specifically custom-made, titratable devices can improve SRBD in adult patients compared to no therapy or placebo devices. Oral appliance therapy (OAT) can improve OSA in adult patients, especially those who are intolerant of continuous positive airway pressure (CPAP). Dentists are the only health care provider with the knowledge and expertise to provide OAT.

The dentist's role in the treatment of SRBDs includes the following:

- Dentists are encouraged to screen patients for SRBD as part of a comprehensive medical and dental history to recognize symptoms such as sleepiness, choking, snoring or witnessed apneas and an evaluation for risk factors such as obesity, retrognathia, or hypertension. These patients should be referred, as needed, to the appropriate physicians for proper diagnosis.
- In children, screening through history and clinical examination may identify signs and symptoms of deficient growth and development, or other risk factors that may lead to airway issues. If risk for SRBD is determined, intervention through medical/dental referral or evidenced based treatment may be appropriate to help treat the SRBD and/or develop an optimal physiologic airway and breathing pattern.
- Oral appliance therapy is an appropriate treatment for mild and moderate sleep apnea, and for severe sleep apnea when a CPAP is not tolerated by the patient.
- When oral appliance therapy is prescribed by a physician through written or electronic order for an adult patient with obstructive sleep apnea, a dentist should evaluate the patient for the appropriateness of fabricating a suitable oral appliance. If deemed appropriate, a dentist should fabricate an oral appliance.
- Dentists should obtain appropriate patient consent for treatment that reviews the treatment plan and any potential side effects of using OAT and expected appliance longevity.
- Dentists treating SRBD with OAT should be capable of

recognizing and managing the potential side effects through treatment or proper referral.
- Dentists who provide OAT to patients should monitor and adjust the Oral Appliance (OA) for treatment efficacy as needed, or at least annually. As titration of OAs has been shown to affect the final treatment outcome and overall OA success, the use of unattended cardiorespiratory (Type 3) or (Type 4) portable monitors may be used by the dentist to help define the optimal target position of the mandible. A dentist trained in the use of these portable monitoring devices may assess the objective interim results for the purposes of OA titration.
- Surgical procedures may be considered as a secondary treatment for OSA when CPAP or OAT is inadequate or not tolerated. In selected cases, such as patients with concomitant dentofacial deformities, surgical intervention may be considered as a primary treatment.
- Dentists treating SRBD should continually update their knowledge and training of dental sleep medicine with related continuing education.
- Dentists should maintain regular communications with the patient's referring physician and other healthcare providers to the patient's treatment progress and any recommended follow up treatment.
- Follow-up sleep testing by a physician should be conducted to evaluate the improvement or confirm treatment efficacy for the OSA, especially if the patient develops recurring OSA relevant symptoms or comorbidities."[143]

27. OZONE THERAPY, BY RACHAELE CARVER MORIN, DMD

BASIC SCIENTIFIC FACTS

- Ozone (O_3) is an allotrope of Oxygen (O_2). An allotrope is a variant of a substance consisting of only one type of atom. It has a NEW molecular configuration and NEW PHYSICAL PROPERTIES. Example: carbon can exist in multiple forms such as: a soft graphite and/or a hard diamond.

- Ozone is created by an energetic reaction that results in an oxygen molecule (O_2) being split into singlet oxygen (O_1). A singlet oxygen then combines with a diatomic oxygen (O_2) forming ozone (O_3). This energetic process is a result of energy produced by: sunlight, lightning, ultraviolet light and corona discharge tubes.

- Ozone is an oxidant and is also referred to as an oxidizer. An oxidizer is a substance that accepts an electron from another substance and is then reduced. It acts as an electron acceptor. It also adds an oxygen atom to the compound being oxidized. In vivo it produces hydroperoxides, lipoperoxides, etc.

- Healthy cells have antioxidant enzymes in their cell membranes, such as: superoxide dismutase, catalase, glutathione peroxidase, etc. There are also antioxidants such as: vitamin C, vitamin E, etc. present in the extracellular matrix fluids, plasma, etc. These antioxidants protect the healthy cells from being oxidized (burned up) by ozone.

- Pathogens such as bacteria, viruses, fungi, and parasites have little or no antioxidant enzymes in their cell membranes. This makes them vulnerable to oxidants. An oxidant (ozone, chlorine, etc.) will destroy the cell membrane of the pathogen resulting in a disinfecting or sterilizing effect. Ozone leaves NO TOXIC BYPRODUCTS like chlorine compounds (trihalomethanes, etc.) leave in vivo or ex vivo. The final breakdown products of O3 are water and oxygen.

- Biofilms are a complex aggregation of structurally and genetically diverse microorganisms growing on a solid surface. Biofilms are found in dental plaque, carious lesions, periodontitis, dental waterlines, etc. The cover story in "THE JOURNAL OF THE AMERICAN DENTAL ASSOCIATION," Vol 140, No 8 978-986 is "Periodontitis: An Archetypical Biofilm Disease" states that "periodontitis is a classic example of biofilm-mediated diseases." The article concluded that, "periodontitis, like other biofilm infections, is refractory to antibiotic agents and host defenses because the causative microbes live in complex communities that persist despite challenges that range from targeted antibiotic agents to phagocytosis." The clinical implications concluded that "the regular delivery of non-targeted anti-biofilm agents may be an effective strategy for treating biofilms, especially if these agents include oxidative agents that dissolve the biofilm matrix." <u>Longevity opinion:</u> This means that ozone could be used in all dental procedures, as it has been proven to eliminate biofilms.

Frequently Asked Questions About Dental Ozone

How does ozone produce therapeutic effects in the Dental Office?

- Ozone is a powerful oxidant. Bacteria, viruses, fungi and parasites have little or no antioxidant enzymes in their cell membranes. Without this protection, ozone oxidizes (burns a hole through) the cell membrane causing it to rupture, resulting in cell death. Healthy cells have antioxidant enzymes in their cell membranes and are not harmed by therapeutic levels of ozone. Water treatment research in Europe has demonstrated that ONE MOLECULE OF OZONE has the oxidizing power of more that 3000 molecules of chlorine. This same research also showed that the ozone killed pathogenic organisms 3500 times faster with no toxic side effects and no toxic byproducts. Medical ozone studies have demonstrated benefits such as improved wound healing, improving the immune system response, and increased oxygen delivery to hypoxic tissues, etc. Velio Bocci, MD, in his book, "OZONE: A NEW MEDICAL DRUG", states, "it is clear that, among complementary approaches, ozone therapy has emerged as the one that is well explainable with classical biochemical, physiological, and pharmacological knowledge."

Are dentists using ozone in their practices now?

- Yes, as reported in the April edition of "Dental Product Shopper", ozone has revolutionized the dental practices of hundreds of Dentists. When ozone is used in Dental procedures it treats the cause of the problem—NOT JUST the symptom. This produces a proactive approach to treatment rather than solely engaging in the routine procedure of damage control.

How are other dentists using ozone for dental treatment?

- Prevention and Protection: Routine use of ozonated water as a pretreatment patient rinse to disinfect their oral cavity. Fill the unit water supply bottles and the Ultrasonic/Piezo reservoirs with ozonated water. This protects you and your staff from aerosol contaminants produced by high speed instruments and water spray from the three way syringe. The unit water lines will also be free of all biofilms when the ozonated water is used in the reservoirs. Ozone performs this disinfection and sterilization and leaves only oxygen and water as byproducts.

- Patient Treatment: In patient care, ozone is utilized in two forms: (1) ozonated water and (2) pure oxygen/ozone gas. Using these two agents in combination allows the dentist to treat all oral infections using only oxygen and water! Regardless of the location or the type of infection ozone is able to treat almost any situation. The ozonated water is the perfect irrigation solution for periodontics and endodontics. For operative dentistry, periodontics and endodontics, ozone gas is used to reach and penetrate areas such as: carious dentin, dentinal tubules, accessory canals and periodontal pockets where no other antibiotic or disinfectant can reach. This is possible because the infection/inflammation is positively charged (acidic) and ozone is negatively charged (basic). Therefore, the chemistry of the infection and/or inflammation attracts the ozone to the area.

Is ozone toxic?

- To reiterate, OZONE IS A STRONG OXIDANT! Because of this extreme oxidant capacity, good ozone hygiene is required. Correctly scavenging the excess ozone gas and preventing it from escaping into the office environment is essential. This aspect is critical because the membranes of the eyes and lungs are very weakly protected by antioxidant enzymes. These are the only tissues that require protection from the dosage levels that are used in dental ozone protocols.

Are there any published studies on dental ozone?

- Yes, there are hundreds of published research studies that use ozone in dental procedures. In the book OZONE: The Revolution in Dentistry, edited by Dr. Edward Lynch and published by Quintessence Publishing Company Limited, there are 132 studies applying ozone treatment to different dental problems (page 78, Table 1). There are hundreds of published articles on the medical uses of ozone. A research article from Scripps Institute, in LaJolla, CA, published in November, 2002, in the journal, "Science", reported that ozone was produced in the plasma cells to kill invading pathogens. This ozone production is a naturally occurring process in our immune systems.

When was ozone first used in dental procedures?

- In the 1930's in Germany, ozone was used for dental procedures by Dr. E.A. Fisch.

How do I learn to use ozone in my dental practice?

The American College of Integrative Medicine and Dentistry (ACIMD) offers "Ozone in Dentistry" courses that are AGD approved for Dental Continuing Education.
- The AGD subject code for Ozone Therapy is #162.
- The ACIMD website is www.ozonefordentisry.com
- Phone 201-587-0222

A Brief Description of Specific Dental Applications

Hygiene Appointments – Protect Patients and Staff
- Patient uses ozonated water as a pretreatment rinse
- Ozonated water is used in the unit water supply bottles
- Ozonated water is used in the Ultrasonic unit water reservoirs
- Ozone gas is used before placing sealants

Operative Dentistry Appointments – Protect Patient, Doctor and Staff
- Patient uses ozonated water as a pretreatment rinse
- Ozonated water is used in the unit water supply bottles
- Ozone GAS is applied to cavity preparations and crown preparations to sterilize the prepared tooth by oxidizing the remaining pathogens and organic materials in the enamel, remaining caries, and dentinal tubules. This produces a pathogen-free oxidized surface that enhances bonding strength and decreases or eliminates post-operative sensitivity.

Periodontal Appointments – Protect Patient, Doctor and Staff
- Patient uses ozonated water as a pretreatment rinse
- Ozonated water is used in the unit water supply bottles
- Ozonated water is used in the Ultrasonic water reservoir
- Ozonated water is used to irrigate periodontal pockets
- Ozone GAS is used to insufflate (blow gas into) the periodontal pockets
- Ozone Custom Trays are used for total saturation (microbaric therapy) of all periodontal tissues AND carious lesions, precarious areas, occlusal grooves, interproximal areas and

margins of existing restorations. This can prevent caries and aid in recalcification of areas that have minimally invasive caries

Endodontic Appointments – Protect Patient, Doctor and Staff
- Patient uses ozonated water as a pretreatment rinse
- Ozonated water is used in the unit water supply bottles
- Irrigate canals with ozonated water to debride the canals and remove biofilm
- Insufflate canals with ozone GAS to eliminate pathogens and oxidize organic materials in the dentinal tubules, accessory canals and lateral canals.

(Information from The American College of Integrative Medicine and Dentistry – www.acimd.net.)

* * *

Rachaele Carver Morin, DMD, graduated from UCONN School of Dental Medicine in 2003 and practices in North Adams, Massachusetts. She is a Dawson Academy Scholar and in 2016 earned her nutrition certificate from the Institute of Integrative Nutrition. She uses her extensive knowledge to educate and treat her patients' complete health through dentistry.

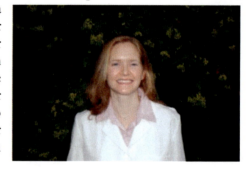

Books Referenced in Blue Boxed Inserts
(In Alphabetical Order)

Bale, Bradley, Amy Doneen, and Lisa C. Cool. *Beat the Heart Attack Gene*. New York: Wiley, 2014, p. 44.

Bell, Weldon. *Temporomandibular Disorders*. 2nd ed., Chicago: Year Book Medical Publishers, Inc., 1986, pp. 1-2.

Campbell, T. Colin, and Thomas M. Campbell, II. *The China Study*. Dallas: BenBella Books, 2006, p. 3.

Cheraskin, E., and W. M. Ringsdorf. *Predictive Medicine: A Study of Strategy*. Omaha: Pacific Press Publishing Association, 1973, front flap.

Corruccini, Robert S. *How Anthropology Informs the Orthodontic Diagnosis of Malocclusion's Causes*. Lewiston: The Edwin Mellen Press, Ltd., 1999, pp. 11-12.

Dawson, Peter E. *Evaluation, Diagnosis, and Treatment of Occlusal Problems*. St Louis: The C.V. Mosby Company, 1974.

Dawson, Peter E. *Functional Occlusion: From TMJ to Smile Design*. St Louis: Mosby, Inc., 2007.

Dawson, Peter E., and John C. Cranham. *The Complete Dentist Manual*. St. Petersburg: Widiom Publishing, LLC, 2017, p. 27.

Fuhrman, Joel. *Eat to Live*. Revised ed, New York: Little, Brown and Company, 2011, pp. 163-164.

Fuhrman, Joel. *The End of Diabetes: The Eat to Live Plan to Prevent and Reserve Diabetes*. New York: HarperOne, 2013, front flap.

Gelb, Michael, and Howard Hindin. *Gasp!: Airway Health – The Hidden Path to Wellness*. CreateSpace, 2016, p. 170.

Glick, Michael, editor. *The Oral-Systemic Health Connection: A Guide to Patient Care*. Hanover Park: Quintessence Publishing Co Inc, 2014.

Hyman, Mark. *The Blood Sugar Solution*. New York: Little, Brown and Company, 2012, pp. 18-19.

Isaacs, Scott. *Hormonal Balance: How to Lose Weight by Understanding Your Hormones and Metabolism*, 3rd ed., Boulder: Bull Publishing Company, 2012, p. 1.

Koufman, Jamie. *Dr. Koufman's Acid Reflux Diet*. Katalitix Media, 2015, p. 4.

Lavigne, Gilles J., Peter A. Cistulli, and Michael T. Smith, editors. *Sleep Medicine for Dentists: A Practical Overview*. Chicago: Quintessence Publishing Co, Inc, 2009.

Lustig, Robert H. *Fat Chance*. New York: Plume, 2012, p. 257.

Mahan, Parker E., and Charles C. Alling, III. *Facial Pain*. 3rd ed., Philadelphia: Lea & Febiger, 1991, p. 193.

Maples, Susan S., and Diana K. DeCouteau. *Blabbermouth!: 77 Secrets Only Your Mouth Can Tell You to Live a Healthier, Happier, Sexier Life*. Michigan: BlabberMouth! Press, 2015, p. 50.

Masley, Steven. *The 30-Day Heart Tune-Up*. New York: Center Street, 2014, pp. 19-20.

McCamy, John, and James Presley. *Human Life Styling*. New York: Harper & Row, Publishers, Inc., 1975, pp. 2-3, 166.

McKeown, Patrick. *The Oxygen Advantage*. New York: HarperCollins Publishers, 2015, p. 68.

Nizel, Abraham E. *The Science of Nutrition and its Application in Clinical Dentistry*. Philadelphia: W. B. Saunders Company, 1966, p. 364.

Park, Steven Y. *Sleep, Interrupted: A Physician Reveals The #1 Reason Why So Many of Us Are Sick and Tired*. New York: Jodev Press, 2008, pp. 4-5.

Perlmutter, David. *Brain Maker*. New York: Little, Brown, and Company, 2015, p. 60.

Roizen, Michael F. and Mehmet C. Oz. *You: The Owner's Manual.* Updated and Expanded Edition. New York: Collins, 2008, p. 5.

Sabbagh, Marwan and Beau MacMillan. *The Alzheimer's Prevention Cookbook.* New York: Ten Speed Press, 2012, pp. 51-52.

Seaman, David. *The DeFlame Diet.* Wilmington: Shadow Panther Press, 2016, pp. 23-24.

Sternberg, Esther M. *The Balance Within: The Science Connecting Health and Emotions.* New York: W. H. Freeman and Company, 2001, p. 13.

Warren, Rick, Daniel Amen, and Mark Hyman. *The Daniel Plan: 40 Days to a Healthier Life.* Grand Rapids: Zondervan, 2013.

ENDNOTES

[1] "What is Integrative Medicine?". Duke Integrative Medicine. https://www.dukeintegrativemedicine.org/about/what-is-integrative-medicine/. Accessed 6 Nov. 2018.

[2] "What is Integrative Medicine?". Duke Integrative Medicine. https://www.dukeintegrativemedicine.org/about/what-is-integrative-medicine/. Accessed 6 Nov. 2018.

[3] "What is Integrative Medicine?". Duke Integrative Medicine. https://www.dukeintegrativemedicine.org/about/what-is-integrative-medicine/. Accessed 6 Nov. 2018.

[4] "What is Integrative Medicine?". Duke Integrative Medicine. https://www.dukeintegrativemedicine.org/about/what-is-integrative-medicine/. Accessed 6 Nov. 2018.

[5] Lean, Leslie, Barnes, et al. Primary care-led weight management for remission of type 2 diabetes (DiRECT): an open-label, cluster-randomised trial. The Lancet Volume 391, No. 10120, p541–551, 10 February 2018

[6] Health Measurement in the Third Era of Health January 2006, Vol 96, No. 1 American Journal of Public Health   Lester Breslow, MD, MPH

[7] Brent Bauer, M.D. Buzzed on Inflammation. Mayo Clinic Health Online Edition July 2014

[8] Dental Caries and Sealant Prevalence in Children and Adolescents in the United States, 2011–2012 NCHS Data Brief No. 191, March 2015 Bruce A. Dye, D.D.S., M.P.H.; Gina Thornton-Evans, D.D.S, M.P.H.; Xianfen Li, M.S.; and Timothy J. Iafolla, D.M.D., M.P.H.

[9] Douglass JM, Li Y, Tinanoff N. Association of Mutans Streptococci Between Caregivers and Their Children. Pediatr Dent 2008; 30(5): 375-87.

[10] Hale FA. "Dental caries in the dog." J Vet Dent. 1998;15(2):79-83

[11] Acs G, Lodolini G, Kaminsky S, Cisneros GJ. Effect of nursing caries on body weight in a pediatric population. Pediatr Dent 1992; 14(5):302-5.

[12] "Dental Caries (Tooth Decay) in Adults (Age 20 to 64)." *National Institute of Dental and Craniofacial Research*, July 2018, Dental Caries (Tooth Decay) in Adults (Age 20 to 64).

[13] Tomoki Maekawa, Jennifer L. Krauss, Toshiharu Abe, Ravi Jotwani, Martha Triantafilou, Kathy Triantafilou, Ahmed Hashim, Shifra Hoch, Michael A. Curtis, Gabriel Nussbaum, John D. Lambris, George Hajishengallis. Porphyromonas gingivalis Manipulates Complement and TLR Signaling to Uncouple Bacterial Clearance from Inflammation and Promote Dysbiosis. *Cell Host & Microbe*, 2014; 15 (6): 768 DOI: 10.1016/j.chom.2014.05.012

[14] Socransky SS, Haffajee AD. Evidence of bacterial etiology: a historical perspective. Periodontol 2000. 1994;5:7-25.

[15] "Periodontal Disease". *CDC*. 10 March 2015.

[16] Turnbaugh PJ, Ley RE, Hamady M, Fraser-Liggett CM, Knight R, Gordon, JI. The human microbiome project. Nature 449p804-10 (2007 Oct 18)

[17] Xuesong He, Xuedong Zhou, Wenyuan Shi. Oral Microbiology: Past, Present and Future. Int J Oral Sci. 2009 Jun; 1(2): 47–58.

[18] Yang NY, Zhang Q, Li JL, Yang SH, Shi Q. Progression of periodontal inflammation in adolescents is associated with increased number of Porphyromonas gingivalis, Prevotella intermedia, Tannerella forsythensis, and Fusobacterium nucleatum. Int J Paediatr Dent. 2014;24:226–233.

[19] Han Yiping W. *Fusobacterium nucleatum:* a commensal-turned pathogen Curr Opin Microbiol. 2015 Feb; 0: 141–147.

[20] Yann Fardini Xiaowei Wang Stéphanie Témoin Stanley Nithianantham David Lee Menachem Shoham Yiping W. Han *Fusobacterium nucleatum* adhesin FadA binds vascular endothelial cadherin and alters endothelial integrity Molecular Microbiology (2011) 82(6), 1468–1480

[21] Elerson Gaetti-Jardim Jr, Silvia L. Marcelino, Alfredo C. R. Feitosa, Giuseppe A. Romito, Mario J. Avila-Campos Quantitative detection of periodontopathic bacteria in atherosclerotic plaques from coronary arteries December 2009, Journal of Medical Microbiology 58: 1568-1575

[22] Bale BF, Doneen AL, Vigerust DJ. High-risk periodontal pathogens contribute to the pathogenesis of atherosclerosis. Postgrad Med J 2017;93:215–220.

[23] Tanja Pessi, PhD; et al, Bacterial signatures in thrombus aspirates of patients with myocardial infarction Circulation. 2013 Mar 19;127(11):1219-28

[24] Tanja Pessi, PhD; et al, Bacterial signatures in thrombus aspirates of patients with myocardial infarction Circulation. 2013 Mar 19;127(11):1219-28

[25] Tanja Pessi, PhD; et al, Bacterial signatures in thrombus aspirates of patients with myocardial infarction Circulation. 2013 Mar 19;127(11):1219-28

[26] J Periodontol. 2009 Jun;80(6):884-91.

[27] J Periodontol. 2009 Jun;80(6):884-91.

[28] J Periodontol. 2009 Jun;80(6):884-91.

[29] J Periodontol. 2009 Jun;80(6):884-91.

[30] Han YW et al., Term stillbirth caused by oral Fusobacterium nucleatum. Obstetrics and Gynecology. 01 Feb 2010, 115(2 Pt 2):442-445.

[31] Orenstein, David." Bacteria may signal pancreatic cancer risk" . https://news.brown.edu/articles/2012/09/periodontic. September 18, 2012. Accessed Nov 6, 2018.

[32] Koufman, Jamie. *Dr. Koufman's Acid Reflux Diet*. Katalitix Media, 2015. p 4.

[33] "The State of Consumption Today". Worldwatch Institute. Retrieved March 30, 2012.

[34] "Fish Consumption: Mercury". Applied Ecology. https://appliedecology.cals.ncsu.edu/fish-consumption/pollutants/mercury/. Accessed Nov 6, 2018

[35] "Mercury in Fish: FAQ". Florida Fish and Wildlife Commission. http://myfwc.com/research/saltwater/health/mercury/faq/. Accessed Nov 6, 2018.

[36] "High Blood Pressure Frequently Asked Questions (FAQs)". CDC. https://www.cdc.gov/bloodpressure/faqs.htm. Accessed Nov 6, 2018.

[37] "Reading the New Blood Pressure Guidelines". Harvard Health Publishing. https://www.health.harvard.edu/heart-health/reading-the-new-blood-pressure-guidelines. Accessed Nov 6, 2018.

[38] "Understanding Blood Pressure Readings". AHA. http://www.heart.org/en/health-topics/high-blood-pressure/understanding-blood-pressure-readings. Accessed Nov 6, 2018.

[39] "Get the Scoop on Sodium and Salt". AHA. https://www.heart.org/en/healthy-living/healthy-eating/eat-smart/sodium/sodium-and-salt. Accessed Nov 6, 2018.

[40] "Sleep Apnea and High Blood Pressure: A Dangerous Pair". CardioSmart. https://www.cardiosmart.org/news-and-events/2015/05/sleep-apnea-and-high-blood-pressure-a-dangerous-pair . Accessed Nov 6, 2018.

[41] "Common High Blood Pressure Myths". AHA. http://www.heart.org/en/health-topics/high-blood-pressure/the-facts-about-high-blood-pressure/common-high-blood-pressure-myths. Accessed Nov 6, 2018.

[42] " Hormonal Causes of Hypertension". MedStar Washington Hospital Center. https://www.medstarwashington.org/our-

services/endocrinology/conditions/hormonal-causes-of-hypertension/. Accessed Nov 6, 2018.

[43] Health, United States, 2011: table 51. End-stage renal disease patients, by selected characteristics: United States, selected years 1980–2010. Centers for Disease Control and Prevention website. www.cdc.gov/nchs/data/hus/2011/051.pdf Updated 2011. Accessed December 20, 2013.

[44] "Diabetes and high blood pressure". Blood Pressure UK. http://www.bloodpressureuk.org/BloodPressureandyou/Yourbody/Diabetes. Accessed Nov 6, 2018.

[45] "Diabetes and high blood pressure". Blood Pressure UK. http://www.bloodpressureuk.org/BloodPressureandyou/Yourbody/Diabetes. Accessed Nov 6, 2018.

[46] "Four Nutrient Deficiencies Every High Blood Pressure Patient Needs to Know". Diet vs. Disease. https://www.dietvsdisease.org/4-nutrient-deficiencies-every-high-blood-pressure-patient-needs-to-know/. Accessed Nov 6, 2018.

[47] Gillogly, Lynne. "How Can Massage and Exercise Improve Your Lymphatic System (Immune System)". Gold Coast Physio and Sports Health. https://www.mygcphysio.com.au/services/articles-useful-info/how-can-massage-exercise-improve-your-lymphatic-system-immune-system/. Accessed Nov 16, 2018.

[48] Seaman, David. *The Deflame Diet*. Shadow Panther Press. April 2, 2016.

[49] F. Berenbaum Osteoarthritis as an inflammatory disease (osteoarthritis is not osteoarthrosis!) Osteoarthritis and Cartilage 21 (2013) 16-21

[50] Fuhrman, Joel, MD. The End of Diabetes. Harper One. 2013. [p 23]

[51] Fuhrman, Joel, MD. The End of Diabetes. Harper One. 2013. *p 16*

[52] Naomi M. Hamburg, Craig J. McMackin, Alex L. Huang, Sherene M. Shenouda, Michael E. Widlansky, Eberhard Schulz, Noyan Gokce, Neil B. Ruderman, John F. Keaney Jr, Joseph A. Vita Physical Inactivity Rapidly Induces Insulin Resistance and Microvascular

Dysfunction in Healthy Volunteers. Arterioscler Thromb Vasc Biol. 2007;27:2650-2656

[53] "All About Your A1c". CDC. https://www.cdc.gov/diabetes/library/features/a1c.html. Accessed Nov 6, 2018.

[54] "Take the Quiz". Voice Institute of New York. http://www.voiceinstituteofnewyork.com/us-patients/. Accessed December 31, 2018.

[55] J.D.B. Featherstone The Continuum of Dental Caries—Evidence for a Dynamic Disease Process. JDR July 1, 2004 https://doi.org/10.1177/154405910408301s08

[56] Featherstone JDB, Chaffee BW, The Evidence for Caries Management by Risk Assessment (CAMBRA®) Adv Dent Res. 2018 Feb;29(1):9-14.

[57] Sherry Shiqian Gao, Irene Shuping Zhao, Steve Duffin, Duangporn Duangthip, Edward Chin Man Lo, and Chun Hung Chu Revitalising Silver Nitrate for Caries Management Int J Environ Res Public Health. 2018 Jan; 15

[58] Dunlap, Tanya. "Prescribing Hydrogen Peroxide in the Treatment of Periodontal Disease". Oral Health. https://www.oralhealthgroup.com/features/prescribing-hydrogen-peroxide-treatment-periodontal-disease/. Accessed Nov 23, 2018.

[59] Hillman, Jeffrey, DMD, PhD. Oral-systemic link and the potential impact of probiotics. Dentistry IQ. https://www.dentistryiq.com/articles/2010/08/oral-systemic-link-and-the-potential-impact-of-probiotics.html. August 31, 2010. Accessed Nov 23, 2018.

[60] Dawson, Peter, DDS. Evaluation, Diagnosis, and Treatment of OCCLUSAL PROBLEMS. The C.V. Mosby Company. St. Louis. (1974).

[61] "NATIONAL SLEEP FOUNDATION RECOMMENDS NEW SLEEP TIMES". https://sleepfoundation.org/press-release/national-

sleep-foundation-recommends-new-sleep-times/page/0/1. Accessed Nov 6, 2018.

62 Cromie, William. "Discovering who lives in your mouth". Harvard Gazette. https://news.harvard.edu/gazette/story/2002/07/harvard-gazette-discovering-who-lives-in-your-mouth/. 2002

63 ADA Adopts Policy on Dentistry's Role in Treating Obstructive Sleep Apnea, Similar Disorders. ada.org October 23, 2017 News Releases

64 Ruth SoRelle Nobel Prize Awarded to Scientists for Nitric Oxide Discoveries Circulation. 1998;98:2365-2366

65 Uncovering The Effects Of Nitric Oxide On The Cardiovascular System. Retrieved Mar 02, 2018 from explorable.com: https://explorable.com/nitric-oxide-in-cardiovascular-system Explorable.com (Nov 17, 2010).

66 Uncovering The Effects Of Nitric Oxide On The Cardiovascular System. Retrieved Mar 02, 2018 from explorable.com: https://explorable.com/nitric-oxide-in-cardiovascular-system Explorable.com (Nov 17, 2010).

67 Lundberg JO1. Nitric oxide and the paranasal sinuses. Anat Rec. Hoboken: 2008 Nov;291(11):1479-84. doi: 10.1002/ar.20782.

68 M.F. Fitzpatrick. Effect of nasal or oral breathing route on upper airway resistance during sleep. Eur Respir J 2003

69 Dawson, Peter E. and John C. Cranham. *The Complete Dentist Manual*. St. Petersburg: Widiom Publishing, LLC, 2017, p. 27.

70 E.P. Harvold. Primate experiments on oral respiration. Am J Orthod. 1981

71 James McNamara DDS PhD Univ of Michigan Center For Human Growth and Development Influence of Respiratory Pattern on Craniofacial Growth International Journal of Orafacial Myology Vol. 10 Number 2

[72] James McNamara DDS PhD Univ of Michigan Center For Human Growth and Development Influence of Respiratory Pattern on Craniofacial Growth International Journal of Orafacial Myology Vol. 10 Number 2

[73] Guilleminault et al UARS and CAP SLEEP, Vol. 30, No. 5, 2007.

[74] Gold, AR, et al. The Symptoms and Signs of Upper Airway Resistance Syndrome. CHEST, 2003;123: 87-95

[75] Christian Guilleminault, Susmita Chowdhuri Upper Airway Resistance Syndrome Is a Distinct Syndrome. AJRCCM Vol. 161, No. 5 | May 01, 2000

[76] The Journal for Sleep Specialists, Oct. 2015

[77] OPPERA Cohort Sleep Apnea Symptoms and Risk of Temporomandibular Disorder. J Dent Res. 2013 Jul; 92(7 Suppl): S70–S77

[78] Paul Macey UCLA 2/16 Sleep apnea takes a toll on brain function JSleep Research

[79] Buckley TM, Schatzberg AF. On the interactions of the hypothalamic-pituitary-adrenal (HPA) axis and sleep: normal HPA axis activity and circadian rhythm, exemplary sleep disorders. J Clin Endocrinol Metab. 2005;90:3106–3114.

[80] Trakada,G, et al. Sleep Apnea and its association with the Stress System, Inflammation, Insulin Resistance and Visceral Obesity. Sleep Med Clin. 2007 Jun; 2(2): 251–261.

[81] Price, Roger. Personal correspondence, 2018.

[82] "Time spent in primary activities and percent of the civilian population engaging in each activity, averages per day by sex, 2017 annual averages". Bureau of Labor Statistics. https://www.bls.gov/news.release/atus.t01.htm. Accessed on Jan 2, 2019.

83 "Snoring, Sleep Disorders, and Sleep Apnea". The American Academy of Otolaryngology – Head and Neck Surgery. https://www.enthealth.org/conditions/snoring-sleeping-disorders-and-sleep-apnea/. Accessed Jan 1, 2018.

84 Zhu Y, Fenik P, Zhan G, et al. Selective loss of catecholaminergic wake active neurons in a murine sleep apnea model. *J Neurosci.* 2007;27(37):10060-10071.

85 Zhu Y, Fenik P, Zhan G, Xin R, Veasey SC. Degeneration in arousal neurons in chronic sleep disruption modeling sleep apnea. *Front Neurol.* 2015;6:109.

86 Rev. CEFAC vol.18 no.1 São Paulo Jan./Feb. 2016

87 Christian Guilleminault, Shehlanoor Huseni, Lauren Lo ERJ Open Research 2016 2: 00043-2016

88 Christian Guilleminault, Shehlanoor Huseni, Lauren Lo ERJ Open Research 2016 2: 00043-2016

89 Huang et al. Pediatric Short lingual frenulum Int J Pediatr Res 2015, 1:1

90 Which Oropharyngeal Factors Are Significant Risk Factors for Obstructive Sleep Apnea? An Age-Matched Study and Dentist Perspectives Nat Sci Sleep. 2016; 8: 215–219

91 Mallampati Score, Wikipedia. https://en.wikipedia.org/wiki/Mallampati_score. Accessed Nov 6, 2018.

92 Kanwar M, Jha R Importance of Mallampati score as an independent predictor of obstructive sleep apnea. European Respiratory Journal 2012 40: P3183

93 Weiss TM, Atanasov S, Calhoun KH.The association of tongue scalloping with obstructive sleep apnea and related sleep pathology. Otolaryngol Head Neck Surg. 2005 Dec;133(6):966-71.

94 Chaubal T, Dixit M Ankyloglossia and its management J Indian Soc Periodontol. 2011 Jul-Sep; 15(3): 270–272.

[95] Kotlow LA. Ankyloglossia (tongue-tie): A diagnostic and treatment quandary. Quintessence Intl. 1999;30:259–62.

[96] Ramanathan Manikandhan, Ganugapanta Lakshminarayana, Pendem Sneha, Parameshwaran Ananthnarayanan, Jayakumar Naveen, and Hermann F. Sailer Impact of Mandibular Distraction Osteogenesis on the Oropharyngeal Airway in Adult Patients with Obstructive Sleep Apnea Secondary to Retroglossal Airway Obstruction J Maxillofac Oral Surg. 2014 Jun; 13(2): 92–98.

[97] William Arnett, DDS, FACD, Jeffrey S. Jelic, DMD, MD, Jone Kim, DDS, MS, David R. Cummings, DDS, Anne Beress, DMD, MS, C. MacDonald Worley, Jr, DMD, MD, BS, Bill Chung, DDS, Robert Bergman, DDS, MSh Soft tissue cephalometric analysis: Diagnosis and treatment planning of dentofacial deformity American Journal of Orthodontics and Dentofacial Orthopedics Volume 116, Number 3 September 1999}

[98] http://epworthsleepinessscale.com/about-the-ess/

[99] Chung F, Abdullah HR, Liao P. STOP-Bang Questionnaire: A Practical Approach to Screen for Obstructive Sleep Apnea Chest. 2016 Mar;149(3):631-8.

[100] Oxygen saturation (Medicine). Wikipedia. https://en.wikipedia.org/wiki/Oxygen_saturation_(medicine). Accessed Nov 6, 2018.

[101] Adrienne S Scott, Marcel A Baltzan, and Norman Wolkove Examination of pulse oximetry tracings to detect obstructive sleep apnea in patients with advanced chronic obstructive pulmonary disease Can Respir J. 2014 May-Jun; 21(3): 171–175

[102] Mohamed El Shayeb, MD MSc, Leigh-Ann Topfer, MLS, Tania Stafinski, PhD, Lawrence Pawluk, MD, Devidas Menon, PhD Diagnostic accuracy of level 3 portable sleep tests versus level 1 polysomnography for sleep-disordered breathing: a systematic review and meta-analysis CMAJ. 2014 Jan 7; 186(1)

[103] Frédéric Roche, Jean-Michel Gaspoz, Isabelle Court-Fortune, Pascal Minini, Vincent Pichot, David Duverney, Frédéric Costes, Jean-

René Lacour and Jean-Claude Barthélémy   Screening of Obstructive Sleep Apnea Syndrome by Heart Rate Variability Analysis. Mar 2018. Circulation. 2018;100:1411-1415 Circulation. 1999;100:1411-1415

[104] Guilleminault et al UARS and CAP(cyclic alternating pattern) SLEEP, Vol. 30, No. 5, 2007

[105] Guilleminault et al UARS and CAP(cyclic alternating pattern) SLEEP, Vol. 30, No. 5, 2007

[106] Guilleminault et al UARS and CAP(cyclic alternating pattern) SLEEP, Vol. 30, No. 5, 2007

[107] Kodentsova VM, Vrzhesinskaia OA, Mazo VK. Vitamins and oxidative stress Vopr Pitan. 2013;82(3):11-8

[108] Charkhandeh, Shouresh. "Prototype device may help predict effectiveness of oral appliance therapy for obstructive sleep apnea treatment". Dentistry IQ. https://www.dentistryiq.com/articles/2015/10/prototype-device-may-help-predict-effectiveness-of-oral-appliance-therapy-for-the-treatment-of-obstructive-sleep-apnea.html. Accessed November 28, 2018.

[109] Joseph A, Ackerman D, Talley JD, Johnstone J, Kupersmith J. Manifestations of coronary atherosclerosis in young trauma victims – an autopsy study. J Am Coll Cardiol. 1993 Aug;22(2):459-67

[110] Dawson, Peter E. and John C. Cranham. *The Complete Dentist Manual*. St. Petersburg: Widiom Publishing, LLC, 2017.

[111] "Complex Regional Pain Syndrome". Mayo Clinic. https://www.mayoclinic.org/diseases-conditions/complex-regional-pain-syndrome/symptoms-causes/syc-20371151. Updated Feb 15, 2018. Accessed Dec 24, 2018.

[112] "Complex Regional Pain Syndrome". Mayo Clinic. https://www.mayoclinic.org/diseases-conditions/complex-regional-pain-syndrome/symptoms-causes/syc-20371151. Updated Feb 15, 2018. Accessed Dec 24, 2018.

[113] "Complex Regional Pain Syndrome". Mayo Clinic. https://www.mayoclinic.org/diseases-conditions/complex-regional-pain-syndrome/symptoms-causes/syc-20371151. Updated Feb 15, 2018. Accessed Dec 24, 2018.

[114] Sleep related bruxism. In: International classification of sleep disorders. 3rd ed. Darien, IL.: American Academy of Sleep Medicine; 2014.

[115] Jeff Rouse DDS The Bruxism Triad Sleep bruxism, sleep disturbance, and sleep-related GERD. Inside Dentistry. May 2010. insidedentistry.net

[116] Dawson, Peter Functional Occlusion from TMJ to Smile Design Mosby 2007 chapter 7

[117] Manns A, Chan C, Miralles R. Influence of group function and canine guidance on electromyographic activity of elevator muscles. J Prosthet Dent. 1987;57(4):494–501

[118] E.H. Williamson, D.D.S., M.S., D.O. Lundquist, D.D.S. Anterior guidance: Its effect on electromyographic activity of the temporal and masseter muscles. June 1983 Volume 49, Issue 6, Pages 816–823

[119] Schellhas KP, Piper MA, Bessette RW, Wilkes CH., Mandibular retrusion, temporomandibular joint derangement, and orthognathic surgery planning. Plast Reconstr Surg. 1992 Aug;90(2):218-29

[120] Schellhas KP, Piper MA, Bessette RW, Wilkes CH., Mandibular retrusion, temporomandibular joint derangement, and orthognathic surgery planning. Plast Reconstr Surg. 1992 Aug;90(2):218-29

[121] Schellhas KP, Piper MA, Bessette RW, Wilkes CH., Mandibular retrusion, temporomandibular joint derangement, and orthognathic surgery planning. Plast Reconstr Surg. 1992 Aug;90(2):218-29

[122] DDS, MS Lisa KingPhD Edward F. Harris, PhD Elizabeth A. Tolley Heritability of cephalometric and occlusal variables as assessed from siblings with overt malocclusions AJO-DO August 1993 Volume 104, Issue 2, Pages 121–131

[123] Gary D. Klasser, DMD, Nathalie Rei, DMD, MSD, Gilles J. Lavigne, DMD, PhD Sleep Bruxism Etiology: The Evolution of a Changing Paradigm J Can Dent Assoc 2015;81:f2

[124] Bhadrinath Srinivasan and Arun B Chitharanjan. Skeletal and dental characteristics in subjects with ankyloglossia. Prog Orthod. 2013; 14: 44.

[125] Dawson, Peter Functional Occlusion from TMJ to Smile Design Mosby 2007 chapter 9-10

[126] Harry Lundeen DDS, Charles Gibbs, PhD. The Function of Teeth, L&G. ISBN 0977151107 2007

[127] Dawson, Peter Functional Occlusion from TMJ to Smile Design Mosby 2007 107-110

[128] Dawson, Peter Functional Occlusion from TMJ to Smile Design Mosby 2007 chapter 26

[129] Dawson and Cranham. The Complete Dentist Manual: The Essential Guide to Being a Complete Care Dentist 1st Edition. The Dawson Academy. 2017.

[130] Dawson, Peter Functional Occlusion from TMJ to Smile Design Mosby 2007 chapter 22

[131] Schellhas KP, Piper MA, Bessette RW, Wilkes CH., Mandibular retrusion, temporomandibular joint derangement, and orthognathic surgery planning. Plast Reconstr Surg. 1992 Aug;90(2):218-29

[132] Christensen, L.V., Rassouli, N.M. Experimental occlusal interferences J Oral rehab July 1995 https://doi.org/10.1111/j.1365-2842.1995.tb01197.x

[133] Dawson, Peter Functional Occlusion from TMJ to Smile Design Mosby 2007 pg. 346

[134] Dawson, Peter Functional Occlusion from TMJ to Smile Design Mosby 2007 chapter 22

[135] E.H. Williamson, D.D.S., M.S., D.O. Lundquist, D.D.S. Anterior guidance: Its effect on electromyographic activity of the temporal and masseter muscles JPD June 1983Volume 49, Issue 6, Pages 816–823

[136] "Sleep Apnea Oral Appliance Information for Patients". SomnoMed. https://somnomed.com/en/patients/somnodent-product-information-for-patients/. Accessed January 1, 2019.

[137] Sleep related bruxism. In: International classification of sleep disorders. 3rd ed. Darien, IL.: American Academy of Sleep Medicine; 2014.

[138] Lavigne GJ, Khoury S, Abe S, Yamaguchi T, Raphael K. Bruxism physiology and pathology: an overview for clinicians. J Oral Rehabil. 2008 Jul;35(7):476-94

[139] María S Commisso, Javier Martínez-Reina, and Juana Mayo. A study of the temporomandibular joint during bruxism Int J Oral Sci. 2014 Jun; 6(2): 116–123.

[140] Jorge A Roman-Blas, Santos Castañeda, Raquel Largo, and Gabriel Herrero-Beaumont. Osteoarthritis associated with estrogen deficiency Arthritis Res Ther. 2009; 11(5): 241.

[141] Lotz, Anne G. God's Story. Nashville: Thomas Nelson. 2009. Page 44-45.

[142] Dawson, Peter. A Better Way. St. Petersburg: Widiom Publishing. 2018.

[143] Council on Dental Practice - Dentistry's Role in Sleep Related Breathing Disorders. ADA. https://www.ada.org/en/member-center/leadership-governance/councils-commissions-and-committees/dentistry-role-in-sleep-related-breathing-disorders. Accessed Nov 29, 2018.

Made in the USA
Coppell, TX
11 November 2022